Gender and Medicine in Ireland
1 7 0 0 – 1 9 5 0

Irish Studies
James MacKillop, *Series Editor*

Collaborative Dubliners: Joyce in Dialogue
Vicki Mahaffey, ed.

Grand Opportunity: The Gaelic Revival and Irish Society, 1893–1910
Timothy G. McMahon

Ireland in Focus: Film, Photography, and Popular Culture
Eóin Flannery and Michael Griffin, eds.

*The Irish Bridget: Irish Immigrant Women
in Domestic Service in America, 1840–1930*
Margaret Lynch-Brennan

Irish Theater in America: Essays on Irish Theatrical Diaspora
John P. Harrington, ed.

Joyce, Imperialism, and Postcolonialism
Leonard Orr, ed.

*Making Ireland Irish: Tourism and National Identity
since the Irish Civil War*
Eric G. E. Zuelow

Memory Ireland, Volume 1: *History and Modernity*
Oona Frawley, ed.

The Midnight Court / Cúirt an Mheán Oíche
Brian Merriman; David Marcus, trans.; Brian Ó Conchubhair, ed.

Modern Irish Drama: W. B. Yeats to Marina Carr, Second Edition
Sanford Sternlicht

Samuel Beckett in the Literary Marketplace
Stephen John Dilks

Gender
and Medicine
in Ireland

1 7 0 0 – 1 9 5 0

Edited by
Margaret H. Preston
& **Margaret Ó hÓgartaigh**

Syracuse University Press

Copyright © 2012 by Syracuse University Press

Syracuse, New York 13244-5290

All Rights Reserved

First Edition 2012

12 13 14 15 16 17   6 5 4 3 2 1

∞ The paper used in this publication meets the minimum requirements
of the American National Standard for Information Sciences—Permanence
of Paper for Printed Library Materials, ANSI Z39.48-1992.

For a listing of books published and distributed by Syracuse University Press,
visit our website at SyracuseUniversityPress.syr.edu.

ISBN: 978-0-8156-3271-9

Library of Congress Cataloging-in-Publication Data

Available upon request from the publisher.

Manufactured in the United States of America

For
Margaret Mac Curtain,
Frances Lundberg,
and
Andrew and James Sneddon

Contents

Figures

Tables

Acknowledgments

We are grateful to various librarians and archivists at the National Library of Ireland, Royal Irish Academy, Public Record Office of Northern Ireland, National Archives of Ireland, and Trinity College, Dublin. Many thanks to all at Syracuse University Press, especially Jennika Baines, who was so helpful. We thank the contributors for their patience and cooperation. We are most grateful to Ciarán Ó hÓgartaigh and Rick Lundberg for their love and support. Our greatest debt is to those persons named in the dedication. Margaret Mac Curtain was engaging, illuminating, and insightful. Andrew and James Sneddon and Frances Lundberg cheerfully shared the book's gestation.

Margaret Ó hÓgartaigh,
Margaret H. Preston
Boston and Sioux Falls, 2012

Contributors

Ciara Breathnach lectures in history at the University of Limerick. Her publications include *A History of the Congested Districts Board of Ireland, 1891–1923: Poverty and Development in the West of Ireland* (2005); *Framing the West: Images of Rural Ireland 1890–1920* (as editor, 2007), and *Portraying Irish Travellers: Histories and Representations* (coedited with Aoife Breathnach, 2007).

Mel Cousins has written extensively on issues concerning the development of social policies in Ireland in the nineteenth and twentieth centuries. He is the author of *The Birth of Social Welfare in Ireland* (2003) and is currently based at Glasgow Caledonian University.

Laurence M. Geary lectures in history at University College Cork. His publications include *Medicine and Charity in Ireland, 1718–1851* (2004); *Nineteenth-Century Ireland: A Guide to Recent Research* (coedited with Margaret Kelleher, 2005); *History and the Public Sphere: Essays in Honour of John A. Murphy* (coedited with Tom Dunne, 2005); and *Ireland, Australia, and New Zealand: History, Politics, and Culture* (coedited with Andrew J. McCarthy, 2008).

Philomena Gorey is a practicing midwife and is completing a doctorate in history at University College, Dublin, focusing on eighteenth-century midwifery.

Greta Jones is based at the Wellcome Centre for the History of Medicine in Ireland at the University of Ulster. She coedited *Medicine, Disease,* *and the State in Ireland 1650–1940* (with Elizabeth Malcolm, 1999) and is the author of *Captain of All These Men of Death: A History of Tuberculosis in Nineteenth and Twentieth-Century Ireland* (2001). She has also published on medical migration, including an article in *Medical History* in 2010 entitled "'Strike Out Boldly for the Prizes That Are Available to You': Medical Emigration from Ireland 1860–1905."

James Kelly, member of the Royal Irish Academy, is Cregan Professor of History and head of the History Department at St. Patrick's College, Dublin City, and university and honorary research professor in history at Queen's University, Belfast. He has published widely on the social, political, and religious history of late-early-modern Ireland. His recent publications include *Poynings' Law and the Making of Law in Ireland, 1660–1800* (2008); *The Proceedings of the House of Lords, 1771–1800* (3 vols., 2008); *Sir Richard Musgrave, 1746–1818: Ultra Protestant Ideologue* (2009), and *Ireland and Medicine in the Seventeenth and Eighteenth Centuries* (coedited with Fiona Clark, 2010).

Elizabeth Malcolm is a graduate of Trinity College, Dublin, and worked in Irish studies at universities in Belfast and Liverpool before taking up the Gerry Higgins Chair of Irish Studies at the University of Melbourne. She has published widely on drink and temperance, mental health, crime and policing, and gender and migration. She coedited the book *Medicine, Disease, and the State in Ireland 1650–1940* (with Greta Jones, 1999). Her latest book is *The Irish Policeman, 1822–1922: A Life* (2006).

Sandra McAvoy coordinates women's studies in University College, Cork. She is a graduate of Trinity College, Dublin, and University College, Cork. Her publications include the articles "Sexual Crime and Irish Women's Campaigns for a Criminal Law Amendment Act 1912–1935" (2008) and "From Anti-amendment Campaigns to Demanding Reproductive Justice: The Changing Landscape of Abortion Rights Activism in Ireland 1983–2008" (2008).

Leanne McCormick is lecturer in modern Irish social history at the Wellcome Centre for the History of Medicine in Ireland, University of Ulster. She has published widely in the areas of female sexuality and the history of medicine in twentieth-century Northern Ireland in *Social History of Medicine* and the *Journal of the History of Sexuality*. Her monograph *Regulating Sexuality: Women in Twentieth-Century Northern Ireland* was published in 2009.

Cormac Ó Gráda is professor in the School of Economics at University College, Dublin. His recent publications include *Jewish Ireland in the Age of Joyce* (2006), *Ireland's Great Famine: Interdisciplinary Perspectives* (2007), and *When the Potato Failed: Causes and Effects of the Last European Subsistence Crisis, 1845–1850* (coedited with Richard Paping and Eric Vanhaute, 2007).

Margaret Ó hÓgartaigh is currently a visiting professor at Harvard Divinity School and was a Fulbright Fellow in Boston. Her publications include *Kathleen Lynn: Irishwoman, Patriot, Doctor* (2006, reprinted in 2011), *Edward Hay, Historian of 1798: Catholic Politics in an Era of Wolfe Tone and Daniel O'Connell* (2010), *Quiet Revolutionaries: Irish Women in Education, Medicine, and Sport, 1861–1964* (2011), and *Business Archival Sources for the Local Historian* (coauthored with Ciaran Ó hÓgartaigh, 2010).

Margaret H. Preston is an associate professor in the Department of History at Augustana College, South Dakota. She published *Charitable Words: Women, Philanthropy, and the Language of Charity* in 2004 and *A Journey of Faith, a Destination of Excellence: The First One Hundred Years of Avera McKennan Hospital* in 2010, which details the Irish Presentation Order's Hospital in Sioux Falls, South Dakota.

Pauline Prior is a senior lecturer in social policy at Queen's University, Belfast. Her research focuses on different aspects of mental health policy, including gender, law, and history. Articles by her have appeared in a variety of journals, including *Éire-Ireland* and *New Hibernia Review*. Her books include *Gender and Mental Health* (1999) and *Madness and Murder: Gender, Crime, and Mental Disorder in Nineteenth-Century Ireland* (2008).

Susannah Riordan lectures in history at University College, Dublin, and has published on the history of sexuality and history of medicine in Ireland. She is currently researching a book on the social history of venereal disease in twentieth-century Ireland.

Oonagh Walsh, professor at Glasgow Caledonian University, was educated at Trinity College, Dublin (BA, PhD), and the University of Nottingham (MA). Her book *Anglican Women in Dublin: Philanthropy, Politics, and Education in the Early Twentieth Century* was published in 2005. Her monograph on the district asylum system in the West of Ireland, *The Connaught District Lunatic Asylum: Land, Power, and Politics in Nineteenth-Century Ireland,* is forthcoming. Her previous posts include a lectureship at the University of Southampton, New College, a senior lectureship at the University of Aberdeen, and senior research fellowship in medical history at University College Cork.

Gender and Medicine in Ireland
1 7 0 0 - 1 9 5 0

Introduction

Margaret H. Preston and Margaret Ó hÓgartaigh

This collection of articles fills many gaps in our knowledge of Irish history.[1] The intersections between gender, medicine, and conventional economic, political, and social history are explored. Gender, it has been argued, is a social construct, whereas sex is defined by biology. However, sex or, rather, the results of sexual activity affect gender relations. Several of the articles discuss the differential levels of censure facing men and women when social and sexual norms are violated.[2] This collection adds to our understanding of the social history of medicine. As well as covering a range of social issues, the essays do not shirk from the analysis of political developments, such as the growing pains associated with the fledging states in Northern Ireland and the Irish Free State in the twentieth century.

The 1999 Greta Jones and Elizabeth Malcolm collection of essays *Medicine, Disease, and the State in Ireland, 1650–1940*,[3] is a role model for this book. Since its publication, the Centre for the History of Medicine in Ireland was established at the University of Ulster and University College, Dublin. The center has given a significant impetus to the study of medicine in Ireland in a historical context. Essays in this collection are drawn from work done at the center.

James Kelly's highly original analysis of eighteenth-century dental practice places the Irish experience in an international context. Extracting information from a wide range of sources, he situates the practice of teeth pulling within a range of other medical services. Teeth pulling was essentially a business affair, with practitioners wildly exaggerating the services they offered. On occasion, they promised no pain but delivered plenty. In his chapter "'I Was Right Glad to Be Rid of It': Dental Medical Practice in Eighteenth-Century Ireland," Kelly avers that the ascendancy of the hospital and of the technicoscientific approach in modern medicine "long sustained" a style of medical history in Ireland "that conceived of it . . . as a story of 'progress and triumph,' in the words of medical historian William Doolin."[4] The commercial environment shaped dental welfare in the eighteenth century. However, as the adoption of the term *dentist* from midcentury to define those who specialized in this area indicates, the practice was also influenced by clinical and scientific developments. The inability of self-taught empirics and journeymen surgeons who had held guild apprenticeships to accommodate more formal learning and increased public expectation encouraged the gradual emergence of dentistry as a distinct branch of medicine.

Greta Jones, in an exploration of a disease that affected thousands in Ireland and millions worldwide, explains the reasons for higher tuberculosis mortality among women in Ireland. In a careful examination of factors outside medicine such as family dynamics, she suggests that women's higher mortality rates may have been related to issues that have not been discussed but that are central to women's lives.[5] In "Women and Tuberculosis in Ireland," Jones explains that "during the late nineteenth and early twentieth centuries Ireland saw a rise in the death rate from tuberculosis," even "at a time when [it] was in decline in the United States and Great Britain. In Ireland, therefore, the experience of tuberculosis was more immediate and vivid than it was perhaps for nations that, although still being affected by the scourge of [the disease], had seen mortality from it decreasing since the middle of the nineteenth century."

Cormac Ó Gráda's analysis of infant mortality in Dublin in the early twentieth century echoes some of Jones's concerns. Using a wide range of sources, Ó Gráda places Ireland's high infant mortality rate in comparative perspective and explains why geography as well as economics dictated this rate. Through mathematical models as well as a wide range of sources from memoirs to British Parliamentary Papers, he suggests in "Infant and Child Mortality in Dublin a Century Ago" that a careful economic analysis of factors such as underemployment as well as appallingly low levels of public-health provision, including the nonavailability of waste disposal, influenced the infant mortality rate. Politicians and engineers were more likely than the medical profession to be able to ameliorate people's lives.[6]

A significant theme of this book is the attempted containment of disease. The landscape of nineteenth-century Ireland was dotted with a whole range of institutions, some of which still remain in the early twenty-first century. Oonagh Walsh's examination of the Connaught District Lunatic Asylum in Ballinasloe, County Galway, provides a convincing explanation for the "moral therapy" advocated in the nineteenth century.[7] Walsh's "Cure or Custody: Therapeutic Philosophy at the Connaught District Lunatic Asylum" ponders "whether asylums were intended to cure or merely to contain." This question "is not entirely facetious": "most institutions for the care of the insane in the nineteenth century faced the 'cure or custody' dilemma." Walsh's chapter examines the types of patients treated in the district asylum at Ballinasloe in the late nineteenth century and explores the means through which medical staff, both nurses and physicians, attempted to meet a governmental imperative to cure and return to society a majority of their charges. Walsh presents a nuanced picture of medical care and the attempts made to coax patients back to full mental health.

Complementing this analysis, Pauline Prior's carefully researched article explains the reasons for committal to Dundrum lunatic asylum (known as the Central Mental Hospital in the early twenty-first century). She explores the gendered attitudes to insanity and the extent to which patients were seen as reformable.[8] Prior's chapter, "Gender and Criminal Lunacy in the Nineteenth Century" makes clear that in 1850 the Central Criminal Lunatic Asylum for Ireland opened its doors to "people previously confined in the prison system." It focuses on the outcome of cases in which women killed men and vice versa and on when the insanity defense was used successfully or not. Prior examines the pattern that developed in order to throw some light on the role of psychiatry in the criminal justice system and on social attitudes to gender, crime, and insanity in nineteenth-century Ireland.

This emphasis on reform is also evident in Elizabeth Malcolm's essay "Between Habitual Drunkards and Alcoholics: Inebriate Women and Reformatories in Ireland, 1899–1919." However, there were contradictions in the approaches to these two groups, as she perceptively notes: "One perceived the 'inebriate' as sick and in need of treatment, hopefully leading to rehabilitation; the other perceived the 'habitual drunkard' as essentially a recidivist petty criminal, requiring punishment, hopefully leading to deterrence." The fundamental question for contemporaries was whether alcoholism was a disease or a vice; it would appear from the evidence accumulated by Malcolm that the latter definition ultimately prevailed.[9] Malcolm explains that the state was regulated by the new Inebriates Act of 1898 (61 and 62 Vic., c.60). "As well as establishing state inebriate reformatories, the 1898 act also made provision for certified inebriate reformatories, which were to be licensed by the state but operated and largely funded by county and borough councils, religious and philanthropic bodies, or private individuals." Malcolm examines the effect of new legislation relating to inebriates.[10]

One of the neglected arenas of Irish history is the work performed by nurses and midwives.[11] Several of the essays in this collection examine this labor from a variety of sources. Philomena Gorey's carefully researched examination of midwifery in eighteenth-century Ireland outlines the attempted medicalization of childbirth as well as the increasing role of certification in medicine.[12] Her comparative approach places Ireland in the context of changing views on childbirth and the role of midwifery in eighteenth-century Europe. In "Managing Midwifery in Dublin: Practice and Practitioners, 1700–1800," she makes clear that the eighteenth century in Dublin was characterized by a transformation in the way a woman's labor and delivery were managed. In 1700, childbirth was an exclusively female event, "bound by culture, tradition, and superstition, where the midwife had a central role." By 1800, "the prescribed norms surrounding childbirth and lying-in had been penetrated by a new breed of male practitioner, the man-midwife, who posed a direct threat to the midwife, whom tradition dictated should be married and older than thirty and should have borne children herself. . . .

[M]idwifery was to become an empirical, clinical skill, a field of expertise where the midwife now had only a marginal role, and the birth experience itself would soon be dominated by institutional, scientific obstetrics." The entrance of men into the field of midwifery was the most significant change in this process, and Gorey assesses that change.

High politics sometimes interacted fruitfully with people's lives, as can be seen in the attempts to "kill Home Rule with kindness." Ciara Breathnach's discussion of the Lady Dudley scheme for district nursing in the West of Ireland shows how aristocratic women could sometimes enhance their status in the community by improving people's lives even though their political perspectives may not have been popular.[13] Local initiatives, as she convincingly suggests, were literally vital in compensating for limited state involvement in public health. This was not unique to Ireland; Lady Rachel Dudley also initiated a district nursing scheme in the Australian outback. This original research on nursing adds to our knowledge of social life in impoverished areas. Breathnach's chapter outlines the attempts the Lady Dudley scheme made in tandem with the Congested Districts Board to organize domiciliary medical care and to improve sanitation in the West of Ireland from 1903 to 1923.

The state affected people's health in complex ways, as many of the chapters of this book illuminate. Laurence Geary explains that although venereal disease may be the "world's oldest infection," attitudes toward it hardly changed in several millennia. In prefamine Ireland, with the state's focus on institutionalization of venereal disease patients, the blame was placed on women because they were seen as "wholly responsible for spreading [the infection"."[14] In "'The Wages of Sin Is Death': Lock Hospitals, Venereal Disease, and Gender in Prefamine Ireland," Geary explains that "[p]rostitution has been designated the second-oldest profession, a premise that confers a certain antiquity on venereal disease, if, indeed, it does not make this disease the oldest human infection. . . . In Ireland, prostitution was never a crime," but society frowned upon it "as a social nuisance, an offense against public decency," a morally objectionable practice, and a public-health issue. Even though the need to control venereal disease in Ireland was a serious concern, nothing was done until the Contagious Diseases Acts in the 1860s. Geary discusses the implications of the conflicting attitudes toward and double standard regarding men, women, sexual relations, and the diseases that sometimes resulted from these relations.

Mel Cousins carefully examines morbidity—that is, the rate of illness in a population—and the effect of a national system of insurance on perceptions of illness.[15] In "'Sickness,' Gender, and National Health Insurance in Ireland, 1920s to the 1940s," Cousins examines "the administration of the Irish national health insurance system in the years after the establishment of the Irish Free State in 1922." He looks "in particular at gender-related issues in the administration and reform of the national health insurance system." He also considers "the implications of this assessment for broader debates about whether data on illness in national health insurance systems can be interpreted as evidence of morbidity or simply as absence from work." With respect to the national health insurance system in Ireland, the chapter discusses "women's (in particular married women's) perceived high claim."

Sandra McAvoy discusses how for Irish women pregnancy moved beyond ill health to fatality. She argues that the lack of sexual freedom as a result of censorship meant that pregnancy was a "death sentence" for some women.[16] In "'A Perpetual Nightmare': Women, Fertility Control, the Irish State, and the 1935 Ban on Contraceptives," McAvoy discusses a sensitive issue from a women's health perspective. One of the most damaging actions taken by a postindependence Irish government was the criminalization of the import and sale of contraceptives under section 17 of the 1935 Criminal Law Amendment Act (1935/6). In effect, the state imposed a prohibition on the most effective methods of contraception apart from abstention. The Fianna Fáil Party introduced this measure with the cooperation of the main opposition parties. This chapter makes clear that a majority of those in decision-making positions within the state and those who influenced them—in particular members of the Catholic hierarchy and Catholic social action movements—remained not only impervious to contemporary arguments about family planning, but also largely unmoved by concerns about those health risks related to pregnancy that could literally be a matter of life or death.

Susannah Riordan's thoughtfully analyzes the impact of various initiatives connected to venereal disease in the Irish Free State in the 1940s.[17] Her essay "'A Probable Source of Infection': The Limitations of Venereal Disease Policy, 1943–1951" explains that "[s]uccessive attempts" in the 1940s to reduce the Irish Free State's venereal disease rates "had fallen victim to internal politics, abrupt policy changes, political dogmatism, and poor drafting." She argues that "throughout the period only two factors remained constant: an unwillingness to challenge the climate of secrecy surrounding these diseases and an adherence to gendered behavioral stereotypes that was politically useful but administratively counterproductive." The social cost for patients was not considered, and the newly formed Department of Health does not emerge well in Riordan's assessment.

In Northern Ireland during the same period, a similar attitude was held. Leanne McCormick's "Prophylactics and Prejudice: Venereal Diseases in Northern Ireland during the Second World War" clarifies that in recent years we have "seen an awakening of interest in the history of venereal diseases in Ireland." This chapter "tackl[es] the overlooked issue of [the disease] in Northern Ireland, focusing in particular on the Second World War years. . . . As the most politically divided, socially conservative, and economically disadvantaged part of the United Kingdom" and an extremely conservative state, "Northern Ireland provides a valuable case study considering how [venereal disease] legislation was implemented at a local level and how local attitudes and beliefs influenced the situation." If the outcome was not so serious, the image of the horrified local government officials, who were convinced that women set out to infect innocent men with these diseases, would be laughable. The impact of sexually transmitted diseases is still being felt in twenty-first-century Ireland and Northern Ireland.

In their seminal book *Medicine, Disease, and the State in Ireland, 1650–1940*, editors Greta Jones and Elizabeth Malcolm suggest that the "social history of Irish medicine is still in its infancy. In compiling this volume, the editors have been constantly struck by the limitations of their knowledge: so many fascinating issues and questions have arisen on which little or no research has been carried out. We hope that the lights shone in this book will give courage to others to continue the exploration of this largely unknown territory."[18] Our own book explores terra incognita and opens up new avenues for exploration. The social history of Irish medicine is no longer in its infancy; it has come of age.

1

"I Was Right Glad to Be Rid of It"

Dental Medical Practice
in Eighteenth-Century Ireland

James Kelly

Medical history long sustained an approach that conceived of the development of the hospital and the emergence of the modern trinity of medical specialists—consultant, surgeon, and general practitioner—as a story of "progress and triumph," in the words of William Doolin.[1] Dentistry is not afforded a prominent place in this grand narrative, but the interpretation imposed on its history is no less intrinsically "whiggish" in that it offers an equivalent narrative of progress from an era of amateur tooth pullers and "surgeon operators for the teeth" to the modern dentist.[2] The reality was more complex, particularly for the formative era of the late seventeenth, eighteenth, and early nineteenth centuries, when the foundations of modern medicine were laid. In Ireland, as in England, "there was no single privileged medicine" because "many types of healing co-existed, overlapping, and clamouring for the public ear."[3] This complexity notwithstanding, the history of dental care in Ireland is particularly opaque because there is no historiography and only a shallow evidential footprint, but the utilization from the 1770s of the term *dentist* to define those who specialized in this area indicates that the eighteenth century was a formative period, though the reality for those in pain or requiring treatment was palpably less encouraging than this qualified positive judgment implies.

Based on what can be recovered, it is clear that dentistry in the early modern period was not the exclusive preserve of the surgeon members of the Guild of Barbers, Surgeons, Apothecaries, and Perukemakers (Guild of St. Mary Magdalene), in whom it was vested by charter in 1577.[4] This is not to suggest that the guild's effort to enforce its legal monopoly into the eighteenth century was entirely in vain; some of the most eminent "operators for the teeth" practicing in Dublin during the first half of the century were prominent members, but the frequency with which that body asserted that only those it licensed were entitled to practice is evidence of its increasing inability to control entry.[5] Matters had always been this way outside the metropolitan area, where surgeons with the requisite skills were seldom available and the local tooth puller was the only recourse of the needy, but the ebbing of the guild's authority in the eighteenth century and its failure even to attempt to enforce specific standards of treatment and care meant not only that empirics and irregular practitioners but also surgeon "operators for the teeth" chose increasingly to function outside its structures. It would be an exaggeration to say that this broader choice resulted in a medical free-for-all, though regulation was palpably deficient, and the boundaries between the trained practitioner, the skillful empiric, and the charlatan were shifting and indistinct. Moreover, dental medicine was not unchanging. It may be presumptuous, based on the adoption of the appellation *dentist* (from the French term *dentiste*) in place of *operator for the teeth* to describe specialist dental practitioners, to conclude that the eighteenth century witnessed the emergence of dentistry as a distinct medical speciality in Ireland, but it did travel some distance along that road. In this initial attempt to map the contours of dental medical practice during that period, there is much that remains elusive. However, it can be established that in Ireland, as in other jurisdictions in western Europe, the eighteenth century witnessed an epidemic of tooth decay that encouraged a small number of surgeons to specialize in dental care, the emergence of a market for dentifrice and other tooth-cleansing agents, and a greater openness to the promotion of dental care in print. Dental practice in Ireland followed the practice in England rather than the more sophisticated French model,[6] with the result that the standard of care available was rudimentary and obliged to compete in a competitive commercial medical marketplace that was as likely to indulge the charlatan who promised a miracle cure as it was to support the honest "operator for the teeth" who did his best with the knowledge and techniques he had at his disposal. Be that as it may, the century generated a greater awareness of the potential of dental medicine and of the merits of the dentist over the tooth puller that was of enduring consequence.

The presence of "teeth" alongside the more expected conditions of consumption, smallpox, and fever on the bills of mortality for Dublin city prepared in the first half of the eighteenth century is a salient pointer as to why dental welfare featured prominently in contemporaries' calculations. "Teeth" did not rival the major contagions (consumption, fever, and smallpox) as a primary cause of mortality, responsible for 15, 22, and 23 percent of the consolidated Dublin bill of mortality for 1712–18, respectively, but a significant 6.82 percent of deaths (1,022 people in all) were accorded a dental origin.[7] The importance of dental morbidity as a cause of mortality had eased somewhat by the 1730s, but returns of 5 percent (119) in 1734–35, 2.47 percent (55) in 1736–37, and 3.68 percent (68) in 1737–38 ensured it remained one of the main identifiable causes of mortality.[8]

Death, of course, was the worst-case outcome of dental morbidity, whose major symptom was pain. Eighteenth-century medical "operators for the teeth" in Ireland and Britain aspired to ease dental pain by extraction, which is why contemporaries were resigned to tooth loss.[9] Bishop Edward Synge of Elphin made this expectation clear in his correspondence with his daughter Alicia. Writing in May 1751 of the "loss . . . of the remaining tooth in mine upper jaw," he observed easily that "I was right glad to be rid of it. It plagued me both in speaking and eating."[10] He was equally philosophical some months later when his daughter anticipated losing a tooth: "I know by sad experience of what consequence it is to preserve teeth, and . . . I fear yours will decay as your good mother's did and mine have done."[11] Synge was approaching his sixtieth birthday when he made this observation, so it is not entirely surprising that he received with such equanimity the news of the loss of a tooth that he was wont to compare to "a bad tenant." His daughter, by contrast, was but eighteen when she experienced troubling dental pain, and Synge's relaxed response suggests that Alicia's experience was not unusual. Commenting on the fact that she had "so many more bad ones," two of which were "condemned," he counseled her "cheerfully [to] submit to . . . the loss of two teeth" and "to take better care of what remain."[12] In offering this guidance, Synge reflected the prevailing ignorance of dental matters even among the well educated. This conclusion is borne out by his earlier advice to his daughter to inquire of her governess "whether she be acquainted with this phrase, *dents de sagasse.* . . . I know the meaning. But have you any of that kind?"[13]

Synge's attentiveness to his daughter's dental health reflected the genuine concern one family member showed another who was in such pain she could not "eat, tho' hungry."[14] Bishop St. George Ashe of Clogher expressed similar emotion in April 1701, when his wife was "in a most grievous distress [with a] violent toothache and swelling in her face." His solution was "prayers," which was probably as useful as the "resolution and patience" that Alicia Synge's governess recommended a half-century later.[15] Some individuals such as Catherine Peacock of County Limerick opted in the late 1740s for the more orthodox but doubtful therapies of bleeding and lancing the gums.[16] Most resorted to the more common palliatives derived from the strong tradition of popular medicine: the different commodities from the realms of food, alcohol, and narcotics that possessed or were perceived to possess analgesic qualities. The usefulness of such compounds depended largely on the patient's perception of their effectiveness, but because recourse to them was essentially a matter of judgment and they were generally self-administered, their employment was in keeping with the practice of self-medication that was a prominent feature of contemporary medical culture. Bishop Synge swore by the combination of "toasted figs to the swell'd gums, and syrup of onions to the ear" when he experienced dental problems: "The former never fail'd to break the swelling, nor the latter to lessen the pain," he counselled.[17] Bishop William Nicolson of Derry vouched for the analgesic qualities of chewing "the root of pellitory of Spain, covered with leaf tobacco" when he was "grievously tortured with the tooth ache" in 1719.[18] Others resorted to the application of poultices or to the consumption of brandy or tobacco to achieve the same result, though the social convention that deemed "the two latter not very decorous . . . for a young damsel" discouraged their use and the use later of the opiate laudanum.[19]

Given the proliferation of patent and proprietary medicines that were heavily advertised in the eighteenth century, it was inevitable not only that remedies for the toothache and other dental products featured prominently in the inventories of retailers of commercial medicine, but also that such medications were commonly appealed to. Because most of them were as ineffectual as Mack's Anodyne fluid, which proved of no assistance to the English diarist Silas Neville in 1767, or "Hongary water," which Catherine Peacock imbibed with equal lack of impact in 1749, a majority of sufferers soon determined on extraction.[20] Some even attempted to perform the procedure themselves, though none followed the example of the eccentric English physician Messenger Monsey, who extracted a painful tooth with a combination of catgut and a pistol, though it could be just as hazardous to trust the local "tooth puller."[21] Catherine Peacock, for example, held long and vivid memories of the "racking pain" caused by a botched extraction performed in 1747 by Cyprian Purcell, a local "jack of all trades."[22] The Reverend William French of Frenchpark, County Roscommon, who ministered in the diocese of Elphin, had a still more excruciating experience in 1751, when, having ventured to a "tooth operator" to deal with "a violent tooth ach[e]," he was obliged to endure "great pain and swelling" when the person in which he vested his trust "pull'd out a sound tooth instead of the diseas'd one; and then in attempting to pull this out too, tore his jaw from his cheek."[23]

It is significant, however, that medical negligence of this magnitude did not scare off Peacock or Parson James Woodforde, who endured an experience comparable to that of William French, because there was sometimes no alternative. Both resorted to their local tooth pullers when further extractions were required, though it is noteworthy that Catty Peacock declined to let Cyprian Purcell "draw her tooth" in 1749 when she required attention.[24] Such caution is comprehensible because some patients did not recover from the injuries incurred—as revealed by the example of William Bull, an attorney and agent based in Dublin, whose death in 1766 was "occasioned . . . by the drawing of teeth" when he did not recover from the injuries incurred.[25] It is not apparent precisely what happened in this instance, but the avoidance of serious injury was an important consideration in persuading those requiring dental assistance to seek out "the best tooth drawer" available[26] and to pay accordingly.[27] Patients were certainly disposed to go to great lengths to locate the best practitioner by the "hazardous" reputation of premodern surgery and, having informed themselves on the respective merits of those available, to opt for the person who was "safe and skilful . . . and not rash."[28] They were prompted to do so also by the appreciating belief in a culture of curing encouraged by the confident claims of the advocates of diagnostic medicine as well as by the evidently self-interested claims of the purveyors of patent and proprietary cure-alls. In this respect, Ireland was comparable to premodern England, of which it has been observed: if it was "a sickness society," it was "equally a medicine society."[29]

The marketing of medicine for every recognized illness, including those of a dental character, was central to the emergence of a consumer society in eighteenth-century Ireland.[30] Yet the increased demand for dental intervention was paradoxically itself a negative consequence of the growth in consumption—specifically the sharp rise in the consumption of sugar, chocolate, coffee, and refined white flour, which was one of the primary causes of a virtual epidemic of tooth decay in the seventeenth and eighteenth centuries.[31] This problem might not have been so serious if the increase in income of which greater sugar, coffee, and white flour consumption and tooth decay were manifestations were matched by the existing medical infrastructure's capacity to provide preventative and interventionist medical solutions and had "craft and oral transmission [not] predominated over formal and organized learning." In Ireland, as in Britain, the provision of dental care, which in practice prioritized extraction over restoration, was assumed primarily by journeymen surgeons and "tooth pullers" who had the nerve, skill, and basic instruments required to perform the function.[32] Had the provisions of the charter of the Guild of St. Magdalene, which stipulated that "noe person shall or may exercise any of the several arts and mysteries of chirurgeons . . . unless admitted first free of the said corporation," been enforced, this task would have been performed only by surgeons who had completed a recognized apprenticeship, but the combination of the guild's weakness and the implications of the so-called Quack's Charter approved at Westminster in 1542, which stated that any person with "knowledge" was at liberty "to practice, use and minister in and to any outward sore, wound, swelling or disease," ensured that unsworn (and, by implication, hardly trained) practitioners were commonplace.[33] The guild sought repeatedly in the early decades of the eighteenth century to inhibit unlicensed practice by sanctioning a penalty of five pounds per month on such practitioners, but it was powerless to enforce its local monopoly and could do little other than acknowledge despairingly that its members were "much imposed upon by . . . [the] foreigners and intruders who take upon them" to practice "without qualifying" according to the guild's rules.[34] The corporation did occasionally prosecute unregistered surgeon practitioners, but this action was already too late to redeem the guild's reputation, which was described unkindly in 1703 as "a refuge for empiricks, impudent quacks, women and other idle persons" from other "trades," who perpetrated "gross errors . . . and barbarous and inhumane practice."[35] Some surgeons conceived that they could better maintain their reputations by establishing a separate organization that would encourage "the true professors of surgery," but Parliament was uninterested, which did nothing for the reputation either of surgeons in general or of those who specialized in dental treatments.[36] Bishop Synge, as usual, captured the reality of the situation when he observed in 1752 not only that "the best surgeons are not . . . the best tooth-drawers," but also that others who had acquired the elusive "[k]nack . . . by practice" had usurped them in the public estimation.[37]

Matters need not have developed in this way had both the Irish Parliament and the Guild of St. Magdalene taken a more direct and interventionist interest in medical regulation.[38] Both were guided in their inactivity by the Westminster legislature's disinterest when they might more profitably have looked to France, where more progressive attitudes had brought about the separation of dentistry and surgery and the emergence of the former as a distinct branch of medicine by the beginning of the eighteenth century. French *dentistes* were indicatively the first in Europe to discourage extraction and to promote the use of toothbrushes, and the advanced character of the dental welfare they practiced and promoted is attested by the books on dentistry published by Fauchard, Geraudly, Bunon, Mouton, Lécluse, Bourdet, Jourdain, and Auzebi. The most influential among these new *dentistes* was Pierre Fauchard (1678–1761), the so-called father of modern dentistry, whose celebrated study *Le chirurgien dentiste ou traité des dents* in 1728 gave the word *dentist* to the world. An encyclopedic account of dental knowledge at the time, *Le chirurgien dentiste* comprised sixty-four chapters and forty-two plates in two substantial volumes. Fauchard's aim was to improve the standard of dentistry and to establish it as a discrete and advanced field of medicine separate from and superior to the empiric "tooth drawers" that were as plentiful in Paris as elsewhere. To this end, he contrived not just to produce a work containing the full store of current knowledge of the physiology and pathology of teeth but also to provide detailed instruction (volume 2) on the most efficient use of the instruments he described, on the making and fitting of prostheses (in which he pioneered new techniques), and on the best therapeutic responses to the range of dental problems, medical and aesthetic, that he described in detail in volume 1 of his study.[39]

As valuable as Fauchard's book was as a source of technical information and guide to best practice, it was no less useful as a source of information on teeth and their development, on dental hygiene, on diseases of the gums and mouth, and on corrective and restorative dentistry because Fauchard was acutely conscious of the aesthetic appeal of good-looking teeth. He was precocious also in identifying heavy sugar consumption as detrimental to both gums and teeth, in recommending limits to its ingestion, in advising that teeth should be cleaned regularly by dental professionals, in identifying the dangers and limits of current practices, and in exposing the limits of contemporary understanding. He was also a relentless critic of the culture of quackery, as he perceived it in Paris, but it is notable that though he aspired to elevate the *dentiste* "above the level of 'empiricism' and quackery," he was "not so different," Colin Jones persuasively argues, not least because he was every bit as "entrepreneurial" as the empirics who were his target.[40]

Be that as it may, Pierre Fauchard's *Le chirurgien dentiste* was a milestone in the development of dentistry. This status was acknowledged by the publication of a German translation in 1733 and of a revised and expanded second edition in Paris in 1746. A further French edition followed in 1786, but no English or Irish edition is recorded. This does not mean that Fauchard's work was unknown in these kingdoms. Edward Worth, the early-eighteenth-century doctor and book collector, secured a copy for the fine library of scientific and medical books he bequeathed to Sir Patrick Dun's Hospital in 1733.[41] Yet the emphasis attached to tooth "drawing" in the British Isles,[42] when compared with the attention that Fauchard, Bourdet, and other French specialists afforded to restoring decayed teeth and advanced technique, indicates that its impact was modest and suggests that Colin Jones's recent assessment that, "in matters dental, the English were way behind the French" was true also of Ireland.[43]

This need not have been the case because there was an identifiable interest in Ireland in improved dental care dating back to the 1680s. The earliest known attempt to respond to this issue was by Charles Allen, whose tract *The Operator for the Teeth, Shewing How to Preserve the Teeth and Gums from All the Accidents They Are Subject To* was published in Dublin in 1686 and 1687. Allen was English, so his presence in Dublin suggests that he was an itinerant dental practitioner and that he used the tract to attract attention.[44] It is not apparent how skillful a practitioner he was or of the level of demand for his services in Ireland, but the attention he afforded the care of teeth and gums, the causes of tooth decay, toothache, teething in children, and the proper use of the "dental pelican" (an instrument for removing teeth) in his pamphlet suggests that he cannot be dismissed simply as a quack, interested merely in making money. That said, his perturbing advice to parents that teething in children might be facilitated by making a cross incision with "a lancer or very sharp penknife" in the gum at the point where the new tooth would emerge was hardly mitigated by his recipe for an exotic pain-easing wash made from figs boiled in whey, plaintain water, honey of roses, and syrup of violets.[45]Allen, it can safely be assumed, followed the practice of most itinerant medical practitioners and moved on once he had exhausted the financial opportunity he identified in Ireland. However, Dublin was a fast-growing city in the late seventeenth and early eighteenth centuries, and because a majority of its residents possessed English ancestry, they were predisposed to look to England for solutions to their dental problems. The range of services available was limited, but it is noteworthy that by the early eighteenth century a heavy emphasis was placed on prosthetics because it was the development of "artificial teeth" by "highly skilled and entrepreneurial master goldsmiths, watchmakers and ivory-turners" in the late seventeenth century that had prompted a "socially- and cosmetically-driven demand" for such products.[46] In dental terms, this meant dentures, and it is notable that in 1707 one could purchase a set of "artificial teeth" that, it was promised, were "put in so neatly," they were impossible to tell from "natural ones." Dental discoloration was another priority; teeth that had become "black and ill-coloured" could be "cleaned and polished."[47]

Dentures and dental discoloration remained abiding concerns for the self-conscious citizenry of Dublin,[48] but the broader health implications of dental neglect presented opportunities for ambitious dental practitioners, who were more skilled than the ordinary tooth pullers. The first to rise to the challenge was Samuel Steel, a licensed "surgeon and operator for the teeth," who commenced practice at the beginning of the eighteenth century and who was based at "the sign of the Surgeon and Tooth Drawer" at Dublin's Essex Bridge when he commenced advertising his services in 1715. He indicated then that, as well as cleaning "black teeth" and fitting dentures "useful to eat with" that could "be worn several years" and kept in overnight, he could extract teeth or "stumps" of teeth and ease toothache. A still more significant detail because it highlights that even reputable practitioners were influenced by the sales methods of irregular practitioners was that by retailing two tooth medications he anticipated the culture of commercial medicine that grew dramatically in the 1720s: a tooth powder, Pulvis Dentifricia, that "cleanses, scowers, and makes white the foulest teeth" and "countered bad breadth of dental origins and the Antiscorbutic Opiat, which, as well as defeating 'most distempers of the teeth,' fortified gums against defluctions, which is the cause that loosens the teeth." Significantly, the latter was applied once a week with a toothbrush.[49]

Steel was an innovative surgeon, alert to new ideas and approaches, which was crucial to his long-term success in the competitive commercial environment then emerging. He certainly appreciated the potential of advertising and of the value of the hyperbolic language of quackery because they were the means by which from 1723 he informed the public of his capacity to "ease . . . tooth ache . . . without drawing" and made prospective clients aware that if they brushed with his "excellent dentifrice, which is the safest and of the best composition, . . . twice a week," they would not only rid themselves of bad breath but also fasten "loose teeth." He also pioneered a superior "new method . . . [of] his own invention"—the details of which he kept secret—of tying dentures in place, in place of his "former method of tying them with silk strings"; this meant that dentures lasting "several years" could "be put into the mouth and taken out again in less than half a minute."[50]

Steel exaggerated the convenience of his dentures, but his marketing was sufficiently effective to enable him to prevail over his competitors. This advantage was most obvious in dentifrice, in which, he maintained, he encountered a number of "pretenders to this art" who were "wholy ignorant of the practice of dentistry."[51] Whether this claim was true or not, Steel demonstrated his skill at attracting notice to the dental service he provided by pioneering the practice in Ireland of illustrating his advertisements with appropriate woodcuts. His initial venture in this direction in 1725 featured a patient sitting on the ground having a tooth extracted (fig. 1.1); assuming this image accurately reflected Steel's method of working, it suggests that he employed a variation on the technique popularized by Fauchard, which was to sit patients on a chair, in place of the traditional stance in which the patient and practitioner sat on the floor with the patient's head between the latter's legs. In response to a competitor's adoption of a comparable image of a man holding an aching jaw in 1729, Steel subsequently opted for the graphic symbol of a molar tooth (fig. 1.2).[52]

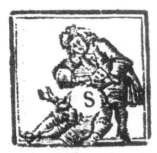
A M U E L S T E E L Surgeon and Operator for the Teeth, living on Ormond Key, oppofite the Cuftom Houfe, Dublin, whofe Experience in drawing Teeth is very well known He gives eafe to the Tooth Ach, and often perfectly cures them without Drawsing, cleans Teeth, be they never fo foul, with Directions how to preferve them. He makes artificial Teeth fo neat, that they cannot be difcovered from natural ones, and as ufeful to eat with as others; for by a New Experiment, they may be worn feveral Years, without being taken out of the Mouth, nor is it any trouble to the Perfon that has them, and much fweeter and cleaner than the former Method of tying them with Silk-ftrings. *N. B.* He has the moft excallent Dentifrice which is the fafeft Compofition for cleaning and fcowering the Teeth, &c.

1.1. Samuel Steel's advertisement in *Dublin Weekly Journal*, 27 August 1727. Courtesy of the National Library of Ireland.

Though Steel used print to market his services in a manner directly comparable to the most skilled retailers of commercial medicine and quack doctors, he was a respectable member of the Guild of Barbers, Surgeons, Apothecaries, and Perukemakers, having served as warden in 1707–1708, and remained sufficiently active in the organization in the interval to stand as candidate in the contest for the mastership in 1729. The fact that Steel registered only four votes (out of a total of sixty-one) in a three-cornered vote attests to the modest size of the dental interest in the guild, but the increased availability of dental hygiene products highlighted that it was already a well-established feature of the fast-growing world of commercial medicine.[53] This increased availability was symbolically affirmed in 1728 when John Audouin, a surgeon who was hanged in Dublin in 1728 for the murder of his servant maid, included his recipe "to make teeth white" in a farewell publication of

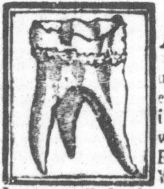AT the Golden Tooth on Ormond Key the Foot Eſſex Bridge, lives Samual Steel Surgeon and Operater for the Teeth, whoſe Abilities in drawing Teeth is well known, having had the Experience of above thirty Years Practice in this City. In many Caſes he gives Eaſe and removes the Pain without Drawing, cleans Teeth from all tartarous and fetid Coagulations, (occaſioned by the Scurvy) which looſen the Teeth, cauſes an offenſive Breoth, and depraved Appetite, with certain and ſure Directions to perſerve them or the future.

He makes artificial Teeth to ſuch Perfection, that the uſe of them, and their likeneſs to natural Ones, has produced Admiration to all wear them by a Method intirely owing to his own Invention. They may be put in and taken out of the Mouth in leſs than half a Minute, and are in no Danger of falling out, they may be worn ſeveral Years with Pleaſure and much cleaner and ſweeter than the old Method of tying with Silk Strings. He has the beſt Antiſcorbutick Powder for cleanſing foul Teeth, and perſerveing them from Scurvy. Note, There are ſome Pretenders to this Practice that are Ignoant of it, but they are eaſily diſcover'd

1.2 Samuel Steel's advertisement in *Dublin Weekly Journal*, 23 August 1729. Courtesy of the National Library of Ireland.

his "choice receipts in physick and surgery, for the cure of diseases."[54] However, Richard Dickson, the most successful retailer of proprietary medicines in Ireland for several decades beginning in the mid-1720s, demonstrated it in a more practical manner by his inclusion of a "specifick tincture," an "antiscorbutic powder" for the teeth, a dental powder, and an unspecified remedy for toothache on the expanding list of nostrums that he offered for sale and by his claim that his "specifick tincture and powder" assisted with all aspects of dental hygiene:

> [It] assuredly preserves the [teeth] from rotting, and those that are a little decayed from becoming worse; makes the foulest teeth as white as ivory, fastens those that are loose, and by often using, utterly extirpates all scurvy-humours in the gums, making them grow up to the teeth again to admiration. It is neither disagreeable to the smell or taste, but really preserves the teeth and gums from all manner of foulness, corruption and putrefaction, and may be depended upon to answer the character here given of it literally and in every respect.[55]

From the early 1730s, Dickson provided his customers with printed directions on how to get the best from products such as the "tincture for the teeth," "powder for the teeth," and "paste for the toothache," all of which he retailed as stock items.[56] Moreover, he keenly followed changes in public taste, for when Thomas Greenough's "celebrated tinctures for the teeth," which received a royal patent in 1743, emerged as the most popular tooth preservative and cure for toothache, Dickson added it to the extensive list of medications he retailed. By the early 1750s, Greenough's Tinctures were firmly established as market leader.[57]

The dominance of the retailers of commercial medicine in the market for proprietary medicine obliged dental practitioners to concentrate on the surgical and prosthetic aspects of dental health. They did not cease selling dentifrice, but, as much as can be figured based on those who can be identified, the most striking feature of this branch of medical activity was the small number of "surgeons and operators of the teeth" who were active at any given time. Samuel Steel's main competitors during his lifetime were William Breach, who was master of the Guild of

Barbers and Surgeons in 1707–1708, and Thomas Osborn (who had "serv'd his apprenticeship" with Breach), an active guild member for twenty years from 1714.[58] Another of Breach's apprentices to make it good was Thomas Allam, who was less active in the guild, but whose distinctive advertisements included an arresting image of a man holding his jaw (fig. 1.3).[59] All had to compete with itinerant operators from England, such as J. Playne from London, who plied for business from Temple Bar in the early 1730s. Significantly, these operators offered little that was not available from the most high-profile Irish practitioners, and it appears, based on the fact that Samuel Steel remained the preference among the social elite, that dental practice evolved but slowly.[60]

With the passing of Samuel Steel and Thomas Allam, a new generation of "operators for the teeth" emerged in the late 1740s and 1750s. Michael Oborn, who was not a licensed surgeon, succeeded to Allam's practice, but though he claimed he possessed the same capacity to draw teeth and to ease "tooth ache without pain or drawing teeth," the extension of an invitation to Charles Williams, a "surgeon and operator for

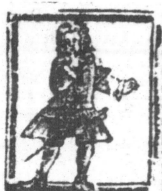

THOMAS ALLAM, Surgeon and Operator for the Teeth, who ferved his Apprenticefhip to the famous *William Breach*, deceas'd, living at the *Little Blue Man*, the corner Houfe in *Golden Lane*, near *Bride-ftreet*, *Dublin*, whofe Experience in drawing Teeth is very well known, and in taking out Stumps to the greateft Perfection. He makes Artificial Teeth fo near that they can't be difcover'd by the fharpeft Eye from natural.

N. B. He has the moft excellent Dentifrice' &c. which is the fafeft Compofition for cleaning and preferving the Teeth, be they ever fo foul, and which often perfectly cures them without drawing.

1.3 Thomas Allam's advertisement in *Dublin Weekly Journal*, 24 January 1730. Courtesy of the National Library of Ireland.

the teeth from London," to succeed Steel suggests that there was far from universal contentment by that date regarding the standard of care that was available. Williams boasted when he was ensconced in the city that he "had the honour of being employed by some of the nobility and gentry," and it is clear from his avowal that he would "attend any, either in city or county[,] who are pleased to favour him with their commands" that he courted upper-class custom. He also contrived to win public confidence by promising (as Allam had done previously) to remove "any tooth or stump however difficult . . . with the greatest ease, safety and expedition" and by claiming that he could do so safely because he used an "instrument . . . of late invention . . . that it is not possible the jaw can be injured by it."[61] Typical of the times, Williams did not reveal the specifications of this "instrument," but such vagueness did not inhibit him from acquiring a reputation as "the best tooth drawer" in Dublin by the early 1750s. When Robert French (1690–1772), justice of the Court of Common Pleas, recommended Williams to Bishop Edward Synge, who had "no opinion of Samuel Steel," Synge advised his daughter Alicia to attend Williams in the belief that "he may be useful to you both in drawing the teeth you must lose, and preserving the rest."[62]

Based on such testimonials, it is apparent that Williams deserved his reputation as "a famous operator for teeth," and he contrived to maintain it by publicizing that he employed the most up-to-date methods. He also retailed dental products; he advertised an "Elixir for the Teeth" for sale in 1747 that "is a certain preservative against decay and rottenness, cures the scurvy in the gums, and in a short time will make the teeth as white as ivory."[63] This claim was sheer hyperbole, but it is indicative of the fact that what attracted customers and paying clients did not always have a sound base—exemplified, perhaps, by Williams's advice to patients not to use toothbrushes: "He is against brushes, and the use of any thing hard or gritty; recommends a sponge, and a linctus which cleans with a kind of lather, without fretting the gums."[64] This advice was accepted as entirely "reasonable," and it is significant that though it contradicted the advice previously given by Samuel Steel, it was consistent with Fauchard's recommendation that gums and teeth should be treated with a sponge dipped in water fortified with aqua vitae and a special paste.[65] It does not appear that Williams was guided by Fauchard's treatise because he acquired the recipe for the paste he retailed at his College Green address from a lesser Italian practitioner, Dr. Guiovani. Indeed, Williams subsequently published a translation of Guiovani's *Treatise on the Disorders of the Teeth and Gums* with "directions for using the liquid paste."[66]

Although Williams may have been prompted to publish Guiovani's tract by his belief in the paste's medicinal efficacy, it is still more notable that he took recourse to a pamphlet to promote the commodity, a print form that the advocates of therapies as diverse as bathing and proprietary medicines employed at this time as a sales medium.[67] His application of the sales techniques favored by the more aggressive retailers of proprietary medicine to dentistry attests to the continuing closeness of the links between Irish "operators for the teeth" and the world of commercial medicine. The fact that he chose to market a dental medication of continental origin was another indicator.

The overwhelming majority of the patent and proprietary medicines offered for sale in Ireland were of English origin, but the mystique attached to exotic-sounding nostrums and the high standing in which eminent European medics such as Herman Boerhaave were held encouraged medical entrepreneurs to seek out their fellows on the continent.[68] Significantly, as in England, few of the dental practitioners in Ireland originated in France, and it is notable also that *none* of the major works on dentistry by Fauchard, Geraudly, Bunon, Mouton, Lecluse, Bourdet, and Jourdain were published in Dublin during the course of the eighteenth century. As Jones has suggested, this neglect of the French may have resulted from the suspicion with which France was regarded within the elite because other European nationalities fared better.[69] Thus, Bartholomew Ruspini, "an Italian surgeon and licentiate of the great medical college and hospital of Bergamo" who visited Dublin in 1753, offered a dental cure-all "made known to him at the said College."[70] However, print was a still more reliable source of new ideas, and it is notable that the fourth edition of the German physician Friedrich Hoffmann's (1660–1742) work *A Treatise on the Teeth, Their Nature, Structure Formation, Beauty, Connection, and Use* was published in Dublin in 1760, including the important section on the "disorders" to which teeth were subject and Hoffman's "remedies" for these disorders.[71] This publication did not make up for the neglect of Fauchard or, indeed, of John Hunter's seminal *Natural History of the Human Teeth*, published in London in 1771, which is now acknowledged as an important work in the "rise of surgery from manual craft to scientific discipline," although, based on the presence of two copies of the first edition in Irish libraries, it possibly did have Irish readers.[72] Be that as it may, most of the small number of dental texts published in Dublin were of English origin, usually by individuals now regarded as "academic lightweights." The most notable was Thomas Berdmore's *Treatise on the Disorders and Deformities of the Teeth and Gums*, which came "illustrated with cases and experiments, intended for general use."[73]

Though the amount of print devoted to the promotion of dentistry was modest, it was still significant, and it attests to the interest in improving the standards of dentistry identifiable in the 1760s and 1770s. It was encouraged, moreover, by an increase in cosmetic dentistry, a feature of the rage for cosmetic enhancement then current, which suggests in turn that Irish consumers were not untouched by the French desire to make the mouth a pleasing feature of the human body. "All manner of cosmetic and medical preparations were marketed" in order to enhance the wearer's aesthetic allure, and because pearly white teeth were as esteemed as a blemish-free complexion and extravagant hair, dentists were as eager as the retailers of commercial medicine to profit from this fashion. A tract published in 1777 for the guidance of young ladies highlighted this goal by including a section on "opiates for preserving and whitening the teeth."[74] Few products were offered for sale solely with this purpose in mind. The Essence of Pearl and Pearl Dentrice developed by Jacob Hemet, the dentist to Queen Charlotte and Princess Amelia, was marketed in traditional terms as a preventative of toothache and tooth decay, a cure for scurvy of the gums, and a sweetener of the breadth, but the tell-tale pointer to the market at which it was targeted is provided by the prioritizing of its capacity to "render" teeth "white and beautiful."[75] Similar claims were advanced regarding "the tincture and dentifrice" sold by Henry Hart, a dentist based at

Crow Street, and Thomas Greenough's celebrated and long-established tinctures.[76]

A positive consequence of the desire for "white" teeth was a greater receptivity to new dental products. This receptivity dovetailed with the surge in the consumption of proprietary medicines in general, which peregrinating quacks such as "the famous Mrs Bernard from Berlin" were quick to cash in on, but it also served as a stimulus to local dental surgeons and encouraged ambitious itinerant practitioners not just to include Dublin in their travels, but also to demonstrate new techniques and skills.[77] The most notable practitioner of this sort was Mr. Davy, who visited Ireland in 1782 (and subsequently teamed up with Mrs. Bernard). Davy was an experienced and adept self-publicist in the tradition of the most successful itinerant quacks of the age, but he was also a skillful "dentist" who advertised his ability to transplant teeth and to fix artificial "teeth, from one to a whole set, by a new and safe method (without giving the least pain) much preferable to any other mode ever before invented." Such a claim was not without precedent in Ireland; Henry Hart had made it known some years earlier that he "makes and fixes from one to a complete set of artificial teeth," reinstates "natural teeth," and performs other complex procedures, but he did so in such a low-key manner as not to encourage confidence in his abilities.[78] Nonetheless, it is apparent that the techniques of those practicing dentistry in Dublin attracted paying customers. Thus, the Dublin businessman Daniel Geale in 1779 paid Edward Hudson, who was the only dental practitioner listed in the Dublin Directory at that moment, £1.2s.9d for a "false tooth" and the still more imposing sum of £6.16s.6d for unspecified work six years later.[79] It was the practice also by the 1780s for groups of rural gentry to travel to Dublin in "a teeth-cleaning party." They may not have had an enormous number of practitioners from which to choose, but the fact that they made the journey with this purpose in mind attests to the emergence, many decades after it had taken place in France, of dentistry as a distinct and recognized branch of medicine. It was during the 1770s that the term *dentist* displaced *surgeon and operator for the teeth* as the appellation of choice of those who pursued this branch of medicine in Ireland.[80]

Practitioners such as Davy and Hart did not conceal their concern at the damage caused to tooth enamel by "the frequent use of instruments and particular powders" that were resorted to in order to correct discoloration and to whiten teeth.[81] Yet the practical reality for those who sought personally to care for their teeth was that their choice of dental powders was limited. The runaway market leader remained Greenough's Tinctures, which was stocked by all of the new generation of ambitious medical retailers who emerged in the 1770s and 1780s. A number maintained that they possessed the exclusive sales rights, but it could be purchased readily from James Hoey, John Magee, Michael Mills, William Wilson, William Bate, Robert Marchbank, Spilsbury and Duignan, and others for between 1s.3d to 1s.7d a bottle during the 1770s, 1780s, and 1790s.[82] It had competitors in Hemet's Essence of Pearl and Pearl Dentifrice, Hamilton's Tincture (both of which were well advertised in Great Britain), and Earlo's Pill and Tincture for the toothache, but because the latter were on average more than twice the cost, they were at an obvious disadvantage in the marketplace.[83]

The most expensive tooth powder of all was produced by Chevalier Bartholomew Ruspini (1728–1813), who had achieved renown in London as the author of "a treatise on the teeth" and "surgeon dentist to . . . the Prince of Wales" in the interval since his visit to Dublin in 1753. He attracted further notice in the late 1780s as creator of a styptic solution that, it was claimed, had "the most salutary effects, both internal and external, in all haemorrhages," but his most lucrative nostrums were a tincture and dentifrice, which were applied with a sponge and a brush, which retailed at eight shillings, one and a half pence in Ireland in the early 1790s.[84] Because of the cost of Ruspini's medications and the hyperbole with which he extolled their merits, satirists and caricaturists mocked him relentlessly.[85] This mockery was more obvious in London than in Dublin, but the perception that he and others like him were motivated solely by greed encouraged skepticism in some quarters, which was reinforced by the knowledge that claims by dentists to possess a "cure for that madness the toothache," gum disease, and tooth decay were egregiously misleading.[86]

As a consequence, even skillful dental practitioners such as James Law, who trained under "the celebrated William Rae" in London before he fixed his plate at Andrew Street, Dublin, in the early 1790s, were singled out. To be sure, Law's claims that he could "manufacture *new gums* and *palates* in a manner not to be distinguished from real nature" as well as fix dentures were imprudent, though he was, as events showed, a talented dentist.[87] Such criticism had little obvious negative impact on a commercial medical culture in which hyperbole and exaggeration were an engrained feature of the sales language. In any event, it ought not obscure the fact that by the early 1790s, as one contemporary noted, "the profession of dentist is becoming very common in this city."[88] Indeed, it was possible at that date (provided one had the money, of course) to choose between Thomas Barralet, who was based on College Green; John McClean, who operated out of a house on Gardiner's Row; James Law, who relocated to Sackville Street in 1794; and various visitors if one required dental work as well as to purchase a variety of creams, dentifrices, and other lotions either to ease toothache or to cleanse teeth.[89]

Dublin was significantly the only location with enough business to allow dentists to set up permanent practices. Belfast, by contrast, was wholly dependent for most of the 1790s on itinerant practitioners from Dublin, Edinburgh, and London, who chose generally not to spend more than a fortnight or three weeks in the city en route to some other location. The situation was comparable in Cork, Drogheda, and Clonmel, as well, it is to be assumed, in other towns, though Limerick seems to have had a resident "surgeon dentist" in 1790.[90] As a result, even those elements of the population who could afford dental welfare often had no option but to attend whichever itinerant quack came along, which could prove problematic. The case of James Bladen Ruspini, the son and "partner" of the celebrated chevalier of the same surname, is instructive in this respect. Having arrived in Dublin in January 1794 to market the "celebrated dentifrice" that had made his father a great deal of money, James Ruspini opened a "warehouse" to meet demand in the capital before setting out for Cork, where his aggressive sales practices (he initiated "prosecutions against eight shop-keepers . . . for daring to vend a spuri-ous kind of tooth-powder in imitation of his") and high prices embroiled him in a price war with the main local medical retailer and obliged him to focus his efforts on "the nobility and gentry" of the city and its vicin-ity.[91] This situation was hardly ideal, but it is indicative of the fact that at the end of the eighteenth century dentistry was still firmly located in a medical culture in which irregulars were a powerful presence.[92]

The eighteenth century witnessed the first steps toward the develop-ment of a distinct dental medical specialism in Ireland. This develop-ment was institutionally part of the process that prompted the major reorganization of the various medical interests that were long embraced within the Guild of Barbers, Surgeons, Apothecaries, and Perukemak-ers. A turning point was reached with the apothecaries' withdrawal in 1745 to form their own guild, and although surgeons remained formally a part of the guild and continued to be admitted to membership, they chose increasingly to "absent themselves." For them, the foundation in 1784 of the Royal College of Surgeons of Ireland represented a more appropriate educational and institutional home for them.[93] Meanwhile, separate from but parallel with these developments, dentistry slowly forged an identity that combined features of the various medical cul-tures of the age.

Dental practitioners in eighteenth-century Ireland were responsible for their own training. This approach did not lend itself to a high stan-dard of dental care, but it was still possible for the reflective practitioner to acquire an understanding of the biology of dental development and the techniques of dental welfare well in advance of that of his prede-cessors by combining what he learned as an apprentice with the new ideas that were transmitted via the fitful stream of publications devoted to dentistry and the occasional visiting practitioner from abroad. On the evidence available, it is apparent—the adoption of the term *dentist* notwithstanding—that in Ireland as in England there was considerable resistance to the embrace of the advanced ideas developed in France and that the predisposition to extract vividly encapsulated in the terms *tooth puller* and *operator for the teeth* proved enduring. At the same time, most practitioners were profoundly influenced in the manner in which they conducted themselves by the burgeoning culture of commercial medicine. This point needs to be made because of the reflexive tendency to dismiss commercial medicine as mere quackery and to overlook the fact that it, as well as the manufacture and sale of a variety of dental tinctures, pastes, and dentifrices, also promoted a method of operating that involved advertising and the sale of proprietary medications that many dental practitioners pursued. Much of what passed for reliable medication in the eighteenth century may well have been ineffective, but it is improbable that all was equally valueless. Moreover, this conclusion can be asserted confidently with respect to dental problems, for although great pain could be inflicted and serious damage done in drawing a tooth badly, such a procedure was still less serious than the consequences of ignoring dental infection, which could be fatal. Indeed, it may be that the decline in the number whose death was ascribed to "teeth" in the Dublin bills of mortality between the 1710s and the 1730s is not unconnected to the activities of dentists such as Samuel Steel and Thomas Allam or to the improved availability of dentifrices.[94]

Yet the situation might have been still better if Ireland had attached more emphasis to training and qualification and been more receptive to the advanced dental techniques and procedures pioneered in France. As it was, at least among those engaged in dental medicine in Dublin, there was some openness in the second half of the eighteenth century to new ideas, which were conveyed through Irish editions of (mainly safe) English texts, and a steady flow of English itinerant practitioners. It is thus not surprising that the situation in Ireland at the end of the eighteenth century can be compared with that in provincial England, which long sustained a network of itinerant dentists.[95] This was the case certainly in Ireland in the early nineteenth century; the situation is less clear-cut for the eighteenth century, probably because the provision was more uneven. What is apparent is that dentistry in the eighteenth century was a mobile and competitive profession, which acted as a stimulus to dentists to improve the service they offered, as indicated by the criticisms directed at those who used amalgams of lead and quicksilver or tinfoil instead of "virgin gold" to fill teeth in the 1820s.[96] Yet it is salutary to note that the patient's experience of the dentist in the early nineteenth century was little different to his experience of the inefficient "tooth puller" in the eighteenth century. When James Pedlow, who lived near Portadown, County Armagh, had a tooth removed in 1834, his experience was comparable to that of William French eighty-three years earlier; he was obliged to endure "three months suffering" because the person who undertook the task tore his jaw so badly it bled for two months.[97]

2

Women and Tuberculosis in Ireland

Greta Jones

During the late nineteenth and early twentieth centuries, Ireland saw a rise in the death rate from tuberculosis (TB). This rise was occurring at a time when the death rate from TB was in decline in the United States and Great Britain. In Ireland, therefore, the experience of TB was more immediate and vivid than it was perhaps for nations that, although still being affected by the scourge of TB, had seen mortality from it decreasing since the middle of the nineteenth century.[1] Mortality from TB in Ireland did not fall until the first decade of the twentieth century, and it remained at a higher rate than in most other European countries for much longer into the twentieth century.[2] The reasons for the particular TB history of Ireland have been discussed elsewhere,[3] so this article looks at a specific phenomenon: the impact of the TB epidemic on women.

The death rate from TB in Ireland throughout the late nineteenth century and much of the twentieth was higher for females than that it was for males.[4] This gender difference is characteristic of other predominantly rural societies. In general, as urbanization increased in Europe, so too did the male death rate from TB, and in cities it usually exceeded the death rate for females.[5] Similarly, as Ireland underwent increased urbanization in the twentieth century the male and female death rates from TB converged. In Northern Ireland, the male death rate overtook the rate for women in the late 1930s.[6] In the twenty-six counties comprising Saorstát Éireann (the Irish Free State), TB death rates for men were higher by the 1940s. But the rural/urban disparity between male and female death rates from TB remained well into the twentieth century. Donnell Deeny calculated rural/urban rates for Northern Ireland for 1929–38 and found the TB death rate was 129 per 100,000 persons for males and 111 for females in urban areas.[7] However, in rural areas it was 91 for males and 108 for females. Similar differentials between males and females in rural areas can be found for the rest of Ireland.[8]

On closer inspection, however, the situation in Ireland was more complicated. A significant contribution to high female TB death rates there was the result of mortality among female textile workers in the north of Ireland. This meant that the industrial Northeast, unlike most urban areas, showed consistently higher TB mortality rates at most age ranges for women than men.[9] William Johnston has noted this phenomenon among female textile workers in Japan during the late nineteenth and early twentieth century. Japan also experienced rising TB mortality, and Johnston goes as far as to attribute Japan's TB epidemic of the late nineteenth century to the rise of the textile industry there and its effect upon women's health.[10]

Experts on TB would have been aware of the male/female disparity throughout most of the period, but there was very little discussion among them about the relatively greater impact of TB upon women. Except for the diseases of childbirth, authorities made few attempts in the nineteenth century to create a statistical picture of women's health or treat it as a separate focus of investigation. At the end of the nineteenth century, this attitude changed. The participation of married women in the workplace was in decline largely due to changes in the economy, but also in part to culture. More rigid definitions of femininity and increasing emphasis on gender separation at work led to doubts about the suitability of certain occupations for women. The failure of infant mortality to decline as fast as other mortality indices in the 1890s also fueled alarm about the effect of industrial work on women's health. Feminists see this trend, justifiably to an extent, as a means of disempowering women by excluding them from the workplace. However, as Joanna Bourke points out in her study of Irish women and work, the rise in earnings among sections of the working classes, making it easier for wives to remain at home, was frequently welcomed by the women themselves. Investing time and energy in home and family was often preferable to the kinds of poorly paid and arduous work available to them outside the home.[11]

The changing attitude to women's work prompted a number of investigations into women's health in an industrial context. Certifying medical officers, who were tasked with enforcing the Factory Acts by carrying out medical inspection of children entering factories, had already noted in mid-nineteenth-century Belfast a higher female mortality from consumption in the linen textile industry.[12] But the first systematic investigations of the northern Irish textile women came with two major government committees of inquiry in the 1890s. E. H. Osborn compiled a report in 1894 on the conditions at work for women and children in the United Kingdom's linen industry, including Belfast and its environs.[13] A female factory inspector, Miss Collet, produced a further report in 1898.[14] Following up these investigations was the *Report of the Belfast Health Commission* in 1908, which described the general health and sanitary condition of Belfast but also drew attention to the high death rate from consumption among women who had worked or were working in linen mills.[15] As such, these reports provided support to what was previously a largely impressionistic view held by medical men in textile regions of the North that women in northern industrial areas had a higher overall mortality from TB than men.

There were various hypotheses about the peculiar susceptibility of women in the textile trades to TB. C. D. Purdon, a certifying surgeon in the Belfast area, attributed much of the problem to inadequately dressed women being frequently doused in water—a characteristic of wet spinning—and then moving from the hot, humid atmosphere of the mill out into the cold. Purdon also reflected a great deal of the moral anxiety produced by the employment of women in the factory. He believed it had led to a loss of domestic skills and consequent deterioration in diet, which affected the health of the whole family as well as that of the female factory operatives.

Modern reflections on the effect of TB in linen factories point, however, to a combination of factors. The workforce in linen was predominantly female; young females in their early teens or twenties were particularly susceptible to tuberculosis.[16] In the Belfast area, a high proportion of those who entered the factory were migrants from the surrounding countryside, some with very little natural resistance to the disease or for whom the stress of migration to the industrial city reactivated an existing, dormant infection. Although Belfast's housing was reasonably good by the standards of other industrial cities or Dublin, these girls were likely to experience crowded workplaces and lodgings, which facilitated the spread of the infection. The debilitating nature of factory work and the shock to the system of entering the mill also weakened resistance.[17] There were, of course, sites of infection in other occupations employing women. For example, as measured by one mid-nineteenth-century report on disease, Dublin's sweated trades, such as dressmaking and finishing shops, produced high TB rates.[18] But, on the whole, cities presented men with more dangers to their health, and as far as can be ascertained, more men than women died from TB in Dublin.

The higher mortality of women from TB in the country remains an unsolved problem. The same is true for rural TB in general. To an extent, the lack of a solution is understandable given that Ireland's TB epidemic was identified in the 1880s as the result of urbanization.[19] Nonetheless, the neglect of rural TB also leads to the failure to identify the particular problems experienced by women. Some interesting suggestions have been made, however, about the causes of women's greater mortality in rural areas. Sheila Ryan Johansson argues that it was a sociostructural problem in which gender played a major role.[20] Patriarchy led to patterns of control of consumption in the rural family that particularly disadvantaged women and resulted in poorer nutrition among them. In the city in contrast, the availability of employment—at least for the young unmarried women—meant that women, even with poor wages, determined their own access to food. The experience of female linen textile workers suggests Ryan's hypothesis does not hold true for all forms of urban employment. It may, however, explain what happened in some situations and certainly, in relating family structure to health, offers interesting lines of investigation. However, until more research is done on patterns of work, wages, migration, family dynamics, and health, we are unable to pinpoint precisely all the possible causative factors leading to greater female mortality from TB in rural areas.

TB affected all age ranges, but it was a disease of young adults in particular. The most common version was consumption—phthisis or TB of the lungs. When TB bacteria lodged in the lungs, it led to their gradual destruction and to death by suffocation and hemorrhage aggravated by exhaustion. Although some survived initial infection, mortality was high, and even when recovery took place, TB could reappear in later years.[21] Tuberculosis of the limbs, joints, and spine, often contracted in childhood, might result in permanent and severe physical disability. In the early nineteenth century, the famous Dublin physician Richard Carmichael argued that consumption was the result of excess and that the rich were thus particularly susceptible.[22] But as the century progressed, better knowledge of TB's incidence in different social classes and the accumulation of the tubercular in the workhouse changed this view. Although no social class was exempt, poor conditions and overcrowding in the home and workplace increased susceptibility. The onset of consumption led to interruption of work or study. Hence, poverty and TB were frequent companions.[23]

For both men and women, the onset of TB in young adults frequently meant that courtship and marriage were overshadowed by the disease. Members of families in which TB was suspected often experienced reduced chances of marriage. For women, pregnancy was likely to exacerbate the symptoms of the disease, which led to increased likelihood of miscarriage. Individuals and families often concealed tuberculosis, in part because of suspicions that it might be hereditary. A great deal of euphemism was employed in referring to the disease; sufferers were variously described as having a weakness of the lungs, general poor health, and susceptibility to colds, persistent cough, stress, and breakdown. Historians are aware that the phrase "traveling for their health" in written materials usually indicates a victim of consumption.

Because adolescent girls were particularly vulnerable, one of the first legacies of TB in popular culture was the romantic picture of youthful female affliction, as a Dublin doctor, Arthur Clarke, summed up in his depiction of the young female consumptive in 1836. Consumption, in his view, "oftenest seems to select its victims in the spring of life or the fullness of maturity . . . seizes upon the best and loveliest of the flock and, while it leads them to a certain sacrifice, adorns them with new and more touching beauties, lending a lustrous brilliancy to the eye, a wax-like delicacy, alternating with a transparent glow on the cheek, as though it would increase by every means 'the bitterness of death to the surviving friends and strew with flowers the dark path which leads to an early and untimely grave.'"[24] Clarke's description represents a feminization of the disease, which can also be seen in depictions of young male sufferers in the early nineteenth century. In spite of the frequent occurrence of the disease in police and military barracks, certain "feminine" qualities—overexercise of the emotions, an artistic temperament, febrile, unstable behavior, and disappointment in love—were considered to render young males susceptible to consumption (or be developed with the presence of consumption). There were, however, other nineteenth-century iconographies of the female sufferer. The cult of St. Therese of Lisieux, who died of consumption at age twenty-four, provided a model of asceticism, suffering borne bravely, and even a cult of the approaching death.[25] Edel Quinn, who was a prominent figure in the Legion of Mary and died of consumption in 1944 at age thirty-seven, was said to have St. Therese's *The Story of a Soul* "constantly in her hands."[26] Some of the descriptions of life in Catholic-run sanatoria in the twentieth century certainly suggest a kind of fusion of religious experience and tuberculosis.[27]

More robust depictions of the female sufferer can be found in a spoof written by one victim of TB about his contemporaries taking the cure in the Swiss resort town of Davos, popular with Irish consumptives. These individuals included "the quiet girl who fades out of the Davos picture and ten years later has a devoted husband and six healthy children" and "the girl who, being allowed half an hour's walk on the Promenade, climbs the Schiahorn and assures you it has done her no harm."[28] In fact, we know little about how the majority of women responded to the disease, but there is a surprising degree of continuity in how their fate was seen by others, in particular the evocation of the poignancy of a young girl's death from tuberculosis. The song the Belfast singer Van Morrison recorded in the 1960s in memory of a young girl who died from TB, though more brutal and honest, evokes quite as much pathos as Clarke's picture of the young female consumptive in 1836.[29]

The vast majority of the sick in the nineteenth century were nursed at home. In spite of women's exclusion from the medical profession until the middle of the nineteenth century and the relative paucity of female doctors well into the twentieth, the majority of day-to-day medical decisions were paradoxically made by women in the nineteenth century. A doctor in attendance was expensive. The poor-law dispensary system in Ireland was by no means confined to the indigent and was increasingly used in the nineteenth century by the nonpauper population. It brought a doctor and pharmaceuticals within the reach of many poorer Irish families. Nonetheless, the housewife frequently decided what preventative measures to use to keep ill health at bay, how to nurse the sick, and what medicine to administer.

A popular belief in the nineteenth century was that TB was the product of "neglected colds"—in fact, the first signs of infection were often a slight fever and raised temperature. This connection led to an emphasis on wrapping up and bed rest at the appearance of coldlike symptoms. But because TB afflicted those in adulthood or on the verge of adulthood and its progression was slow, especially in the case of respiratory TB, the sufferer might conceal his or her symptoms or self-medicate. Only at diagnosis or if the afflicted collapsed would intensive home nursing follow. Home nursing was more likely than not because the consumptive was unpopular in general hospitals owing to the long progression of the disease and poor chances of recovery.[30] The very poorest with little or no home support often ended up in the workhouse infirmary. For this reason, by 1900 the workhouse inmate had the highest incidence of TB of any of the other occupational classifications in public-health reports. For most people with TB, however, until the development of the sanatorium system—and even after that—nursing took place in the home.

The advice of mothers to daughters, sister to sister, and female friend to female friend was an important transmission belt for information about treatment and may have carried as much weight as the opinion of the dispensary or attending doctor—though very little examination of this phenomenon has been done. As literacy and access to printed culture increased in the nineteenth century, so too did the sources of medical information to the woman of the house. Medical information could be found in almanacs, often the only literature in a poorer home, or in books on domestic management for the more literate and better off. Many of these publications bowdlerized scientific medical knowledge. An enterprising publisher might very well scan the pages of the *Dublin Quarterly Journal of Medical Science,* available from 1832, for the latest fashionable treatments. A successful almanac would be reprinted regularly, and updating the medical knowledge in it was not a high priority. Almanacs and manuals of domestic management could survive for many years in a home, which produced the effect that much of the knowledge about the treatment of TB was the medical science of a previous generation.

Johnson and Oldham's Housekeeper's Almanac: A Manual of Domestic Medicine and the Treatment of Disease, published in Dublin in 1872 by a firm of dispensing chemists, advised the use of counter irritants, emetics, and bleeding in the treatment of consumption.[31] Even by 1872 this advice was old-fashioned. By the 1860s, it had been superseded in medical circles by the climatic treatment of TB, which advised travel to find the weather and air quality that might effect a cure. Inhalation of iodine, a fad that swept Dublin medical circles in the 1830s and that Arthur Clarke described in his 1836 pamphlet, similarly remained popular to the end of the nineteenth century in spite of the revolution in understanding the cause of TB brought about by Robert Koch's discovery of the TB bacterium in 1882. Patent-medicine advertisement also exercised an effect on treatment. Though some patent medicines advertised in newspapers were also found in the pharmacies of workhouses and dispensaries, many were of dubious value and even fraudulent.

Treatment in successive generations rested upon what mother dispensed, and it included medical advice from the doctor, commercially advertised patent cures, almanacs and domestic-management books, advice from relatives and friends. Even when the family almanac had disintegrated into dust, memory of the treatment remained, which some-times produced confusion about oral and folk tradition. For example, the Johnson and Oldham manual of 1872 and other similar publications of the time advertised linseed oil as a patent medicine suitable for the treatment of consumption. In 1972, linseed oil is listed as a traditional Irish folk remedy against consumption.[32] "Folk cures" were conversely sometimes turned into commercial products. A tobacconist in Belfast in the late nineteenth century was reputed to sell cigarettes made from mullein leaves, and mullein is listed as a cure for TB in folklore collections. In *Treatise on Consumption of the Lungs* (1726), which advertised itself as exemplifying the latest "scientific medicine," Edward Barry similarly includes the old folk remedy of drinking milk in which snails have been boiled. This cure resurfaces in 1904 as what Dr. H. S. Purdon describes as "an old north of Ireland cure" for consumption in an article he wrote for the *Ulster Journal of Archaeology*.[33] But Purdon's gardener, who told him of this cure, might very well have acquired the knowledge from written sources utilizing Barry's work rather than from an authentic, unbroken oral tradition.[34]

It is important to see medical publications, including manuals on domestic health, in the context of the marketplace or the competition for patients. Medical professionals regarded their treatises and articles as advertisement of their knowledge and an aid to recruit patients and therefore, it was hoped, to supplement their income. Though they often belonged to "schools," they would generally hedge their bets and append to their work a wide variety of possible cures—just in case. However, health manuals written for women by medical professionals or voluntary charitable organizations often conveyed moral and social messages along with medical "expertise." This was one reason why qualified women doctors soon entered the field of providing medical knowledge and health advice to women. Much of their motivation was similar to that of their male colleagues, but it was sometimes driven by anxiety at what they felt was the limited appreciation of women's lives by doctors and even some professionals' outright antifeminism. With the rise of first-wave feminism in the late nineteenth century, handbooks of medical advice to the housewife became contested territories.[35]

The available cures and treatments in the nineteenth century were eclectic and varied in origin. This was particularly the case with TB, from which recovery was possible, but no understanding existed of how or why it went into remission. As a consequence, TB encouraged a great deal of entrepreneurship in finding treatments from which medics, patent-medicine vendors, dispensing chemists, and medical entrepreneurs in general benefited. Even well into the twentieth century, when understanding of the disease had considerably advanced and a medically approved regime of treatment had emerged, doctors recognized the psychological dimension of disease and sometimes recommended medicines of doubtful efficacy simply for the hope they inspired.[36] Families would also persist with dosages of valueless concoctions as part of remembered family tradition. Patent-medicine vendors continued to package optimism about survival to the hopeless.

The age in which scientific understanding of TB took a giant step forward was when in 1882 Robert Koch identified the bacterium that caused TB. The spread of understanding of the significance of this finding among the general public was surprisingly slow. By the 1890s, however, the majority of medical professionals were convinced of the validity of Koch's conclusions and TB's infectious nature. There was no effective cure for TB until the advent of therapeutic drug treatment in the 1940s, but the fact that it was now seen as an infectious and not constitutional disease forged a consensus around the most appropriate hygienic regime to combat it. By 1900, a program of recommended measures had emerged, including segregation of the infected and the provision of separate laundry and eating utensils. Medical advice demanded that the home and workplace were to be kept dust free and that the sputum of those infected by TB be destroyed; in addition, measures against spitting in public were enacted by Dublin Corporation and other local government agencies. Nutritious food and rest were recommended for the patient, as well as a regime of exposure to fresh air by opening windows or wheeling the patient's bed outside.

The fight against nineteenth-century epidemic diseases such as typhus and cholera had already created an infrastructure of government and local-authority services. Looked at from the perspective of the nineteenth century, much of the early effort against TB was an adaptation of existing practices developed by these agencies to combat the "fevers"—disinfection of the sick room by public-health officials, extended notification of disease, and isolation of the patient. The public-health measures enacted to bring about decline in epidemic disease, such as water provision and nuisance removal, also had a strong impact on the nineteenth-century domestic environment and hence particularly on women. The campaign against TB, launched in most countries in the 1890s, was the motor for further changes in expectations of what was considered an acceptable domestic environment. It refocused attention on women's role in cleansing and regulating the domestic space.[37]

Historians have noted the extra pressure that the hygienic regime for combating TB put upon women.[38] It also became clear, as the campaign progressed, that the burden of providing separate sleeping accommodation, constantly changing bed linen and utensils, and providing nutritious food for the tubercular was too great for many working-class homes. In these circumstances, free sanatorium treatment for the poor became the ideal sought by campaigners against TB. Charitable provision proved inadequate, however, and the state increasingly became involved in building and subsidizing sanatoria and sanatorium treatment. TB was also the spur to early-twentieth-century housing reform— the provision of houses built and rented from local government—with the aim of reducing overcrowding and therefore slowing down the rate of infection. By the twentieth century, TB increasingly brought the state into medical provision and social reform.

Voluntary sanitary societies had grown in the nineteenth century as agents of domestic reform. Composed largely of middle-class women volunteers, they gave advice to women about the home nursing of fever patients, diet, cleanliness, and so on. They engaged in visits to the sick and campaigned for improvements in water supply and sewage and against adulterated food. In this capacity, many of their members were among the first women elected to local government positions at the end of the nineteenth century. These women were agents of sanitary reform, but they also illustrate the distance that existed between the life of the poor and the assumptions of Victorian sick nursing. Much of their advice was framed in ignorance of the realities of working-class life.[39] In the fight against TB, the Women's National Health Association (WNHA), founded in 1907, was the most visible and dramatic example of this kind of engagement against tuberculosis. Formed, staffed, and directed by women, it became engaged with issues of child and maternal health and, above all, with Ireland's TB problem.

The WNHA has sometimes been seen as a kind of protofeminist group and its leader, the Liberal home ruler Lady Aberdeen, wife of Ireland's viceroy, as a heroine of the struggle against TB. However, much of the credit for the fight against TB should be given to the largely male and doctor-led National Association for the Prevention of Tuberculosis, at whose suggestion the WNHA was founded and who continued to work closely with it and guide its deliberations. The patronage of Dublin Castle and Lady Aberdeen's public profile propelled the WNHA to prominence in these years and led to the WNHA's becoming the leading organization dedicated to the fight against TB in Ireland before the First World War. Its roots were firmly in the late-nineteenth-century tradition of voluntary fund-raising and woman-to-woman transmission of hygienic advice. Nonetheless, although the WNHA had a traditional view of women's role, it was the type of organization that propelled women to importance in national issues and thereby accelerated the movement toward their political emancipation, as Patricia Hollis demonstrates in her study of women in nineteenth-century politics.[40] Peamount Sanatorium, founded by Lady Aberdeen outside Dublin in 1912, was one of the few mixed-gender sanatoria that had a woman chief medical superintendent.[41] Women also shared in the expansion of professional opportunities created by the increasing public-health focus on TB, usually through nursing—the TB dispensary nurse became an increasingly familiar figure in the twentieth century. Rarer were women specialists and consultants. Dorothy Stopford-Price, who specialized in childhood TB and was an early advocate of BCG vaccination, is a remarkable exception.[42]

The state's increasing involvement in dealing with TB was a feature of the twentieth century. This involvement was tied up with the introduction of the insurance system in 1911 in Britain and Ireland, which gave the insured access not only to unemployment benefit, but also to health care. Included was a sanatorium benefit paid to those undergoing treatment. Grants were made to local government from the central insurance fund, and councils were allowed to levy a local rate to provide publicly built and operated sanatoria and TB dispensaries. Women benefited from these developments, patchy and inadequate as they were in the first decades of their operation. However, although insurance was supposed to be "gender blind," it was introduced initially in industrial occupations, which meant that only a small number of female-dominated sectors of employment—such as textiles—was covered. For most women, health care was not available under the insurance scheme, so a stay in a sanatorium necessitated falling back upon the poor law.

Though benefits to dependents were gradually introduced, the discourse on TB revolved around the important issue of the cost to a family of removing the main breadwinner, usually male, for sanatorium treatment. Though sanatorium benefit made up some of the shortfall, it was never sufficient to meet the full costs of losing the main wage.[43] This was a real and significant issue for a family. However, concentration on this problem has tended to disguise hidden economic costs borne by women, including the extra strain of managing the budget during the husband's hospitalization. In addition, if the woman was the patient, the costs and difficulties of having to replace her labor in the home also acted as a deterrent to her entering the hospital that was quite as compelling for the family as losing the main wage.

Moreover, TB hit women working in the informal and often "hidden" economic sector. Cross-referencing the TB outpatients at Sir Patrick Dun's Dispensary in the center of Dublin with the 1901 census yields the example of a woman age thirty attending for consumption in 1906. According to the 1901 census, the house she gave as her address was relatively prosperous, comprising two apartments, each with eight rooms. One household consisted of an unmarried forty-two-year-old woman whose religion was Church of Ireland. She taught a kindergarten and at the time of the census lived with a servant age twenty-two and a child of twelve who was boarding with her. The appearance of TB in the house would have brought both teaching and boarding to a stop at least temporarily.[44] Similarly, at the other end of the social spectrum were widows with children who took in lodgers to make ends meet and women who did washing or dressmaking or who baked for their neighbors to increase the family income.[45] Even the suspicion of TB would signal the ruin of the business.[46]

By the 1940s, the campaign against TB had moved considerably beyond the assumptions made by Lady Aberdeen and her ladies with their sympathetic but essentially didactic and "top-down" approach. Their belief that the key to Ireland's good health lay largely in the hands of its women had undergone significant change. Failures in housing, the relative lack of generosity in provision of sanatorium allowances, and the strains of nursing the tubercular in the working-class home became a focus for radical reformers in the Ireland of the 1940s. The continuing death toll from TB, which rose during the Second World War, was seen as a result of social inequality rather than of failures in the domestic hygienic regime. A view arose that the solution was political not individual. No amount of good advice or training in hygiene could by itself overcome the disease, which could be tackled only by greater state commitment of resources to the problem. In both parts of Ireland, this change in view resulted in a concerted effort by the state and public-health authorities to increase allowances and free treatment and to expand the infrastructure of TB services.

The state's increasing involvement produces an interesting question for feminist historians. Jacques Donzelot, for example, sees the state's greater assumption of what traditionally was seen as the male breadwinner's responsibility as a kind of feminization of public policy. He describes the effect as an attack on patriarchy, a process that altered the balance of power in the family in favor of women. Hence, he suggests that women were "collusive" in the change toward greater government and state involvement in health and family regulation.[47]

This interpretation is open to challenge. Women's attitudes to the state's involvement in regulating family life were a great deal more hostile than Donzelot's interpretation allows,[48] as is illustrated by the history of tuberculosis. Jurisdictions north and south made substantial efforts to reach the tubercular in the twentieth century. There were some outstanding successes in doing so, particularly in Northern Ireland after 1945.[49] But in spite of these successes, a significant proportion of the TB afflicted shunned contact with the authorities and avoided the sanatorium and the dispensary. A Donegal TB dispensary doctor estimated in 1941 that there were 125 notifications of TB patients to the register but 111 deaths without registration in his area. Calculations at the time suggested that registration of TB sufferers in Dublin in the late 1930s was only 54 percent of the recorded deaths from the disease.[50] The facts that the registered number of those suffering with TB (registration was not compulsory in Ireland) was sometimes smaller than the number of those dying from the disease unregistered in an area and that among the deceased were those who were quite unknown to the public-health authorities always disturbed the government.[51] Added to this problem were patients who were in contact with the public-health authorities but who turned down an offered place in a sanatorium for which there were waiting lists during most of the twentieth century.

In 1944, officials of the Department of Local Government and Public Health in Dublin examined the records of a total of 1,006 patients (653 alive and 353 patients deceased from TB). Of these patients, 38 percent had refused treatment. Revealingly, 42 percent of women offered a place turned it down, as opposed to 35 percent of men. Subsequent surveys in Northern Ireland for 1947–48, 1950–51, and 1955 show a diminishing number of refusals, influenced probably by more generous allowances for sanatorium patients and by a greater aura of optimism about recovery in the age of therapeutic drugs. But they do not show an appreciable difference in refusal rates between men and women.[52]

Women were therefore quite as resistant to institutionalization as men, though the reasons they gave reveal some difference. In the Dublin sample, 42 percent of the total sample did not give any reason for refusal, but, of the remainder, dislike of the institution was offered in 26 percent of the cases, 17 percent cited economic hardship, and 10 percent family affection.[53] Rather more women than men gave family affection as their reason, and slightly fewer gave dislike of the institution; slightly more women appeared to be prepared to accept the discipline and drawbacks of sanatorium life. More men than women appear in the very small category who were characterized as incorrigible or eccentric, but this left quite a few intolerably insubordinate women or, as they were described by one public-health official, "stupid stubborn patients."[54] Economic hardship appeared to be as important for women as for men,[55] covering not just single women who worked, but a substantial proportion of married women.[56]

It is precisely the case of refusals and avoidance that point to another important but neglected aspect of the story of women and TB. Historians have concentrated a great deal of their attention on the public world of wage rates, housing provision, government and local-authority expenditure, and professional medical care and advice. These important subjects had an impact on women and the home. But although this public world was not entirely male, it was a sphere to which Irish women had only limited access throughout much of this period. In contrast, we know relatively little about the inner dynamic of families with TB. Yet the evidence suggests that this dynamic was a major factor in determining the course of the campaign against tuberculosis. Impressionistic accounts exist, generally from the adult, educated, and articulate. They often point to stigma and concealment by the family as a whole and sometimes a closing of ranks against medical authority. Sanatorium survivors tell of a distance growing up between them and their families after a period of separation.[57] Apart from these accounts, however, we know very little about the effect on the family of having an afflicted member in their midst, in particular a child.[58] Yet much of the history of TB is the history of the family—its economics, its domestic management, the decisions taken, the emotional impact, and attitudes to medicine and disease. It is a story in which women played a leading role.

3

Infant and Child Mortality in Dublin a Century Ago

Cormac Ó Gráda

The scholarly literature on infant and child mortality in Europe before the First World War is already considerable.[1] This chapter's contribution is to address familiar issues in a new setting with new data. Dublin's high mortality rates a century or so ago are well documented. At the time, they attracted a great deal of attention from officials, commentators, and politicians and helped sustain a long-lasting campaign for improved public-health measures, in particular the provision of cleaner water and better sanitary facilities. Others, however, saw the city's poverty and the poor quality of its housing stock—private poverty rather than public squalor—as the main reasons for its high death rates.[2]

This chapter's main analytical focus is a subpopulation living in a part of the city now largely encompassed by the postal district Dublin 4, a relatively affluent area in the southeastern part of the city. A century ago this area constituted the suburban township of Pembroke. Their ethnic, confessional, and socioeconomic diversity make Pembroke households an interesting group to study. I seek to assess the relative importance of socioeconomic, cultural, and environmental factors in accounting for the variation in infant and child mortality between households in Pembroke a century ago.

However, I begin with a review of conditions in the city as a whole in the decades before the Great War. An analysis of aggregate censal and civil registration data supports impressionistic accounts of high mortality but also suggests some slight improvement over time. I then place Pembroke in this period in context, describe the Pembroke database, and provide an econometric analysis and outcome.

Arguments about the relative importance of poverty and public health are a common feature of studies of infant and child mortality.[3] Victorian and Joycean Dublin's water and sanitary facilities were probably no worse than those of many other cities at the time. Indeed, Dublin had been a leader in the public provision of clean water. The ambitious Vartry reservoir scheme ended Dublin's dependence on supplies from the Royal and Grand canals in the 1860s. Moreover, though the city relied on the river Liffey as its main sewage outlet until 1906, more than two decades earlier a royal commission of inquiry into Dublin's sewerage disposal had found that "the existing system of sewerage, although a cause of nuisance by polluting the river, could not be made wholly answerable for the high rate of mortality," and by the early 1890s the city had "an extensive and well-built system of street drains."[4] Plans to provide a main drainage system had been mooted from midcentury, but vested interests delayed implementation. The scheme that was eventually adopted, largely modeled on London's, was designed to carry the sewage of the city and outlying districts in large drains along the Liffey to the Pigeon House for treatment and disposal.[5]

Poverty's role in accounting for Dublin's high mortality a century ago is strongly implied by the significant variation in death rates by socioeconomic class and area. In 1909, for example, the overall death rate in Dublin's relatively affluent southern suburbs was 16 per 1,000, whereas in North City No. 2 District, composing part of the inner city to the north of the Liffey, it was 24.7 per 1,000. And in Dublin Registration District as a whole (i.e., Dublin and suburbs) in the mid-1880s, the death rate in households headed by "hawkers, porters, laborers" was nearly three times that in households headed by "merchants and managers, higher class." Dublin's high mortality rate is explained in part by the high proportion of casual, unskilled laborers making up its labor force. In table 3.1, the considerable mortality gap between rich and poor is captured by the age distributions of deaths by class in the mid-1880s and the 1900s.

Table 3.1

The Age Distributions of Deaths (%) by Socioeconomic Group in the Dublin Registration Area, 1883–1887 and 1901–1910

A. 1883–1887

| Class | Total | Age in Years | | | | | |
		0–4	5–19	20–39	40–59	60–79	80+
I	2,295	10.1	5.1	12.2	18.3	38.0	16.3
II	7,709	24.4	9.6	19.1	17.8	22.5	6.6
III	12,694	37.2	11.1	15.9	18.9	14.9	2.0
IV and V	27,555	34.3	7.9	15.5	19.5	19.7	3.0
I–V	50,253	32.4	8.8	16.0	19.0	19.8	3.9

B. 1901–1910

| Class | Total | Age in Years | | | | | |
		0–4	5–19	20–39	40–59	60–79	80+
I	3,406	5.0	2.0	9.5	19.8	41.6	22.1
II	14,059	18.4	8.0	18.0	20.7	26.6	8.3
III	19,910	29.9	8.1	16.4	22.5	20.2	2.9
IV and V	53,287	34.7	6.8	15.1	19.9	20.5	2.9
I–V	90,662	30.1	7.1	15.6	20.6	22.2	4.5

Note: I = professional and independent class; II = middle class; III = artisans and petty shopkeepers; IV = general service class; V = workhouse inmates.
Source: Weekly Returns of Births and Deaths (yearly summary), 1883–87; British Parliamentary Papers 1914, vol. XV, Cd. 7121, "Supplement to the 47th Report of the Registrar-General Containing . . . Cecennial Summaries," xlix.

Not only was congested and rundown housing a good proxy for low income, but it also seriously constrained the benefits of investments in municipal water supply and sewerage schemes. Poor, overcrowded housing meant blocked water closets, a lack of heating and proper food, inadequate hygiene, damp walls, contaminated water, and antisocial behavior.

Ethnoreligious differences have also been invoked in accounting for Dublin's poverty and the ensuing high mortality: "The Irish were held to be more dirty than the English and, lest there be any misdirected imputation, the Protestant cleaner than the Roman Catholic."[6] The impact of religion or culture per se on mortality has not been quantified, however. Elsewhere it clearly played a role: a century ago mortality in European Jewish communities was lower and fertility in Catholic communities higher than predicted by income or socioeconomic status alone.[7] In Dublin, a municipal official attributed the "healthy offspring and low infant mortality" of the city's small Jewish community, in part at least, to the monthly mikva ritual practiced by its womenfolk in specially provided facilities in Tara Street baths.[8] (I have analyzed the infant and child mortality rates of Dublin's Jewish community elsewhere.[9])

In Dublin, the Catholic and Protestant communities were not segregated as they were in Belfast, but they tended to live rather separate lives. As throughout Ireland, schools, hospitals and other charitable institutions, voluntary organizations, and social and sporting clubs—of which there were many—tended to be organized along denominational lines.[10] Political affiliation was also largely determined by religion. This sense of separateness is well reflected in novelist Elizabeth Bowen's memoir of childhood in middle-class Dublin in the 1910s:

> It was not until the end of those seven winters that I understood that we Protestants were in a minority, and that the unquestioned rules of our being came, in fact, from the closeness of a minority world. Roman Catholics were spoken of by my father and mother with a courteous detachment that gave them, even, no myth. I took the existence of Roman Catholicism for granted but met few and was not interested in them. They were simply "the others," whose world lay alongside ours but never touched.[11]

The relative importance of religion, economics, and neighborhood in accounting for the differences in mortality levels between Catholic children and those of other faiths remains an unresolved issue, however.

The bleak image of late Victorian and Joycean Dublin that emerges from the historiography is easily justified. In no other city in western Europe on the eve of the First World War did one-third of households live in one-room tenement accommodation (such housing was categorized as "fourth class" in the census reports). The overcrowded tenements, rooms in what were formerly the homes of some of Dublin's richest families, dated mainly from the late Georgian era. Dublin's poverty was exacerbated by the weakness of its industrial base and the lack of employment opportunities for most women outside the home. And mortality in Dublin was indeed high by western European urban standards.[12]

Yet snapshot depictions of the city tend to overlook any improvement that took place. Poor as Dubliners seemed (and *were*) on the eve of the Great War, they were better off than Dubliners of the previous generation. This difference is reflected in trends in housing conditions and wages. In 1881, 42.7 percent of households lived in fourth-class housing, but in 1861 the proportion had been 46.7 percent. Dublin's housing problem was therefore less the lack of improvement in the city as a whole than the persistence of thousands of one-room tenement units in its festering core. Such tenement units constituted the bulk of Dublin's fourth-class housing in these decades, and their number declined only slowly (23,360 in 1881; 19,342 in 1891; 20,564 in 1911).[13]

Critics on the left and right repeatedly accused the city's elected officials of doing little about the housing problem.[14] There certainly was plenty of jobbery and corruption to complain about, yet not even the corporation (city government), overwhelmingly nationalist in composition from the early 1880s on, was impervious to pressure. It began to act in the 1880s, rehousing a total of 2,447 people in the Liberties. It marked time in the 1890s but rehoused more than 4,000 individuals between 1900 and 1913. This number may not seem much for a city of more than 300,000 people. And yet, for all the corporation's poor reputation, the 1,385 units municipally housed by 1914 represented the highest proportion of inhabitants so accommodated of any city in the United Kingdom.[15]

Some progress was also made on other fronts. The corporation's sanitary officers vigorously pursued, fined, and named those found guilty of trading in adulterated food, which seems to have had some effect. They also sought to improve sanitary conditions in the slum areas. The use of flush toilets spread rapidly after 1880. Between 1880 and 1882, the number of flush toilets in Dublin rose from 743 to 15,000, and two decades later privies were almost a thing of the past. A serious drawback was that in tenement housing toilets were located outside and shared between several families, which in practice restricted their use to men and older boys. In order to minimize vandalism and the transmission of disease, corporation workmen set yard toilets in asphalt and rid them of all woodwork. The corporation also made strides in the closing down of dangerous housing, refuse removal, the control of slaughterhouses, and health inspections. Recalcitrant landlords were also fined and named.[16] Much more might have been done had the corporation's tax base not been constrained by the retreat of so many middle-class residents to the suburbs and by the remaining middle-class residents' reluctance to pay more.

Wage data offer another plausible gauge of changes in material well-being. A series describing the nominal daily wage earned by (unskilled) Dublin building laborers suggests a rise of about one-half between the early 1880s and the eve of the Great War.[17] Moreover, these data suggest that the gap between British and Dublin nominal wages narrowed in the construction sector between 1880 and 1914.[18] Because the cost of living probably fell somewhat over this period, a bigger rise in relative living standards is indicated.[19]

How high was mortality in late Victorian and Joycean Dublin? In Ireland, the civil registration of births, marriages, and deaths began late, in 1864. As if to compensate, almost from the outset the registrar general produced a wealth of detail, including weekly data on births and deaths in Dublin for publication in the local newspapers. Beginning in 1880, cross-tabulations of deaths by age, gender, socioeconomic status, and district were also analyzed at length in the annual reports of the city's chief medical officer.[20] Even in Dublin, however, the registrar general's data for the early years are unfortunately subject to considerable underenumeration, as is evident from the fact that until 1877 the total number of burials in the city's main cemeteries[21] exceeded registered deaths in Dublin Registration District. The ratio of registered deaths to burials jumped abruptly in 1879, when new legislation required the cemetery authorities to forward burial data to the registrar general.[22] Between 1880 and 1914, the ratio of registered deaths to burials hovered between 1.15 and 1.2. The ratio of infant to total deaths was also nearly constant over the same period (average 0.184, coefficient of variation 0.06). The president of the Dublin Sanitary Association was probably justified in claiming in 1890 that "probably at the present time the accuracy of the Dublin registration is as nearly perfect as care and labour can make it."[23]

If that was the case, it means that the overall death rate in greater Dublin (i.e., the city and neighboring townships) declined in these years (tables 3.1 and 3.2).[24] The cross-tabulation of deaths by social class in table 3.1 reflects the broad categories employed by the Irish registrar general at the time. It suggests that the life expectancy of those in the top three classes rose significantly between the mid-1880s and the 1900s, whereas that of the poor improved only marginally. Because the share of the poor in the total population rose, life expectancy overall did not rise much.[25] By the same token, table 3.2 shows that mortality in Dublin was higher than in Belfast in the 1880–1910 period, but that the gap was narrowing over time.

What of infant and child mortality? Here infant mortality in year t (IM_t) is defined as registered deaths of children less than one year in year t divided by the number of births in the same year. Child mortality is defined analogously as registered deaths of children ages one to five years in year t divided by five times the number of children ages one to five years. The latter is approximated by five times the number of births in year t multiplied by ($1 - IM_t$). These admittedly crude definitions suggest that Belfast's advantage over Dublin also held in the case of infant mortality and the mortality of children one to five years old.

How did infant and child mortality in the city change over time? The trends in the prewar period, as reflected in the registrar general's figures, are shown in tables 3.3 and 3.4. Although the results suggest that in Ireland trends were more muted than in Britain, the declines in Dublin are worth noting. A significant narrowing in the gaps between Dublin and Belfast over these decades is also implied, particularly in the 1900s. Both aggregate and infant and child mortality trends from around 1880–1914 thus corroborate the impression gained from wage and housing data.

Table 3.2

The Death Rate in Dublin and Belfast, 1881–1911

A. *Greater Dublin*

Year	Population	Recorded Deaths	Death Rate (per 1,000)
1881	311,672	9,424	30.2
1891	316,313	9,195	29.1
1901	349,019	9,571	27.4
1911	371,936	9,118	24.5

B. *Belfast*

Year	Population	Recorded Deaths	Death Rate (per 1,000)
1881	207,671	4,911	23.6
1891	255,922	6,537	25.5
1901	351,083	7,738	22
1909	386,756	7,028	18.2

Sources: W. E. Vaughan, *Irish Historical Statistics: Population 1821–1971*, edited by A. J. Fitzpatrick and W. A. Vaughan (Dublin: Royal Irish Academy, 1978), 28–29; *Thom's Almanac*, various years; *Returns of Births and Deaths in Dublin*, various years.

Some context may be useful here. In England and Wales, the decline in early child mortality preceded that in infant mortality by several decades. The infant mortality rate dropped sharply in both urban and rural areas from 1899 on. The universal character of the fall suggests a common cause and also argues against the specifics of water supply and sewage disposal in particular areas.[26] Robert Woods has stressed that the English pattern of a decline in early childhood mortality in the late nineteenth century, followed by a rapid drop in infant mortality from the beginning of the twentieth, was not unique.[27] In Dublin, too, the decline in child mortality seems to have preceded that in infant mortality.

Woods interprets these findings as suggesting that "a number of universal factors, operating alone or in a synergistic fashion, seem to have been at work and to have had a significant and immediate effect."

Table 3.3

Infant and Child Mortality in Dublin and Belfast, 1880–1914

| | Infant Mortality (per 1,000) | | Child Mortality (per 1,000) | |
Period	Dublin	Belfast	Dublin	Belfast
1880–84	186.5	149.7	175.5	n/a
1885–89	176.6	148.1	167.6	n/a
1890–94	169.1	167.4	132.4	93.1
1895–99	175.0	161.6	157.0	122.7
1900–1904	164.4	149.3	123.4	107.2
1905–1909	146.6	139.1	104.6	92.8
1910–14	147.9	137.6	116.4	98.9

Note: "Child mortality" refers to ages 1–5.
Sources: W. E. Vaughan, Irish Historical Statistics: Population 1821–1971, edited by A. J. Fitzpatrick and W. A. Vaughn (Dublin: Royal Irish Academy, 1978), 28–29; Thom's Almanac, various years; Returns of Births and Deaths in Dublin, various years.

Table 3.4

Infant and Child Mortality (%) with Respect to Wife's Age at Marriage and Marriage Duration in the Dublin Registration Area, 1901–1911

| | Marriage Duration in Years | | | | | | |
Wife's Age at Marriage	0–4	5–9	10–14	15–19	20–24	25–29	30–34
< 20	13.2	20.6	23.5	26.8	30.0	32.1	27.8
20–24	11.3	16.4	19.9	22.9	26.1	28.7	22.9
25–29	9.6	13.8	19.5	21.3	26.2	25.6	20.5
30–34	11.3	17.0	20.1	25.8	24.9	28.3	22.0
35–39	12.3	18.8	31.8	27.8	23.2	25.7	25.0
40–49	13.0	19.5	28.9	30.4	26.0	29.6	25.2

Source: Data derived from 1911 Census General Report (Dublin: His Majesty's Stationery Office, 1911), 502–27.

He doubts whether cleaner milk alone could have produced such a radical decline in infant mortality but suggests an important role for fertility control; indeed, he speculates that "the general effects of family limitation on the course of European demographic change . . . may provide a counter to the long-established wisdom associated with transition theory, in which infant mortality decline in particular acts as a spur to fertility control."[28] This mutual causation adds to the difficulties of formally identifying the determinants of variations in either fertility or mortality.

Much of the research into infant and child mortality patterns in Great Britain and the United States a century ago is based on information gleaned from the censuses of 1911 (Great Britain) and 1900 (United States) because in both cases special surveys of marital fertility yielded data on the number of children ever born and the number surviving in each household inhabited by a married couple. The reporting of deaths was retrospective and confined to couples cohabiting on census night, but it has generally been deemed sufficiently accurate for both cross-sectional and time-series inferences.[29]

The 1911 Irish census, conducted on the night of 2 April 1911, is well known to be problematic in another respect, however. A glance at its age distributions reveals an implausibly large increase in the numbers of men and women in their sixties and seventies between 1901 and 1911. The increase in apparent survival rates was largely a by-product of the Old Age Pensions Act of 1908.[30] In the absence of civil registration before 1864, hard evidence of age, particularly in more remote and poorer regions, was not always available. Claimants suspected that census declarations of age might be used in processing pension claims, and this suspicion affected the 1911 census. Deliberate age misreporting was widespread in Ireland in 1911. It was less common in urban areas than in rural areas, however, and married women were less likely to lie than were widowed or single women. This factor was fortunately unimportant in the two subpopulations analyzed here.

Cross-tabulations of data from the Irish census of 1911, which included a survey very similar to those in Great Britain and the United States, are reported in tables 3.5 and 3.6. Table 3.5 describes the association between infant and child mortality in the Dublin Registration District (the city plus suburbs), marriage duration, and the wife's age at marriage. Wives' age at marriage is inferred from age in 1911 and marriage duration. Note the familiar U-shaped relation between the death rate and age at marriage at all durations and the implication that children born to very young and older mothers were at greater risk. These outcomes seem plausible, as does the association between marriage duration and mortality.

In table 3.6, the finding that mortality varied with fertility is also sensible. "Spacing" of children seems to have reduced mortality: compare the high mortality rates for big families at marriage durations of 0–4, 5–9, and 10–14 years in figure 3.1. This finding corroborates the

Table 3.5

Family Size, Percentage of Children Dead within Family, and Marriage Duration in the Dublin Registration Area, 1901–1911

No. of Children	Marriage Duration in Years					
	0–4	5–9	10–14	15–19	20–24	25–29
1	7.1	9.6	11.0	14.9	16.8	20.7
2	11.2	11.3	14.1	19.4	18.3	20.7
3	16.4	13.4	15.8	18.1	19.2	18.8
4	27.1	16.4	16.1	18.0	21.2	24.1
5	32.0	22.7	17.7	19.9	22.5	22.0
6	—	25.6	20.9	21.4	22.1	24.3
7	—	27.9	24.9	22.1	26.8	26.6
8	—	44.9	30.6	23.8	25.6	28.3
9	—	44.4	31.3	27.8	27.8	30.5
10	—	—	37.4	34.5	30.6	31.6
11	—	*	47.9	34.2	33.3	33.0
12	—	—	40.3	40.5	34.6	36.0
13+	—	—	54.9	44.6	44.8	41.8
Avg.	10.9	16.5	20.8	23.9	27.3	29.3

Note: Asterisk [*] indicates fewer than twenty deaths.
Source: Derived from 1911 Census General Report (Dublin: His Majesty's Stationery Office, 1911), 502–27.

Table 3.6

Marriage Duration and Child Mortality (% Dead), 1911

Marriage Duration in Years	Ireland	County Boroughs	Dublin	England and Wales
< 1	6.9	6.2	6.3	7.2
1	6.1	7.9	7.9	7.8
2	7.9	9.9	9.7	9.0
3	8.4	11.4	11.3	10.1
4	9.3	13.1	12.2	11.0
5–9	11.2	16.2	16.5	13.8
10–14	14.0	20.3	20.8	17.3
15–19	16.0	22.8	23.9	19.5
20–24	17.9	26.5	27.3	21.4
25–29	19.6	28.9	29.4	22.7

Source: Data derived from *1911 Census General Report* (Dublin: His Majesty's Stationery Office, 1911), table 165, and the 1911 census of England and Wales.

link between fertility and mortality emphasized by historical demographers David Reher and Robert Woods.[31] Note, too, however, that when there were many children, the death rates peaked at the marriage duration of 10–14 years. Perhaps some long-married parents "forgot" to report early births that had failed to survive.

The mortality data are therefore tarnished to some extent by both age misreporting and underenumeration. In mitigation, the outcome of the census is consistent with the registrar general's findings. Bear in mind that the latter include all births, whereas the census tables exclude the children of single parents, who were at far greater risk. Comparing 1911 Dublin mortality rates with rural Irish and English rates also offers some reassurance because it implies—plausibly—that in Ireland as a whole mortality rates were slightly lower than in England, but in Dublin and other Irish cities mortality rates were unusually high.

In the econometric estimation that follows, the analysis is confined to married women younger than fifty, which should eliminate most of any bias resulting from either omitted deaths or age exaggeration.

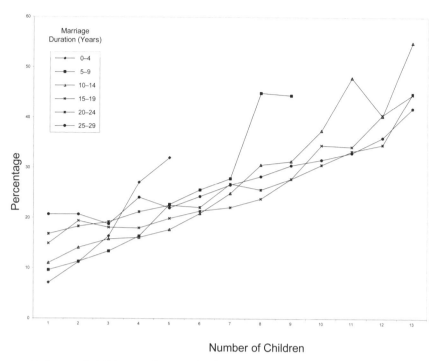

3.1. Infant and child mortality (%) by family size and marriage duration, Dublin registration area (from 1911 census).

The main focus from this point is infant and child mortality in Pembroke Township. The township, which got its name from the fact that most of the area it encompassed was part of the estates of the earl of Pembroke, became part of Dublin city proper only in 1930 but formed part of the Dublin Registration District in the decades covered in this study.[32] The database used here is taken from the manuscript enumeration forms of the 1911 Irish census. It contains 2,649 married couples, 471 of whom had never had children. The remaining 2,178 had already produced 9,091 children between them, though more than one in six (1,628) of these children had died before census night. The deaths were very concentrated in a small number of families. Forty-five percent of the total took place in 9 percent of the families, who suffered three or more infant or child deaths.

Pembroke was located to the southeast of the city proper, its 650 hectares broadly overlapping with the modern postal district Dublin 4.

Its status as a separate municipality freed its taxpayers of the burden of cross-subsidizing the old city's poorer inhabitants. Though disproportionately middle class, the township was mixed in both confessional and socioeconomic terms. It contained both working-class neighborhoods and some very opulent streets, such as Ailesbury Road.[33] Pembroke's population rose from 20,982 in 1871 to 29,294 in 1911.

In confessional terms, Ireland a century ago was overwhelmingly Catholic,[34] but it contained districts where the non-Catholic presence was significant. Pembroke is a good example of the latter type of district. This characteristic is reflected in the database used here, where nearly one-third of the households are non-Catholic. Of this group, most (22.8 percent) subscribed to the Episcopalian Church of Ireland; Presbyterians and other non-Catholics accounted for 3.3 percent and 5.6 percent, respectively, and 2.6 percent of the couples included a Catholic and a non-Catholic.[35] It should be noted that religious affiliation counted for much more in the period discussed than in modern semisecularized Ireland. Religious observance was the norm for members of all churches, and the ratio of clergy to laity was very high.[36] Another feature of Pembroke was its high proportion of immigrants, either from abroad (mainly Great Britain) or from elsewhere in Ireland. Of this proportion, 13.8 percent of the fathers in the database and 13.5 percent of the mothers were born abroad, and 28.9 percent of the fathers and 29.7 percent of the mothers were born elsewhere in Ireland than Dublin.

The socioeconomic gap between Catholics and non-Catholics in Pembroke was very wide. Catholic couples accounted for 95 percent of all couples living in tenements. Catholic households contained a median of 1.7 people per room, compared to a non-Catholic median of 0.87. Catholic men accounted for 89 percent of the laborers, 78 percent of semiskilled workers, 63 percent of those in skilled occupations, 43 percent of the clerks, and 32 percent of those in professional occupations.

In terms of housing quality, Pembroke fared much better than the city proper, being closer to its rival township of Rathmines in this respect than to Dublin proper. Yet Pembroke also contained many tenement dwellings and one-room apartments. In terms of occupational break-down, Pembroke was also closer to Rathmines than to the old city. It was more mixed socially and economically and more industrial than Rathmines. Nearly one in three of its labor force was an unskilled worker, and these workers included dockers, gardeners, fishermen, and seamen. Its main industrial plant, the Irish Glass Bottle Company, located in Ringsend, employed more than three hundred men at the time.

Though Pembroke is a relatively small area (three square miles), it has been divided up into five districts here in the quest for purely local and neighborhood effects: Sandymount, Ballsbridge, Donnybrook, Ringsend, and "Inner Pembroke." Ringsend was poorest: 42 percent of its labor force was unskilled, and only 1. 3 percent in top occupations such as land agent, barrister, or stockbroker. In Sandymount, only 11.4 percent were in the former category, but 23.1 percent in the latter. Note, however, that although the gap in infant and child mortality rates between Ringsend (20.9 percent) and Sandymount (14.3 percent) was significant, Ringsend was fortunate in this respect compared to the poorest districts of Dublin proper. Table 3.7 provides cross-tabulations of fertility and mortality by religion, occupational status, and district.

Note that the omission of some households from a particular cohort owing to migration or death may lead to some selection bias. The death or absence of a parent could well influence the life chances of surviving children. This chapter ignores this type of problem.

The database used here consists of Pembroke households in which neither husband nor wife had been previously married or had already produced one or more children before census day.[37] Age at death of nonsurviving children is not given, and so the analysis (like analyses of Britain in 1911 and the United States in 1910 given earlier) must necessarily treat infant and child mortality together. The database contains 2,178 couples who had already produced at least one child by 1911.[38]

The objective is to explain at least some of the variation in infant and child mortality in the pre-1911 period. It must be emphasized that the task is complicated by the lack of precise measures of some of the likely determinants of mortality and by the endogeneity of one or more

Table 3.7

Religion, Class, Fertility, and Mortality in Pembroke, 1901–1911

Occupation	Number	Children Born	Children Dead	Death Rate (%)	Children per Couple
I	411	945	89	9.4	2.3
II	534	1,514	210	13.9	2.84
III	354	1,326	226	17.0	3.75
IV	486	1,892	390	20.6	3.89
V	847	3,368	710	21.1	3.98
Religion					
Catholic	1,736	6,533	1,265	19.4	3.76
Church of Ireland	605	1,612	231	14.3	2.66
Presbyterian	88	266	40	15.0	3.02
Mixed	68	226	34	15.0	3.32
Other	149	445	58	13.0	2.99
District					
Donnybrook	431	1,467	243	16.6	3.4
Ballsbridge	333	1,039	176	16.9	3.12
Ringsend	949	3,800	796	20.9	4.0
Sandymount	454	1,297	185	14.3	2.8
Inner Pembroke	482	1,488	228	15.3	3.09

Note: Occupation codes: I = elite occupations such as accountant, surgeon, land agent; II = white-collar workers and traders; III = skilled workers; IV = semiskilled workers; V = unskilled occupations.

The omission of some households from a particular cohort owing to migration or death may lead to some selection bias. The death or absence of a parent could well influence the life chances of surviving children. This chapter ignores this type of problem.

Source: 1911 Census General Report (Dublin: His Majesty's Stationery Office, 1911).

of the explanatory variables. The socioeconomic covariates include an indices of men's occupational status ranging from category I (elite occupations such as accountant, surgeon, land agent) through II (white-collar workers and traders), III (skilled workers), IV (semiskilled workers), and V (unskilled occupations such as laborer or gardener) and indices of housing quality provided in the census itself (the number of rooms and the number of house points—that is, the class of house, whether one, the highest grade of accommodation, or four, the lowest grade—two indices provided in the census itself). Culture is represented by religion (Church of Ireland, Presbyterian, Other Nonconformist, and Mixed). The duration of marriage and the ages at marriage and places of birth of husband and wife are also given.

In modeling infant and child mortality, the number of children dead (CDEAD) or the proportion of children dead (PDEAD) are probably the most obvious candidates for dependent variable. The analysis here, however, relies instead on the mortality index devised by Samuel Preston and Michael Haines for their classic study of infant and child mortality in the United States a century ago.[39] This index is also in Eilidh Garrett and her colleagues' study of mortality in England.[40] The index is the ratio of actual child deaths (as given in the census for all mothers in the database) to expected deaths. Expected deaths are obtained by multiplying the number of children ever born to a mother by an expected child mortality level for the relevant marriage duration group (0–4, 5–9, 10–14, 15–19, 20–24, 25–29, and 30–34 years). The use of marriage duration categories controls for how long children have been exposed to the risk of dying. Here the expected averages are based on the Coale-Demeny Model Life Table Level 13.5, which is consistent with e_o = 49.8. The choice of level is not crucial, however, because the index values are proportional. The index is normalized at the value of one.

One of the advantages of the Preston–Haines mortality index is that it "encrypts" marriage duration and marital fertility. Using CDEAD or PDEAD would have required a measure of fertility as a covariate insofar as large families increase the pressure on household resources. However, mortality also influences fertility through the so-called replacement effect. Finding suitable instruments to finesse this endogeneity problem is not easy. However, the Preston–Haines index seems to offer a way out in this instance because it is fertility adjusted.

Two variables are included as measures of exogenous pressures at the time when infants and children were most at risk. The first is the gross emigration rate in the first four years of marriage (EMR). EMR rose from 10 per 1,000 in 1876–80 (for marriages of 30–34 years duration) to 16.9 per 1,000 in 1881–85 and fell thereafter, reaching 7.2 per 1,000 in 1906–10 (for marriages of 0–4 years duration). The second background covariate included here is the child mortality rate in Greater Dublin during the first four years of marriage (CMR); it is included to capture the shifting incidence of risks such as the prevalence of infectious diseases. This measure, too, fell over time, but with a blip in 1896–1900 (see table 3.3).

Table 3.8 describes the marginal effects produced by three specifications. The signs on most of the covariates are as expected. Living in a tenement increased risk, whereas being born in a Presbyterian household reduced it; the offspring of professional couples had better survival chances, and those living in the poorer neighborhood of Ringsend had worse. The outcomes leave a role for geography, culture, and socioeconomic influences. All faiths other than Catholicism were associated with lower mortality, with the infants and children of Presbyterians and other nonconformists being least at risk. The results also show that mortality was subject to a steep socioeconomic gradient. The impact of housing proxies comes across when the block of occupational categories II to V is excluded, but including both blocks swamps the impact of housing quality. The coefficient on the interaction term *ringprot* suggests that the children of non-Catholics in Ringsend were at particular risk. And, for some unknown reason, living in Sandymount affected the hazards facing the children of semiskilled and unskilled workers (IVsandy and Vsandy) differently. Overall, the most robust outcome is that in Pembroke the impact of socioeconomic status, as measured by occupational group, was much stronger than that of religious affiliation.

This preliminary analysis of infant and child mortality in Dublin a century or so ago began with a survey of trends in the city as a whole based on published censal and civil registration data. Such data highlight the impact of urbanization and socioeconomic status. Individual-level data for the southern suburb of Pembroke confirm the role of "culture" but imply that, if anything, economic factors influenced the life chances of infants and children even more. Perhaps this conclusion

Table 3.8

Mortality in Pembroke: Marginal Effects, 1901–1911

Variable	dy/dx	dy/dx	dy/dx	Mean
II	.0860	.0975*		.1912
III	.2825	.2901*		.1388
IV	.4753	.4854*		.1847
V	.4178	.3938*		.3378
Household with 1 domestic servant			−.0418	.3174
Tenement	.1144	.1050	.0922	.1585
Number of rooms in household			−.0295	4.642
Lodging house			−.1111	.0818
Church of Ireland	−.2594*	−.2784*	−.3423*	.2178
Presbyterian Church	−.2761	−.3167	−.3974	.0326
Mixed	−.1252	−.1435	−.2028	.0257
Other	−.3359	−.3615*	h−.4170*	.0565
Age of wife at marriage		.0200*	.0202*	35.92
EMR	.0314			
CMR	.0053*	.0042*	.0043*	138.4
Husband rural*	.1208	.1032		.2872
Wife rural*	−.1709*	−.1935*	−.1898*	.3006
ringsend		.0378	.0739	.3704
IVsandy	.6707*	.6877*	.4647	.0156
Vsandy		.5563*	.6430*	.0188
ringprot	.4541*	.4476*	.4769*	.0781
Number of observations	2176	2176	2177	
Prob > F	0.000	0.000	0.000	
R-squared	0.050	0.055	0.049	
Adj R-squared	0.043	0.047	0.043	
Root MSE	1.147	1.579	1.582	

Note: ringprot, IVsandy, and Vsandy = interaction variables referring to Ringsend, Sandymount, and occupational categories IV and V.

Source: 1911 Census General Report (Dublin: His Majesty's Stationery Office, 1911).

can be reached in part because the proxy used for culture—religious affiliation—is a poor one. Regression analysis also pointed to the influence of location, though the study area of Pembroke is too small for this effect to have much scope. This study is also inevitably constrained by the imprecise nature of some of the covariates used. More research is needed at both the intensive and extensive margins.

4

Cure or Custody

Therapeutic Philosophy at the
Connaught District Lunatic Asylum

Oonagh Walsh

To ask whether asylums were intended to cure or merely to contain is not entirely facetious: most institutions for the care of the insane in the nineteenth century faced the "cure or custody" dilemma. Despite an extensive program of asylum construction throughout Great Britain and Ireland,[1] there appeared to be little consideration of a coherent treatment system that would make best use of this newly available resource. Although most institutions constructed after the 1820s reflected the broad principles of moral treatment—rooms were adapted to allow for leisure activities, grounds were extensive and landscaped, and physical restraint, in straw-filled cells or by mechanical means, was discouraged—only a few opened with a clear conception of how the patients might be medically restored to health. Despite the fact that the medical profession itself promoted the belief that the only way to treat patients was in large, purpose-built establishments that could offer medical expertise, only a few "mad doctors" in the early nineteenth century actually proposed specific new treatments.[2] In this new branch of a medical profession that was becoming increasingly specialized, therapies emerged largely on an ad hoc basis rather than as a coherent strategy to care for increasing numbers of the mentally ill. The other principal body behind the expansion of the asylum system—government—had varied reasons for encouraging a faith in institutional care, reasons that often had little to do with the most appropriate forms of treatment. This chapter seeks to examine some of the patient groups treated in the Connaught District Lunatic Asylum at Ballinasloe, County Galway, in the late nineteenth century. It also explores the means through which medical staff, both nurses and physicians, attempted to meet a governmental imperative to cure and return to society a majority of their charges.

Having begun on a rather gloomy note, I should now say that the very great majority of those involved in patient care, be they the physicians who offered treatment or the government officials who provided funding for the system, sincerely wished for the cure and rehabilitation of the insane. In Ireland, the only individuals who explicitly stated that they saw asylums as custodial institutions were the managers of jails and workhouses, who wished to transfer their own long-stay lunatic inmates to the new asylums. Local communities' attitude, however, was rather more complex, and in the case of Ballinasloe it is surprising how readily ordinary people made use of the institution. They clearly viewed it as a public resource, turning to the Connaught District Lunatic Asylum in the hope of a cure for their relations or as a source of respite care for often very violent individuals. Indeed, some saw in the opening of the asylum a convenient means of disposing of troublesome relatives or as a way of smoothing the path toward sole ownership of family land, although the majority appears to have viewed the asylum as a means through which disturbed or distressed individuals could be cared for and, they hoped, cured. The surviving letters from relatives to the resident medical superintendent reveal ongoing concern and contact from the relatives of incurable patients stretching over forty years and more and a clear acceptance that the asylum represented a standard of care that could not be offered at home.[3]

The Ballinasloe asylum was constructed when moral therapy held full sway, and therapy's effects were to be felt at all levels within the institution, from the organization and outfit of the buildings themselves to the directions given to the medical and nursing staff.[4] The *Bye-Rules and Regulations for the Government of the Connaught District Lunatic Asylum* of 1853 demonstrated a benevolent attitude toward the patients and demanded effort and attention that might be difficult to achieve even today.[5] Rule 2 is worth quoting in full:

> They [the attendants] are never to use harsh or intemperate language to Patients, but should, by steadiness, kindness, and gentleness, contribute to that system of moral government, upon which the value of the Asylum depends. No Keeper, or Nurse, shall at any time deceive, terrify, or irritate by harsh language, by mockery, by mimicry, or by allusion to any thing ludicrous in the present appearance or past conduct of any of the Patients. The Keepers shall not indulge or express vindictive feelings, but considering the Patients as utterly incapable of restraining themselves, shall forgive all petulance or sarcasm, and treat with equal tenderness those who give the most and the least trouble. Keepers and Servants are expected to be willing, not only to encourage but join, the Patients in all harmless amusements in which they may be inclined to engage.

Given that many of the nursing staff (of which more later), male and female, were ill educated (a surprising number in the mid–nineteenth century were illiterate) and had a lesser status than other general nurses, the standards expected of them were high. Not all fulfilled these expectations, of course, and the board of governors' minutes are burdened with instances of nurses fined for insubordination, carelessness, and drunkenness.[6] Nevertheless, it does indicate both an understanding of the vulnerable nature of the patient body and a determination to ensure as far as possible that the patients enjoyed the sort of dignified consideration that should be every citizen's right. For example, it is interesting that a specific injunction was laid down against mocking the patients: because many patients suffered from delusions and behavioral peculiarities that would easily make them objects of ridicule, it was far-sighted indeed that the management insisted on such high standards of behavior from the staff. Nursing staff were in fact being asked to expose themselves to abuse and verbal ill treatment but were not allowed to retaliate. The demand for enlightened treatment of the insane was a priority at Ballinasloe: the injunction to "conduct themselves towards [the physician] with the utmost respect" was made only in Rule 10, following specific instructions on shaving patients (on Tuesdays and Saturdays), cutting their hair ("constantly"), and keeping them clean and tidy.

As mentioned earlier, among the few groups who were somewhat unconcerned with the curative power of asylums were the workhouse and jail managers. Throughout the century, they made constant use of the Dangerous Lunatics Act (DLA) of 1838 (1 & 2 Vict. c.27) to have inmates removed from their institutions and placed in the nearest district asylum.[7] The DLA's powers had huge and largely negative implications for both the asylums and the patients committed to them. In the early years of the nineteenth century, there were no voluntary admissions as we understand them today: every patient had to be committed on the evidence of another person, very often a family member. There were two methods of committal to Irish asylums: in the first instance by straightforward application to an asylum and in the second through admission under the DLA by warrant of the lord lieutenant. The act applied only to Ireland and allowed quite exceptional powers of committal to ordinary citizens. Any person could make an unsubstantiated allegation of insane behavior against another, and on the basis of this alone the individual could be arrested, brought before two justices of the peace, examined by a medical officer, and, if judged insane, committed initially to jail and thence to the appropriate district lunatic asylum. Moreover, proof of insane behavior did not have to be provided, and although some patients were independently witnessed threatening or actually committing an assault, the majority was not. Allegations ranged from physically striking a complainant with fists or tools to threatening or abusive language and to a mere peculiarity of manner or expression. The point of the act was that the patient be classed as dangerous to self or others, and the accusation against him or her required that he or she be "discovered and apprehended . . . under circumstances denoting a derangement of mind, and a purpose of committing an indictable crime."[8] Ireland was therefore the only country in this period to make a legal link between insanity and criminality, and it was an association that had a detrimental effect on those who fell under its provisions.

Another major problem with the DLA was the fact that many of the alleged lunatics processed under it spent periods of up to twelve months in jail before being transferred to the asylums, thereby further strengthening the perception that they were primarily criminals rather than individuals laboring under mental illness. Moreover, the lengthy stay in prison often weakened family ties, with the effect that patients who came from jail, especially those suffering from genuine mental distress, often arrived with little information regarding place of birth or residence, details of next of kin, or even basic information as to age and occupation. Many patients committed under the DLA were not, in fact, suitable cases for treatment and should never have been admitted. However, the DLA's far-reaching powers were such that the asylum physician had no power to refuse anyone brought under its auspices, regardless of their actual state of mental health. The consequent overcrowding was part of the reason for Ireland's massive overexpansion in asylums. The act also had obvious and serious consequences for any campaign to rehabilitate the mentally ill because a large proportion of the asylum population were incurable. In 1876, the inspector, J. Nugent, noted:

As a rule, I consider the great majority of the Patients to require Asylum care, and that due supervision which can only be received in a regularly organised Institution for the insane; but I must say I observed many who it appears to me were placed here unnecessarily—harmless idiots and utterly demented and aged persons, who, with little or no trouble, could be well looked after in Workhouses. Of 97 admissions in the course of the twelve months just expired, I find no less than 79 were effected by Magistrates' Warrants, the parties being represented, or rather deposed to, as dangerous, when the reverse would seem to be the case, they being quiet and inoffensive on reception here. I cannot but think that Justices of the Peace too frequently exercise the powers vested in them without due consideration, the result of which is overcrowding Asylums, and the subsequent necessity of costly enlargements, which the expense of maintenance is double. A female without feet, was transferred a day or two ago from a Poorhouse, under Police armed escort, and thinly clad, no less than 46 miles. The Master of the Union would have acted correctly had he applied to the Board in the first instance. The rate-in-aid was intended for Lunatics in the proper meaning of the term.[9]

Recent work in asylum history has added considerably to our knowledge of the patient experience and of the various uses made of asylums by local communities.[10] However, the nursing staff's experiences and their responses to the changing face of psychiatric treatment have received rather less attention. Part of the reason for this neglect may be the peculiar invisibility of such staff, despite their numbers, and in particular the relative lack of written records that directly reflect their lives. The survival of individual archives in Ireland, as in Britain, has been very much a matter of chance: some psychiatric hospitals have had the good fortune to have administrative personnel who have taken some steps to protect and preserve records; the records at other hospitals have simply been abandoned or destroyed for no particular reason. Even in the worst-case scenarios, however, we still have published sources to turn to, and the annual inspectors' reports as well as the various parliamentary commissions give us a more than fair idea of patient treatment, admission, discharge, and death rates as well as the introduction and modification of therapeutic regimes. If we add to this the discussions that take place in journals such as the *Dublin Journal of Medical Science,* we can build up a pretty solid picture of patient and physician life in the Irish district asylums. But one cohort is largely absent from this picture, and that is the nursing staff. Without at least, say, the board of governors' minute books, we catch only glimpses of the nurses, and even then they rarely appear in their own right in the way that patients emerge from committal warrants and case books or in the way the physician's own authoritative voice rings clear from the monthly report or the prescription books or the case notes. We are often (quite rightly) shocked when we discover during our research the many patients who spent lifetimes in the asylum—the longest stay I have discovered at Ballinasloe to date is forty-seven years—yet we do not as often reflect on the nursing staff who spent the whole of their adult lives literally in the asylum and outlasted the majority of the patients as well as medical and administrative staff. In the nineteenth century, the senior as well as most of the rank-and-file nursing staff lived in accommodations on the asylum grounds, and it was only well into the twentieth century that they were routinely allowed to live in their own homes or approved accommodation in the town of Ballinasloe. Like domestic servants, nursing staff were allowed an afternoon off per week, but this free time was frequently suspended for infractions of the asylum's many rules or because of emergency admissions. In the busier Irish institutions, such as the Richmond Asylum in Dublin, nursing staff left the institution only for their annual holidays and were otherwise permanently resident in the asylum.

Nursing staff were at the forefront of patient care at Ballinasloe, as in the other district asylums. They were required to report at regular intervals to the matron[11] and physician on patient behavior and to draw the attention of senior staff to any sudden change in a patient's condition. They also administered prescribed medicines, purges, and special diets, and they crucially were responsible for the application and removal of restraint, supposedly only on order of the physician, but frequently in fact on their own authority. They thus came into the most frequent and most direct contact with the patient body and had to deal directly with the consequences of gross overcrowding. The most important aspect of the large admission of incurable cases may be its impact on the formulation of medical therapies in the asylum and their implementation by the nursing staff. Implementation of therapy operated in several ways. In the first place, staff were so occupied with the literal supervision of patients that implementing any sort of therapeutic regime was difficult. Attendants had to get patients up in the mornings; help those who needed assistance with washing, dressing, and feeding (several patients required spoon feeding at each meal, and the attendant was required to record the quantity of food eaten every time); get them out of the wards and refectory to their work in the fields or to supervised recreation in the day rooms; and then complete the process again at dinnertime and suppertime. Getting the patients to bed in the evenings was a lengthy and often frustrating task and had to be performed to a strict timetable. As the century advanced, and the asylum became intolerably overcrowded (in November 1900, for example, Ballinasloe had 1,165 patients in an accommodation designed to hold 840), there was a staff–patient ratio of one attendant to twenty male patients and one nurse to fifteen female patients.[12] Although this figure might not seem to suggest that staff were actually overwhelmed, the reality was that the asylums were badly understaffed. The ratio includes *all* nursing staff—that is, the attendants and keepers who were on night duty as well as those who were on day duty—thus leaving a much smaller number to deal with a large patient body in each half of the day, many of whom required one-to-one attention for reasons of incapacity, violence, or delusions that would not allow them to eat alone or to dress themselves. Nursing staff throughout the nineteenth century, then, had responsibilities far beyond the medical care of their charges. With some limited assistance from the patients themselves and the very few general maids employed in the asylum (a grand total of one maid in 1895), nurses had charge of changing beds—a daily occupation in the wards with "wet and dirty" patients—and caring for and counting bed linen to and from the laundry; assisting in dressing and feeding patients as necessary; supervising work parties of patients in the building and on the asylum grounds; organizing and participating in asylum dances, games of tennis, rugby, and cricket; and supervising large numbers of patients in the exercise yards. This range of responsibilities far exceeded those required for any other branch of nursing and ensured that staff were kept fully occupied in Ireland's asylums. Ironically, the asylum could not recruit additional staff because it had no accommodation to offer them. However, it was unable to refuse to accept patients admitted under the DLA, so the number of patients continued to increase.

There is a curious disparity at Ballinasloe, but one that is not likely unique to it, between the management and staff's aspiration toward a high rate of cure and the lack of a strategy to achieve it. The case notes, committal warrants, board of governors' minutes, and the physician's report continually reiterate the importance of curing patients but place less emphasis on the means through which this cure might be achieved. Of course, until the introduction of drug therapy, psychosurgery, and psychotherapy in the mid–twentieth century, there was often little that could be done for many patients. The physician's role (at Ballinasloe, the resident medical superintendent was Dr. John Fletcher from 1874 to 1904) was often that of observer, and recommendations regarding improvements to mental health were based on years of experience of patients suffering from similar afflictions rather than on any specific therapy. If a medical therapy may be said to have existed at Ballinasloe (or at the other Irish asylums), it was one that took a holistic approach to illness and attempted to restore patients through as far as possible a regime of relative quiet, physical labor appropriate to age and strength, and a reasonably nutritious diet. In at least one category of patient, this procedure had positive results.

One of the most important "therapies" for many patients was the opportunity to rest physically. This therapy was particularly vital for married women, many of whom were exhausted by a continued round of pregnancy and nursing. In common with women admitted with puerperal insanity in England,[13] many women in Ireland became ill as a result of malnutrition, miscarriages, and a poor standard of care following deliveries.[14] A rest of only a few months in an asylum, with the benefit of a good diet and relief from continual worry regarding the care of families, was often enough to restore them to both mental and physical health. At Ballinasloe, this therapy was also regarded as a crucial element in the curative process, and women admitted with puerperal insanity in particular were prescribed the "extra diet" as well as plenty of rest. Male patients on the ordinary diet were slightly better fed than the women. Both sexes enjoyed an identical menu of a pint of tea with eight ounces of bread for breakfast; one quart of soup made with six ounces of beef, scotch barley, and potatoes, with eight ounces of bread for dinner four days a week or a quarter stone of potatoes with one-third of a quart of milk the other three days, and six ounces of bread with a pint of cocoa for supper. The male working patients also received an additional eight ounces of meal and one-third of a quart of milk made into stirabout (porridge) for breakfast. However, those in need of extra nourishment could be prescribed the "hospital diet," which included extra "bread, milk, tea, eggs, wine, or any other articles the Physician may deem advisable." Women admitted with puerperal insanity or indeed young married women of childbearing years in general tended to be prescribed the hospital diet in a clear attempt to build them up physically. Once they were reported to be less agitated and to have gained weight, they were on the road to release.

This approach resulted in higher discharge rates for young women than men and to a greater degree of indulgence while such women were in the asylum.[15] The physician was likely to note disapprovingly when male patients refused to take part in organized sports and work parties (discussed later), but women were more often treated leniently and allowed somewhat more latitude with regard to their participation in activities in the asylum. The early evidence from Ballinasloe may suggest that women patients were regarded as more curable than men, not least because their illnesses were in many cases the result of all too frequent childbearing and poor diet. Even when they were diagnosed with the same illness as men, they were more likely to be presented as curable. For example, two women admitted within weeks of each other in 1895 were diagnosed as suffering from "mania," a catch-all category for a range of symptoms and behavior. Their committal warrants further note however that one, a thirty-five-year-old mother of "several children," was anemic and had "suffered from puerperal mania some time ago and never recovered." The other, a forty-year-old mother of six, was described as "debilitated." Both women recovered swiftly and were discharged within months of admission. Indeed, medical staff regarded a diagnosis of "anaemic" as significant, believing that it could trigger mania in susceptible individuals, such as the twenty-eight-year-old woman admitted in 1899. Like the two women described earlier, she was prescribed bed rest, the hospital diet, and gentle exercise in the asylum grounds and was released some seven months later.

Despite a widely acknowledged connection between reproduction and depression or breakdown, the diagnosis of puerperal insanity was not always made, even when other evidence might seem to suggest it. A thirty-eight-year-old woman was admitted to Ballinasloe in September 1899, suffering from what was called "mania." She was a mother of nine children and was committed under the DLA. After she had been in the asylum for eight months, her husband removed her on ten-pounds bail—she does not appear to have been readmitted. Another mother of eight children, following threats to kill her children, was admitted that same year. She was described as anemic, but after only three months in the asylum, where she was on the hospital diet, she, too, was discharged. Although the vast majority of patients were paupers, with no means of support (the average number of paying patients at Ballinasloe was two per annum and until the end of the century, when the asylum had expanded greatly, very rarely rose above three in any one year), even relative prosperity could not necessarily protect against incessant childbearing. A woman admitted in August 1899 was diagnosed with puerperal insanity following the birth of her fourteenth child three weeks earlier. Her husband was a schoolmaster, but she was described as suffering from the general weakness that was a perhaps obvious consequence of having borne fourteen children by the age of forty-five. The prognosis for women admitted with puerperal insanity or indeed with mania following delivery was generally very good, and they tended to be discharged as cured within months or at most a year.

The standard of medical care within the Ballinasloe asylum was generally good, although much of the attention was inevitably focused on curing physical illness rather than mental. Despite the massive overcrowding and the appalling ratio of physician to patient—as late as 1899 there was only one resident medical superintendent, with two medical assistants, for a patient body of 1,130—efforts were made to protect and improve the inmates' physical well-being. Indeed, the physicians, in the absence of any specific strategy to cure their patients' psychological conditions, appear to have expended much of their energy in attempting to heal their charges' bodies. The case notes make a careful record of changing mental states but also record the efforts made to improve physical health. For many of the patients, the treatment they received at Ballinasloe was the first medical intervention of their lives. One male patient, admitted in 1899, had a hernia so large that it hung to his knees. Although the physician noted that it appeared to be causing the man little discomfort, he operated on him and prescribed a truss to relieve this dreadful injury. Many patients arrived at the asylum in poor physical condition, and the case notes suggest a great deal of anger on the physician's part that individuals already disadvantaged through their illness should continue to be treated cruelly. In 1897, a sixty-two-year-old man was admitted from Roscommon Workhouse, where he had attempted suicide by cutting his throat nine days earlier. On his arrival at Ballinasloe, he was "in a very filthy condition from the Strokestown Workhouse Hospital. . . . [I]t [the wound] was only dressed once he says: it has been pouring out pus which is matted into his beard and giving out an almost intolerable stench." The man had returned from America "with a considerable sum of money which the relations wheedled out of him," and in response to his state he had attempted suicide. He remained deeply depressed and suicidal until his death in the asylum in March 1902.[16]

This case was typical of many from the late nineteenth century and encapsulates the therapeutic philosophy, such as it was, of the medical profession within the asylum system. The case notes are detailed, but there was an obvious absence of any coherent strategy directed at the individual and his or her recovery such as became common in the twentieth century. Part of the reason for this absence, once again, is the gross overcrowding in the asylum. Simply catering to the physical needs of the large patient body took up most of the staff time, making tailored regimes the preserve of small, private institutions or of the small number of psychiatrists operating privately at the end of the nineteenth century. That is not to say that Dr. Fletcher did not have a vision for his patients and their care. On the contrary, it is clear from his records that certain general strategies were on routinely used to encourage and assess recovery.

The first strategy involved a concern with the patient's physical health—an obvious enough concern for the asylum physician, of course, but one that apparently had a particular importance for Dr. Fletcher, as indicated in the asylum reports he wrote. In the first place, he made a clear connection between an improvement in bodily health and an improvement in mental health—a linkage that modern psychiatrists also stress. He also made a much less secure but much more dangerous connection between the presence of an illness such as epilepsy and insanity. In this assumption, he was not unique, as some of the categories used to explain illness suggest. The asylum inspectors consistently noted throughout the nineteenth century the significance of poverty in precipitating certain kinds of mental collapse and regarded such linkage as especially important in the case of women. In general, the medical profession employed several different categories under the two broad headings "moral" and "physical" in determining the causes of insanity. The physical subdivisions are straightforward: intemperance, cerebral diseases, and bodily injuries.[17] The moral causes include "grief, fear, and anxiety"; "religious excitement"; "study and mental excitement"; and "poverty and reverse of fortune," a category under which women appeared in greater numbers than men. Patients admitted with physical causes of mental impairment tended to form the core of the long-stay inmates: in particular, those who had suffered brain damage as a result of fever or injury and those diagnosed with congenital mental disability would never be deemed "recovered." The best they could hope for was their eventual removal by relatives.

One of the most interesting of the incurable groups was epileptics. Although obviously not insane, they were regarded as legitimate subjects for admission. A lack of understanding of the causes of epilepsy generated a great deal of fear in the general population, with a suspicion of supernatural possession that lingered well into the late nineteenth century. Epileptics were also significantly disadvantaged in that they found it difficult to keep employment given the unpredictable nature of their fits. It was the study of epilepsy that ironically led to two major experimental treatments for mental illness—insulin injections and electroconvulsive therapy—in the 1930s, but there was no therapy devised for epileptics in asylums, despite the fact that they were not in the majority of cases mentally ill.[18] The attitude of the medical profession toward this group was interesting. Although epileptics did not usually present with symptoms common to many of the other patients (some did), the physicians accepted that they would become long-stay inmates of the asylum and appeared to presume that they would become increasingly erratic in their behavior. There does not seem to have been any consideration of the impact of institutionalization upon individuals who were otherwise in good mental health, and this view is in contrast to the attitude often displayed toward nonepileptic patients. In short, the physicians operated on the knowledge that epileptic patients would not be discharged, and as a consequence they duly noted increasingly insane behavior by them as the years went by. Three patients, each admitted in 1897, followed a similarly stereotypical pattern:

March 8, 1897 [presentation of dates as given in the original documents]: Patient has been taking fits for the past 17 years. He used to work in England: He has no recollection of the circumstances immediately preceding his admission but from the police account appears to have been in a state of epileptic furor [*sic*].

June 11, 1897: Becomes somewhat excited and restless after fits gets up and is restless and so falls and hurts himself. Beyond a somewhat defective memory he does not appear to be otherwise insane. . . .

Nov. 12, 1898: Is constantly subject to epileptic fits and then violent and destructive. Is undergoing rapid mental deterioration: is confused and incoherent cannot grasp a question and answer it coherently; is easily irritated: talkative garrulous and somewhat exalted religiously. Died in asylum.[19]

❋

March 27, 1897: Patient on admission had a depressed & sullen look, answered questions with the slow, laboured, & monotonous voice of an epileptic. . . .

June 11, 1897: Is much improved of late in bodily health is helpless after fits but rarely violent or troublesome . . .

March 4, 1900: Quarrelsome, feverish and irritable: often subject to fits: mentally unchanged. . . .

August 26, 1902: He remains a determined epileptic works a little quietly in a groove but if disturbed or irritated rushes to the fray with the ungovernable fury of reckless rage. Is sullen and stubborn and never admits he is wrong in anything . . .

July 14, 1905: Does no work always irritable and quarrelsome very troublesome in the stage of excitement before fits brutally ferocious when vexed: will not answer me now so I end the interview. Died in asylum, March 26, 1912.[20]

✳

May 12, 1897: . . . he has been calm rational and coherent save that he has had fits every week or so. . . .

June 11, 1897: Has had two or three attacks of epilepsy since last note. After the fits he becomes violently excited with religious delusions of exaltation and hallucinations and sometimes refuses his food. . . .

Nov. 19, 1897: Is frequently subject to fits and becomes excited and incoherent during them. At other times he is quiet and rational. . . .

Oct. 27, 1898: The intervals between the fits become shorter and the reduction of mental power and maniacal excitement in the post Epileptic stage seems to increase gradually. He has not so clear a grasp of his position and former affairs as he possessed some time ago. . . .

March 6, 1901: Frequently stupored from fits and remains help-less in bed: is delusional and hypochrondriacal and shows no tendency to improve. . . .

Feb. 7, 1902: Spends a great deal of his time in bed. Is always stupid confused and incoherent; frequently hurts himself falling in fits: is steadily deteriorating. . . .

July 15, 1904: Very dull. Gets fits weekly at which point he loses power for a day or so. Gets excited before the fits. Eats well and sleeps well. . . .

July 15, 1905: Absolutely unimproved: often in fits before and after quarrelsome irritable and ready for fight. . . .

June 18, 1907: Is quite unimproved: talkative inconsequent and very quarrelsome fighting fiercely on the least provocation. Died in asylum, June 17, 1908.[21]

These few cases (and there are many more) follow the same sort of pattern. Epileptic patients were most often admitted under the DLA, with accusations of violent behavior following a fit. What the observations in the asylum indicate, however, is that many of these patients became disorientated and confused immediately before or following a fit and were easily provoked into violence. Their committal was then straightforward, and their incurable condition made it unlikely that they would be released unless relatives volunteered to care for them. However, it is what happened to them after admission that is most interesting. Despite the frequent note at the start of their records that they are not insane or delusional, they are without exception eventually diagnosed as suffering from severe mental illness, including "visual and auditory hallucinations," "religious delusions," and "persecutory manias." Modern medicine claims no link between epilepsy as an indicator of mental illness, but the Ballinasloe physician appears to expect it as a developmental aspect of the affliction. An association is made between fits that increase in number and a deterioration of mental ability, to the point that any peculiarities in behavior are described as "[an] inevitable progression." It can certainly be argued that epilepsy had an exhausting effect on sufferers and that frequent fits may have left some in a depressed state, but that is a different proposition from claiming that epilepsy could turn a sane individual into one who exhibited distressing and severe forms of mental illness.

So what sort of therapy did the Ballinasloe asylum offer to its patients? As far as modern medical practice is concerned, very little. There was no drug therapy beyond the administration of wine and brandy, principally as part of an improving diet. Morphine was occasionally used to calm violent patients but was not prescribed for more than one or two cases per year. Mechanical restraint and physical seclusion, which had been an important part of a coercive therapy in early-nineteenth-century asylums, was now (officially at least) rarely used at Ballinasloe. Medical interventions were routinely made, but in order to cure physical ailments as opposed to mental. Thus, operations were performed on patients admitted with existing medical conditions, including tumors, hernias, old fractures, hare lips, and various ophthalmic diseases. The physician also attended to injuries received in the asylum itself and routinely treated those suffering from burnings, stabbings, bruises, and breaks, self-inflicted as well as the result of assaults by other patients. Dr. Fletcher was quite an innovative physician and saw important possibilities in research into patient illness. To this end, he attempted to perform post mortems in the asylum but was hampered by a lack of appropriate facilities. Nevertheless, in 1898 the asylum inspector noted that Dr. Fletcher was pressing ahead despite the unsuitable conditions:

During the period under review the cause of death has been verified by post mortem examination in 29 cases [out of a total of 51 deaths that year]. This speaks volumes for the energy and enthusiasm in the cause of science displayed by the Medical officers, having regard to the fact that the dead house is nothing but a small shed, with neither the accommodation nor the surroundings necessary for the pursuit of pathological study. May we hope that in the near future a room will be provided fitted with those appliances for scientific work now generally found in similar institutions.[22]

The efforts made to restore the mentally ill came down largely to a modified form of moral therapy, especially in relation to cheerful and constant occupation. The vast majority of the patients at Ballinasloe were agricultural laborers and farm servants, and the management sought to ensure that these people were employed on the asylum grounds in a range of tasks. From a meager 11 acres of poor land in 1833, the Ballinasloe asylum grew to 171.5 acres of farmed land in 1898, with a suggestion in that year that if the farm were doubled in size, the asylum could be largely self-sufficient. Patients went to the fields in large work parties, and their labors there were regarded not merely as a cost-saving exercise, but as a vital part of their recovery. Year after year the inspector remarked favorably on the beneficial effect such work had on the patient body, especially on the depressed. Indeed, a willingness to work was regarded as a crucial part of a patient's rehabilitation, and the attendants and the physician kept a careful record of how well an individual completed set tasks. Another key test of improving mental health was a willingness to take part in games and entertainments, with scrupulous notes again taken on those who disrupted sports or refused to obey rules. On an obvious level, an ability to engage with other patients and with staff through these activities did indeed indicate an even temperament (depressed patients were, for example, incapable of interacting socially in the asylum). But it was also a way of persuading patients back into a social world from which they had been cast, involuntarily or otherwise, and of creating a bridge between the secluded world of the institution and the world beyond its walls.

5

Gender and Criminal Lunacy in Nineteenth-Century Ireland

Pauline Prior

The Central Criminal Lunatic Asylum for Ireland (now the Central Mental Hospital) was opened in 1850 to cater to a group of people previously confined in the prison system. These people both had committed a crime and had a mental disorder. An analysis of the information held in convict and medical records for these people reveals a highly gendered landscape especially in relation to homicide. Regardless of the motive for the crime—domestic dispute, land dispute, or random violence—the insanity defense was used successfully by men who killed women but rarely by women who killed men. In this discussion, some of these cases are examined within the context of lunacy policy in Ireland and against a background of current academic debates on the historical roots of services for mentally ill offenders in Ireland and elsewhere.[1]

Ireland in the nineteenth century was subjected to waves of legislation in relation not only to crime and punishment, but also to vagrancy and lunacy.[2] Although some of this legislation was aimed at controlling unruly elements in society, some had the more positive aim of providing services for people with a mental disorder. After a somewhat shaky start, these services developed rapidly during the century. After the publication of the report of the Select Committee on the Aged and Infirm Poor of Ireland in 1804, which found little being done for "idiots or insane persons," Sir John Newport, member of Parliament for Waterford, attempted unsuccessfully to introduce legislation for the building of four asylums.[3] A few years later, Robert Peel, chief secretary for Ireland from 1812,[4] ordered an investigation into institutions with lunatics as inmates.[5] It was carried out by Foster Archer, the inspector of prisons, and showed that only nine of the thirty-two counties in Ireland had any provision for lunatics. Dublin was best served, with a private asylum, St. Patrick's, and plans for a public asylum. There was also a public asylum in Cork. Elsewhere the only public provision was within workhouses and prisons, but it was grossly inadequate and unsuitable for individuals suffering from a mental disorder. This evidence was brought before the 1817 Select Committee on the Lunatic Poor in Ireland and led to the Lunatic Asylums (Ireland) Act of 1817.[6]

This act was the first of many laws that contributed to the establishment of a network of publicly funded district lunatic asylums throughout the country.[7] The first district asylum in Ireland opened at Armagh in 1825, and seven more opened within the following ten years. By the middle of the century, there were ten district asylums dotted throughout the country, providing more than three thousand beds in total. The second wave of asylum building, more vigorous than the first, took place between 1852 and 1869, when twelve more district asylums opened. These asylums were bigger than those built in the first half of the century owing to the ever-increasing demand for places from the public. By 1900, there were twenty-two asylums in Ireland, providing more than sixteen thousand beds.[8]

It was within the context of these developments that the Central Criminal Lunatic Asylum for Ireland was built at Dundrum on the outskirts of Dublin (the asylum is hereafter referred to as "Dundrum"). The actual decision to open this establishment was made by the 1843 Select Committee on the State of the Lunatic Poor in Ireland.[9] It was influenced by the evidence presented by Dr. Francis White, inspector of prisons, who later became the first inspector of lunatics in Ireland. He had received complaints from managers of prisons and asylums about the presence of criminal lunatics in their institutions. The problem was also causing concern in England at this time. Since the opening of two criminal wings at Bethlem Hospital in 1816, there had been an ongoing debate on the value of having a separate establishment for this group of patients. This debate exploded onto the public arena in 1843, when Daniel McNaughten attempted to kill Sir Robert Peel, the British prime minister. This debate influenced the decision to establish separate institutions for criminal lunatics. Dundrum opened in 1850, and a similar institution for England opened at Broadmoor in 1863.[10]

A number of interesting facts emerges from an examination of the age and gender of criminal lunatics admitted to Dundrum in the first fifty years of its existence. Of the 823 admissions, only 21 percent were women, reflecting the pattern evident elsewhere—in historical and current statistics—of the underrepresentation of women in crime statistics.[11] The age profile was similar for both men and women, with 66 percent of the women and 65 percent of the men between twenty and thirty-nine years of age at the time of their admission.[12] The predominance of men and the concentration of admissions in the age range of young adulthood were patterns echoed in the district asylum population, a fact that Mark Finnane attributes to the Land Acts, which had left many young men dispossessed of their farms.[13] The religious composition of the patient population reflected that of the general population (although the non-Catholic proportion was slightly higher than expected): 80 percent Roman Catholic, 18 percent Protestant and Presbyterian, and 2 percent unknown.[14]

These people had one thing in common—poverty. Like the occupants of district asylums, workhouses, and prisons, they were predominantly from the lower socioeconomic layers of Irish society. Because there is no record of income for patients, their literacy levels and occupational backgrounds are taken as descriptors of socioeconomic status. The literacy levels in Dundrum were lower than those in the general population, but they reflected the general trends. As shown by both Mary E. Daly and Joseph Lee, literacy levels rose steeply in Ireland during the second half of the century after the establishment of a national school system in 1831.[15] More than half of the Irish population was illiterate in 1841, but by 1900 this proportion had dropped to one-sixth. In Dundrum in 1874, 41 percent of patients were completely illiterate, 16 percent could read and write well, and 43 percent could read or write "indifferently."[16] The patients' occupations for the same year, 1874, show that many of them came from lower-income groups—with 83 percent of patients describing themselves as agricultural laborers or as having no occupation. The remaining 17 percent had worked in skilled jobs such as shoemaking, weaving, and carpentry.[17] A decade later the literacy level had improved. The inspectors commented in the annual report of 1886 that only one-third of the 178 patients was illiterate, with the others able to read and write. This shift corresponded with a lower number of patients from an agricultural background—just less than 50 percent—and a higher number from skilled occupations and from the security forces.[18] In an analysis of Dundrum statistics for the longer period of 1850–1995, Pat Gibbons and his colleagues found a similar occupational pattern—an overrepresentation of unskilled laborers and an underrepresentation of professionals or business owners. Among those found "unfit to plead," 51 percent were unskilled laborers, 45 percent were tradesmen or farmers, and 4 percent were professional or business people.[19] Among those found "guilty but insane," the pattern was even more pronounced—65 percent were unskilled laborers, 27 percent were tradesmen or farmers, and 8 percent were professional or business people.[20]

The opening of Dundrum in the mid–nineteenth century provided a real alternative to the death penalty (or penal servitude) for those who had committed serious crimes in Ireland. As argued elsewhere, it was theoretically accepted by both lunacy institution and prison authorities that for some people treatment rather than punishment was the appropriate response to criminal behavior.[21] However, as argued by scholars such as Joel Eigen and Roger Smith in relation to England, it was not always easy to implement this theory in practice because of the complex relationship between insanity and crime.[22] The difficulty involved in distinguishing "disease" from "vice" (as a cause of a particular crime) was highlighted in many articles in the *Journal of Mental Science* (the forerunner of the *British Journal of Psychiatry* and the main source of medical knowledge for Irish psychiatrists). For example, Dr. S. W. North, visiting medical officer to the York Retreat, England, wrote in 1886, "While groups of acts, in themselves criminal, may be, and often are, the direct outcome of insanity—acts of destruction, murder, arson, every form of violence, and the acts of lust and appetite—that which calls the passions into play being disease not vice. The same motives may influence an insane as a sane man. Investigation alone will prove their character, and in which category the act should be placed."[23] In other words, it is impossible to classify certain actions as sane or insane. It all rests on the question of culpability. Legal systems in Ireland and the United Kingdom, though different now, are based on a common intellectual tradition. One of the early legal landmarks occurred in 1800, when former army officer James Hadfield attempted to kill King George III in London by shooting at him as he sat in the royal box at Drury Lane Theatre.[24] Fortunately for the king, Hadfield did not succeed, but he was arrested for attempted murder. He had been discharged from the army on the grounds of insanity. His main delusion was that God was going to destroy the world. In an effort to have himself killed (by execution) without committing suicide, which he regarded as a mortal sin leading to damnation, Hadfield decided to kill the king. Owing to the brilliant oratory of his defense lawyer, he was not executed. This case created a new set of rules for pleading "not guilty on the grounds of insanity" and introduced the practice of presenting medical evidence to the court. Within a month of Hadfield's trial, the Criminal Lunatics Act of 1800 was passed at Westminster.[25] This act also applied to Ireland.

The next legal landmark was the case of Daniel McNaughten, who shot and killed Edward Drummond, private secretary to the British prime minister, Sir Robert Peel, in 1843. He had meant to kill Peel because he suffered under the delusion that he was being persecuted by the Tories. He was found "not guilty on the grounds of insanity" and sent to Newgate Prison until "Her Majesty's pleasure be known."[26] Many people were unhappy with the verdict, judging it to be too lenient. After a heated public debate in the press, the Law Lords developed a set of rules for future cases, rules that became known as the "M'Naghten rules." These rules state: "[To] establish a defence on the grounds of insanity, it must be clearly proven that at the time of the committing of the act, the party accused was labouring under such a defect of reason, from disease of the mind, that he did not to know the nature and quality of the act he was doing; or if he did know it, he did not know that what he was doing was wrong."[27] In Ireland, the first two laws governing the outcome of trials in which the offender was deemed to have a mental disorder were the Criminal Lunatics Act of 1800, already referred to, and the Lunacy (Ireland) Act of 1821. Before 1800, the verdict had been "not guilty," and the accused was allowed to walk free, having been acquitted completely of the crime. In the 1800 act, the verdict became "not guilty on the ground of insanity," and the offender was sent for a period of indefinite detention subject to the "pleasure" of the monarch or of the lord lieutenant for Ireland. This verdict remained in force until 1883, when there was a major change in the form of the Trial of Lunatics (Ireland) Act. With this legislation, the verdict became "guilty but insane," with no change in sentencing. In the act's words, "The jury shall return a special verdict to the effect that the accused was guilty of the act or omission charged against him, but was insane as aforesaid at the time when he did the act or made the omission."[28]

In a retrospective analysis of patients admitted to Dundrum from 1850 to 1995, Pat Gibbons, Niamh Mulryan, and Art O'Connor found that before 1910 the insanity defense was used successfully by an average of five patients per year. Of the 437 cases explored (for the complete period), 81 percent were male, and 19 percent were female. The average age for males who used this defense was thirty-seven years and for females thirty-four. Crimes against the person predominated as the "index offense," with a significant gender difference in relation to homicide. Although both men and women had been almost equally involved in murder (53 percent of men and 59 percent of women in the cases covered), almost half of these women had killed children. After 1910, the number of people admitted to Dundrum using this defense decreased to one per year, with the greatest reduction among women. As Gibbons and colleagues argue, this reduction was most probably owing to a change in social and legal attitudes to infanticide, making it easier for the court to be more lenient and to find an alternative solution for these cases.[29]

Discussions on cases (especially those in which murder was alleged) in nineteenth-century medical literature show that the final judgment as to whether an offender was a criminal or a lunatic was more often influenced by legal arguments than by medical opinion. Disputes between legal and medical experts on specific issues were rooted in a difference of approach to the questions of guilt and responsibility. Whereas lawyers sought to determine if offenders knew what they were doing and that it was morally wrong, doctors sought to prove the presence or absence of a disease.[30]

An examination of medical records and official reports on Dundrum for the period 1850–1900 reveals some interesting offending patterns. More than half of the patients had committed serious crimes—murder, manslaughter, and assault; 31 percent of women and 32 percent of men in Dundrum had committed murder or manslaughter.[31] Most of these women had killed children, whereas the men had killed other men, women, and children. The remaining patients had committed less serious crimes. The largest group—37 percent of women and 22 percent of men—had been involved in theft, some of which was minor. In contrast to people tried for murder or manslaughter, who were usually sent to Dundrum directly from the court, many of those involved in minor crimes had been sentenced to imprisonment in the first instance and transferred from prison to Dundrum only after they exhibited signs of mental disorder and became difficult to manage within an ordinary prison.

The courtroom was the arena in which the crucial distinction was made between those offenders who were "mad" and those who were "bad." At a time when the death penalty was in use, a successful insanity defense was regarded as a positive outcome, even though it might lead to an indefinite sentence. What is of particular interest to the discussion here is that the overall effect of legal deliberations—especially on cases in which murder was alleged—was to produce a particular pattern of sentencing that was highly gendered. Whether the unsoundness of mind that relieved the criminal of responsibility for the crime was caused by imbecility, dementia, delusion, or impulse—all conditions used in court to plead insanity—it was found most often in women who had killed children and in men who had killed women. It was almost never found in women who had killed men.[32]

Today, men outnumber women in general crime statistics throughout the world, and this pattern does not change when the crime is related to a mental disorder. A similar pattern operates in relation to homicide in general, with more men than women convicted for murder and manslaughter. Although male-on-male homicide is more common statistically, the number of male-on-female homicides is significant.[33] Judging by police records on reported crime, this pattern was also well established in nineteenth-century Ireland, with most of the male-on-female homicides taking place within the family network.[34]

It is extremely difficult to put exact numbers on these crimes because of the problems surrounding crime statistics in nineteenth-century Ireland. From my own research and that of Carolyn Conley, Mark Finnane, Elizabeth Malcolm, Ian O'Donnell, and William Wilbanks, it is clear that the majority of both perpetrators and victims of homicides were male and that in crimes where women were the victims, the perpetrators were likely to be male.[35] In other words, although men who killed men were in the majority, a substantial number of men killed women.[36] Because official crime statistics do not give the level of detail required to make an accurate judgment of how many men killed women, we have to rely on partial statistics derived from detailed police reports for some periods. The records of the Royal Irish Constabulary (RIC) on "outrages reported to the constabulary office" reveal the names of more than one hundred men who killed their wives between 1838 and 1892 and almost the same number of men who killed other female relatives.[37] The victims included mothers, daughters, sisters, aunts, and female in-laws. These records also show that many of the cases did not reach court and that of those that did, some perpetrators received the death sentence, but for many the death sentence was reduced to penal servitude for life, and some received short sentences or were sent to Dundrum as criminal lunatics.

The inspectors of lunacy in Ireland give one explanation of wife killing in the report on Dundrum for 1855:

The most frequent kind of homicide among the men is wife murder. . . . This fact, at first sight, might seem to argue less constancy, fidelity and tenderness with the male sex; but there are strong causes to explain away, or, at least, reduce the force of the conclusion; for it is well known, that, occasionally, among the first and most marked symptoms of the disease with lunatics may be reckoned a mistrust and aversion to members of their own family, and to those particularly with whom they had been united by the strongest ties of affection, and who, if physically weaker, in case any control is attempted, are most exposed to suffer from their violence.[38]

This comment reflects the medical argument that the killing of a wife or close relative could be symptomatic of a mental disorder—in other words, the crime was a manifestation of a preexisting mental condition that emerged in the pressurized environment of the home.[39] However, it is also a highly gendered and incorrect view of the situation. The "most frequent kind of homicide" in Ireland was not "wife murder"—in fact, most homicide victims were male.[40] However, men who murdered their wives (or indeed any member of their family) had a higher than average probability of putting forward a successful insanity defense.

It would also be wrong to assume that the medical profession in Ireland suggested a direct link between insanity and the potential to kill. In fact, the opposite was true, as is evident in the writings of Dr. Michael Corbet, the medical superintendent at Dundrum. In the annual report in 1864, he wrote: "As to the homicidal propensity among the insane, or a predisposition to kill for the mere object of killing, we apprehend it to be of the rarest occurrence. The act, when preconceived, appears to us to be almost uniformly directed against an individual alone, and to result from some lurking ideas or fancy of an actual or intended wrong."[41] In other words, it is very rare for someone with a mental illness to kill, and when it happens, it is usually not random. Rather, the perpetrator perceives the victim as a threat—real or imaginary. This is usual not only in cases where there is evidence of an existing mental disorder, but also in cases where the crime takes place during what the medical and legal professions called "temporary insanity" or "transitory frenzy."[42]

In cases where the impulse to kill or to commit a violent act was linked to alcohol consumption, lawyers and doctors did not always agree whether this factor removed or reduced responsibility for the crime or not. In relation to a case in Scotland in 1883, that of "George

Miller, age twenty seven, a native of the North of Ireland . . . who had killed a man . . . but could recall nothing that had occurred," Dr. David Yellowlees of Glasgow Royal Asylum commented as follows on Miller's acquittal on the grounds of insanity: "There can be little doubt as to the correctness of this opinion, though some may demur to the complete exculpation of a man who wilfully drank to excess after so many warnings as to the dangerous condition which drinking induced."[43] An exploration of the cases in which men had killed women while in a state of intoxication confirms the concern Dr. Yellowlees raised. These men were known to be violent when they had drunk too much, yet they were excused of responsibility for their crimes on the basis of their alcoholic state. Some were acquitted completely, some were given short sentences, and a few were sent to district asylums or to Dundrum. For example, James McM., a publican from Belfast who killed his wife, Margaret, age thirty, "while in a state of intoxication," was sentenced to imprisonment for twelve months. The RIC report gave jealousy as the motive for the crime.[44] In the same year, John S., a rag gatherer from Cork, killed his wife by stabbing her in the neck "with a sharp pointed poker" during a quarrel. He, too, was "under the influence of drink" and was acquitted.[45] Similarly, in 1884 John McC., a mechanic from Belfast, killed his forty-year-old wife, Catherine, after a bout of drinking. She "died from the effects of injuries inflicted by her husband, who flung her down stairs, thereby fracturing her skull." The police reported that though he had been drinking, he was "not intoxicated" at the time of the crime. He was acquitted of her murder.[46]

All of these crimes highlight not only the link between intoxication and domestic violence, but also the relative leniency of the judicial system in relation to men's violence against women. Does this leniency show an acceptance of domestic violence (directed toward women) in the Irish courts? Conley thinks not. She quotes from a Limerick newspaper and from assizes reports to back up her claim. "The *Limerick Reporter* used the headline 'Shocking Outrage' for a story about a fisherman who had struck his wife in the head with a pewter pot." However, Conley does suggest that the involvement of alcohol in a violent attack made it less serious in the eyes of the law.[47] It is clear that the concept of masculinity in nineteenth-century Ireland incorporated behavior that was both violent and irrational. Though violence was not condoned, it was accepted as a likely outcome of male drinking patterns.

It is very difficult in retrospect to reconstruct the arguments used in court cases because of the loss of so many of the court records in the Custom House fire in 1921 and the selective coverage of cases in newspapers and other sources.[48] However, there are indications in police records that the men who received lighter sentences or were acquitted were seen as neither dangerous nor deliberately cruel. For men regarded as dangerous or deliberately violent, two very severe outcomes were possible—an indefinite sentence to confinement in Dundrum as a criminal lunatic or a sentence to execution by hanging. The crucial element in the decision to accept the insanity defense was the evidence presented to the court that the crime had taken place as a result of a "transitory frenzy" during a period of "temporary insanity" that could be a symptom of an existing mental disorder or could be brought on by either intoxication or epilepsy (see table 5.1).[49] For example, Michael G., a farmer from County Tipperary, was sent to Dundrum in 1883 for killing his thirty-five-year-old wife, Maria. According to the police report, "She died from the effect of injuries inflicted by her husband Michael. The deceased who was in a delicate state of health was lying in bed when her husband came into the house under the influence of drink. He dragged her out of bed and violently assaulted her. Several slight wounds were found on her body as well as two large burn marks. These injuries combined with the shock to her enfeebled system caused almost immediate death. The outrage is solely attributable to drink."[50] Here we see the police report pointing the court toward an explanation of the crime that in other cases got the accused man off with a light sentence. However, the post mortem examination of her body indicated not only that this man was dangerous when drunk, but that this final act of violence against his wife was part of a pattern of continuous abuse also linked to his overindulgence in alcohol. This information led to the conclusion that he was dangerous but not responsible for his actions. Another famous case in which alcohol was involved was that of Dr. Terence B., a dispensary doctor who shot his wife in their home in 1886. He was

Table 5.1

Wife Killers Found to Be Insane at the Time of the Crime
(Selected Cases), 1850–1900

Name	County	Cause of Crime/Diagnosis	Year(s) in Asylum*
Patrick M.	Down	Chronic mania	1867–91
Andrew D.	Leitrim	Delusions	1870
William H.	Tyrone	Insanity	1873
Daniel C.	Cork	Insanity	1879
Michael G.	Tipperary	Alcoholic frenzy	1883
John C.	Tipperary	Insanity	1884
Dr. Terence B.	Galway	Delirium tremens	1886–92
James C.	Louth	Delusions	1887
Michael R.	Waterford	Insanity	1887
John D.	Tipperary	Insanity	1887
Darby L.	Galway	Insanity	1889
William I.	Westmeath	Insanity	1891
Allan S.	Antrim	Melancholia	1892–99
Alexander McM.	Antrim	Alcoholic frenzy	1893
Michael F.	Longford	Dementia	1894
James McD.	Fermanagh	Insanity	1895
John McD.	Roscommon	Delusions	1897
John C.	Donegal	Insanity	1898

* Dundrum or a district asylum or both.
Sources: Medical records, Central Mental Hospital (formerly Central Criminal Lunatic Asylum), Dundrum; police records and individual convict files, Misc. Files, National Archives of Ireland, Dublin.

found to be insane at the time of the crime owing to a "tranzitory [*sic*] frenzy" brought on by his alcohol consumption.[51]

Another common denominator emerged in reports on cases where the insanity defense was successful: jealousy as a motive for the fatal attack on a wife—jealousy based on an alleged infidelity. In cases where it was accepted that the wife had not been unfaithful, the husband's jealousy was viewed as delusional and symptomatic of a mental disorder. In 1870, Andrew D., a farmer from Leitrim, killed his wife by stabbing her

Table 5.2

Matricide: Men Found to Be Insane at the Time of the Crime (Selected Cases), Ireland, 1850–1900

Name	County	Cause of Crime/Diagnosis	Year(s) in Dundrum
Patrick McC.	Cork	Imbecility	1869–91
Edmund H.	Kilkenny	Insanity	1890
John K.	Longford	Deafness and dumbness	1892
James M.	Galway	Insanity	1892

Sources: Medical records, Central Mental Hospital (formerly Central Criminal Lunatic Asylum), Dundrum; Royal Irish Constabulary, *Return of Outrages,* and individual convict files, National Archives of Ireland, Dublin.

with a knife. The police reported that "he laboured under an unfounded suspicion of his wife's infidelity."[52] Similarly, in 1887, James C., a baker from County Louth, killed his sixty-year-old wife, Mary Anne, on a public road near Ardee. According to the police report, "[H]er skull was fractured and she received other injuries which caused immediate death. The weapon used was an iron hammer. It is believed that jealousy was the cause of the crime."[53] Both men were found to be insane and sent to Dundrum (see table 5.1). These men and others like them were viewed with some leniency within Dundrum, and the medical superintendent often presented pleas for clemency to the lord lieutenant. For example, in the report of 1855, one such man is referred to: "The lunatic labours under a disadvantage in one respect; for, though acquitted of a moral crime, he may still become the penal sufferer by a more lengthened confinement. Amongst other instances under our cognizance, as illustrative of this view, we shall refer to . . . a man in the Central Asylum, who it was proved whilst labouring under maniacal excitement from jealousy towards his wife in consequence of her supposed freedom of conduct, committed homicide."[54] Some of these men were discharged home and some to district lunatic asylums, depending on their state of mind and their families' willingness to have them return home.

There is something particularly shocking about a son who kills his mother. Police records from the nineteenth century show that this crime was fairly rare—as it continues to be today. An analysis of RIC records for the period 1838–1900 revealed the names of eight men who had killed their mothers, one who had killed a stepmother, and one a mother-in-law.[55] All of the men lived with their mothers, a fact showing their financial interdependence. In most cases, the place of residence was the family farm. Two of the mothers were in their fifties, but the others were in their seventies. Of the eight men, four were found to be insane at the time of the crime and sent to Dundrum on an indefinite sentence; one was sentenced to death, but his sentence was later reduced to penal servitude for life; two received prison sentences; and one committed suicide.[56]

Two of the killings were particularly gruesome, and there is some indication in their files that the men were intellectually disabled as well as mentally unstable at the time of the crime (see table 5.2). Edmond H., a laborer from Kilkenny, killed his seventy-five-year-old mother, Mary, in 1890.[57] This case was tragic not only because the crime was particularly vicious, but also because the cause of the dispute had nothing to do with the mother. According to the report in the *Kilkenny Journal*, Edmond was a fisherman who also worked on his wife's family farm. His anger knew no bounds when his mother-in-law sold the farm, and he threatened to kill her. However, no one could have predicted that he would turn his anger toward his mother and murder her.[58] Equally vicious was the crime committed by James M. from County Galway, who killed his seventy-year-old mother, Mary, in 1892. She was described in police records as a farmer, and we can assume that her son worked and lived on the farm with her.[59] Both men were sent to Dundrum as criminal lunatics, as were two other men who committed the same crime—Patrick McC. and John K. From the information available on Patrick McC., we know that he was from County Cork and that he killed his mother, who was a widow, in 1868. We do not know from the records what age this woman was, but she owned a farm and "died from the results of frightful injuries inflicted on her head with a hatchet" by her son Patrick. Because he was one of the patients transferred from Dundrum in the 1890s, we can track his asylum career. He was described in medical notes variously as "very treacherous and violent," "quiet, amiable and stupid," and as suffering from "imbecility or moral insanity." The phrase *moral insanity* was often used to describe individuals of "weak intellect" who were regarded as not being able to distinguish right from wrong. Patrick McC. remained in Dundrum until 1891 (twenty-three years in confinement), when he was transferred to Cork District Asylum, which indicates that authorities probably saw him as someone who might be dangerous. However, by the time he was discharged, this danger had apparently passed because he was described as "quiet, [with] chronic dementia."[60]

Just as Patrick was leaving Dundrum, another man who had killed his mother was about to be admitted (see table 5.2 for both): John K. from County Longford, who killed his seventy-year-old mother, Catherine, in 1892. She was also described as a farmer. At the time of the crime, she had refused to give her son money for clothes. He was "deaf and dumb and said to be not quite sane." He attacked his mother "with a shoemaker's knife and inflicted several incised and punctured wounds about her face and head."[61] This woman had probably done her best for this son, whose disability would have marked him out as outcast in a society that had little tolerance and no support services for men like him. Unfortunately for her, as she became frail, he became powerful, with terrible consequences for both of them.

Academic literature on crimes committed by women highlights the relative absence of women from statistics on the murder of adults.[62] When women do become involved in this crime, their victims are usually spouses or close relatives. Even then, their contribution to the statistics on spousal or family murders is low when compared with the statistics for men. Theoretical explanations of the low rate of adult homicide committed by women include notions of weakness and compliance.[63] This weakness is usually conceptualized as emanating from a lack of opportunity and physical strength, which leads to a state of fear of retaliation from those with more power (physical and legal), epitomized in male figures in both private and public spheres. The compliance may derive from fear in some cases, but it may also be based on realistic judgments on the impact of criminal behavior on the woman herself and on her children. The loss of a mother to the criminal justice system, now as in the past, leads almost certainly to the placement of children under the protection of the state, which often means a lifetime of care away from the family of origin.

Women in nineteenth-century Ireland were engaged in very similar crimes to those reported elsewhere in the academic literature. They had a much lower rate of participation in crime than men; their highest visibility in crime statistics was in relation to crimes against property, and when they engaged in killing, their victims were usually children.[64] However, women did kill adults—men and women. Here, the focus is on women who killed men. Although it is not possible to give an overall figure for the nineteenth century, convict records and RIC *Returns of Outrages* reveal the names of at least thirty women who killed a man between 1840 and 1900.[65] Some killed husbands, some killed brothers or other relatives, and some killed neighbors.

Of the thirty cases explored for this study, seven women were found guilty of murder and sentenced to death; of these women so sentenced, three were executed, and the sentences for four of them were reduced to penal servitude for life (see table 5.3). Sixteen of the thirty women were found guilty of manslaughter or assault and sentenced to imprisonment—sometimes with the additional condition of penal servitude or hard labor—for periods of time ranging from four months to life (see table 5.4). As with men who killed women, the severity of the sentence depended on the circumstances of the death and the responsibility for the crime attributed to the woman offender. The remaining six women were arrested for the crime but were either acquitted or discharged owing to lack of evidence.[66] Finally, only one woman was found "guilty but insane": Mary R., a nurse from Galway who killed a man in her care in 1887.

Mary R.'s crime was unusual in that the man she killed was neither a relative nor a neighbor; he was her patient. Mary was a thirty-year-old widow with four children. She was employed by the victim's family to look after him when he became seriously ill with "typhus fever." Michael D., the patient, was being cared for in his home. Other

Table 5.3

Women Convicted of Murdering a Man and Sentenced to Death (Selected Cases), 1850–1900

Name	Victim	Weapon/Cause of Death	Sentence	Time Spent in Prison
Honora S.	Cousin	Beating	Death: Executed April 29, 1853	1852: 8 months
Bridget S.	Cousin	Beating	Death: Executed April 29, 1853	1852: 8 months
Margaret S.	Neighbor	Pistol	Death: Executed May 27, 1870	1870: 3 months
Elizabeth B.	Husband	Pistol and knife	Death: Reduced to PS for life	1881–91
Catherine D.	Cousin	Blunt instrument	Death: Reduced to PS for life	1884–98
Catherine D.	Husband	Poison	Death: Reduced to PS for life	1884–98
Mary B.	Brother	Knife	Death: Reduced to PS for life	1886–95

PS = penal servitude in prison

Sources: Transportation database and General Prison Board, Royal Irish Constabulary and convict records, all at the National Archives of Ireland, Dublin.

members of his family were in the house on the night of the crime—his mother, two brothers, and a sister-in-law. All had shared a drink of whisky with the nurse before retiring to bed. In the middle of the night, they awoke to the sound of screams from the kitchen. There, they found Michael lying dead on the floor very near the fire, with Mary R. dancing around him, saying she had cast out a devil. When the case came to court, the legal team defending Mary concentrated on the connection between alcohol consumption and "transitory frenzy" or "temporary insanity" rather than introducing any arguments about the casting out of devils or evil spirits. These arguments were used elsewhere in the legal system as mitigating circumstances in other murders committed during the 1890s. They were successful in two instances—that of the Doyle family, in which a thirteen-year-old boy with an intellectual disability

Table 5.4
Women Convicted of Manslaughter or Assault for Killing a Man, 1850–1900

Name	Victim	Weapon/Cause of Death	Sentence	Time Spent in Prison
Margaret B.	Husband	Knife	20 years PS	1879–90
Kate S.	Bailiff	Stone	18 months HL	1879
Margaret K.	Husband	Stool	6 months HL	1880
Ann M.	Cousin	Gun and kicks	12 months prison	1880
Mary L.	Husband	Spade and pitchfork	PS life	1881–92
Catherine L. (15 years old)	Father	Spade and pitchfork	10 years PS	1881–88
Margaret O'N.	Cousin	Stone	14 years PS	1885–95
Mary S.	Neighbor	Oil lamp	6 months HL	1889
Lizzie B.	Stranger	Knife	3 years PS	1894–96
Mary B.	Husband	Deep cuts to head	4 months HL	1889
Mary W.	Son-in-law	Deep cuts to head	4 months HL	1889
Johanna N.	Son (age 15)	Asphyxia	5 years PS	1891
Margaret M.	Stranger	Knife	12 months prison	1891
Mrs. R.	Husband	Oil lamp	5 years PS	1892
Maria H.	Husband	Hatchet	10 years PS	1893
Lizzie McA.	Stranger	Umbrella point	4 months prison	1894

PS = penal servitude in prison
HL = hard labor in prison
Sources: Transportation database and General Prison Board, Royal Irish Constabulary, and convict records, all at the National Archives of Ireland, Dublin.

was beaten to death by his mother and siblings because they thought him to be a "changeling," and that of the Cunningham family, in which an adult son was also beaten to death by his father and brothers because they thought "the Devil was in him."[67] The arguments were not successful in the case of Bridget Cleary, the twenty-six-year-old woman burned to death by her husband and family.[68] Many members of the judicial system were very skeptical about excuses based on superstition. This defense was successful only if the superstitious statements continued to be expressed for some time after the crime was committed, making it possible for a psychiatrist to reconceptualize them as delusions.

In the case of the nurse Mary R., the court was told that she had consumed almost a half bottle of whisky, which therefore likely led to a period of "temporary insanity" during which she killed the man in her care. Mary was sent to Dundrum for an indefinite period of confinement, to be released "at the Pleasure of the Lord Lieutenant." Luckily for her, she quickly recovered her sanity and was discharged after four years of confinement as a criminal lunatic. She later immigrated to the United States to join other members of her family.[69] Mary was regarded throughout the trial and her confinement in Dundrum as a "good" woman, and the label of criminal lunatic removed responsibility for the crime from her shoulders.[70] The case was tragic and shocking, but the verdict was not controversial. What is interesting is that Mary R. seems to be the only woman for whom the insanity defense was used successfully in a case where a woman killed a man. There may have been others, but for the moment they remain invisible, possibly the result of missing case records.[71]

To understand the significance of the absence of the insanity defense in cases where women killed men, we can look briefly at some of the other cases in which women appeared before the courts for this crime. As with modern-day statistics, very few women were involved in the killing of men; only three women were executed (for any crime) in Ireland during the period 1850–1900. These three women were found guilty of the murder of two men in disputes over land. In County Clare in 1853, Honora S., her husband's brother Richard, and his wife, Bridget, were hanged for the murder of Richard's brother James in a dispute over the ownership of a farm.[72] In the second case, Margaret S. and her brother, Lawrence, from King's County, were hanged in 1870 for shooting Patrick D., a neighbor, with whom they were in dispute over a right of way to a bog.[73] Three other women were found guilty of murder and were sentenced to execution, but their sentences were reduced to penal servitude for life, with all being released after an average of ten years in prison. Two of the women had killed their husbands, and one her brother. Some of these killings could be described as "impulse killings" similar to those in which men killed their wives and pleaded insanity. In addition to the women sentenced to death, others were sentenced to long periods of penal servitude for killing men, most of whom were their husbands.[74]

What is interesting about these cases is that the circumstances were not dissimilar to those in which men had killed women. In some cases, there had been an obvious dispute leading to a fight; in some there was alcohol involved; and in some there was known domestic violence. For some of these situations, the plea of temporary insanity or "transitory frenzy" could have been used. However, this study has uncovered no evidence that the insanity defense was put forward in these cases. These women were considered rational and therefore responsible for their actions. It seems that it was easier for society to see them as "bad" rather than "mad" when they committed the ultimate crime not only of questioning the authority of the male (husband, brother, or employer), but of destroying him.

Clarice Feinmann argues in her feminist analysis of current crime that patriarchal societies tend to categorize women "according to the degree to which they fit the role of either Madonna or whore."[75] The good woman fits the traditional role and supports her husband and the other male members of the family. For this role, she is respected both within the household and in society at large. The bad woman, in contrast, "destroys man and brings pain and ruin," and for this she has to be controlled within the family and punished by society if she steps out of line. This characterization seems to have been the case in Ireland during the nineteenth century.

By providing one institution for criminal lunatics—the Central Criminal Lunatic Asylum for Ireland at Dundrum—the authorities hoped to divert people who were not responsible for their crimes toward a treatment regime that would contain and perhaps cure them. It also provided an alternative legal route for people who otherwise might have been given the death penalty. Irish psychiatry (represented by the Inspectorate of Lunacy and the doctors working in Dundrum) was in a very good position to play a leading role in diverting people, regardless of gender, from punishment they did not deserve. However, it is clear from medical and convict records that courts called psychiatrists only to confirm social stereotypes. These stereotypes included a view of men who killed women and of women who killed children as probably "mad" rather than "bad"—resulting in consistent efforts by the legal and medical profession to divert them into the asylum system. They also included a view of women who killed men as "bad" rather than "mad"—resulting in little or no attempt by the same professionals to save these women from the death penalty or prison. In other words, medical knowledge was not used to challenge stereotypes, but rather to uphold a system of patriarchy.

This brief discussion on Dundrum also reveals some of the social attitudes to crime and insanity during this period. People who committed crimes were reported to the police, but not all were brought to trial. The police often found it difficult to find witnesses who would testify in court, especially in cases where a murder had taken place. It is also clear from police records that some crimes were regarded more seriously than others. A domestic dispute between a man and his wife, though it might have led to her death, was not always regarded as a serious crime. Premeditation or the man's prior violence made the crime more serious. The crime that had the highest chance of achieving the death penalty was a killing that was related to a land dispute. This pattern of punishment was true for women as well as for men. In fact, the only women executed during the second half of the nineteenth century were involved in killings that were land related.

Social attitudes to insanity during the nineteenth century were characterized by fear and ignorance. The solution to the problem of insanity in a family was to banish the afflicted person to the nearest district asylum. The double stigma of having a family member labeled as a criminal and a lunatic was one that many families could not endure. Records from Dundrum show not only that many of the men and women who had been involved in serious crime left Ireland (usually for the United States) immediately on discharge, but that members of their immediate families had to do so also.[76]

This study of criminal lunacy in the past raises many questions about the present. Does the current system of dealing with offenders with a mental disorder continue to be biased by gender and social status? Is psychiatry merely a tool of the legal system, or does it have any power in its own right in these cases? What kind of a life can a person have after "doing time" in Dundrum or a similar establishment?

6

Between Habitual Drunkards and Alcoholics

Inebriate Women and Reformatories in Ireland, 1899–1919

Elizabeth Malcolm

In June 1899, the County Clare prison in Ennis, which had been built in 1815 and closed in the 1880, was reopened as a state inebriate reformatory, regulated by the new Inebriates Act of 1898 (61 & 62 Vic., c.60).[1] The reformatory provided accommodation for thirty male and thirty female inmates, sentenced by the courts for drink-related offenses, and was administered by the General Prisons Board.[2] As well as establishing state inebriate reformatories, the 1898 act also made provision for certified inebriate reformatories, which were to be licensed by the state but operated and largely funded by county and borough councils, religious and philanthropic bodies, or private individuals. In May 1903, the Lodge retreat for fifteen paying female Protestant inebriates, which had been established in a private house in Sydenham Avenue, East Belfast, in 1902 by the Irish Women's Temperance Union, was certified under the 1898 act.[3] In March 1906, another certified reformatory, St. Patrick's, was opened in Waterford town for thirty male Catholic inebriates. St. Patrick's was located in a former convent in Hennessy's Road, and members of an English religious order, the Congregation of the Divine Pastor, operated it and occupied part of the building.[4] In December 1908, St. Brigid's reformatory for sixty-six female Catholic inebriates, situated in a disused prison in Wexford town and staffed by

the Sisters of St. John of God, was also licensed.[5] These certified reformatories, unlike the Ennis state reformatory, were overseen by one of
the lunacy inspectors based in Dublin Castle.[6]

Throughout the nineteenth century, numerous therapeutic, charitable, educational, custodial, and punitive institutions were established
in Ireland. General and specialist hospitals proliferated in all the major
cities, along with infirmaries in towns and dispensaries in rural areas.
By the early 1850s, Ireland had some 140 hospitals, with beds for
around 9,000 patients; and by the late 1870s, there were more than
1,000 dispensaries, staffed by 804 doctors and 217 midwives, annually
treating some 670,000 patients.[7] From the 1820s, a network of state
lunatic asylums spread throughout the country, eventually numbering
twenty-two, plus a criminal lunatic asylum at Dundrum in Dublin; by
the mid-1890s, they housed around 13,600 patients.[8] During the 1840s,
163 workhouses were erected, which at their peak in 1851 were accommodating more than 217,000 paupers and continued to accommodate
around 50,000 for the next thirty years.[9] Asylums and workhouses operated in conjunction with prisons. After transportation of convicts over-
seas largely ended in 1853–54, Ireland had nine convict prisons, housing
nearly 3,900 convicts, with a further 5,700 prisoners serving shorter sentences in 137 local jails and bridewells.[10] In addition, by 1880 there were
fifty-six industrial schools, containing 5,700 children, most of whom
had been apprehended for vagrancy and begging.[11] In 1906, a borstal at
Clonmel, County Tipperary, was added to the juvenile detention system,
with accommodation initially for 54 young male offenders.[12]

Such institutions and others multiplied during the nineteenth century not simply because more were built to house greater numbers, but
also because they became more specialized, catering in separate premises for carefully defined and segregated groups, classified usually by
sex, age, class, religion, nature of offense, or type of disorder.[13] Thus, in
many respects, the opening of four small institutions between 1899 and
1908 specifically for Catholic and Protestant men and women labeled as
inebriates either by themselves and by their families or by the courts was
hardly a major innovation. Nevertheless, these reformatories had novel
features that are revealing; they can tell us much about contemporary

attitudes to chronic drunkenness and in particular to "deviant women." Moreover, unlike Irish prisons, asylums, and workhouses, many of which operated for more than a century in the same premises and all of which also catered to drunkards, the four Irish inebriate reformatories had closed within twenty years of their establishment. Why they did not endure when so many other specialist institutions did is one of the questions this chapter addresses.

Like the temperance movement itself, the concept of specialist inebriate institutions had originated in the United States. As early as 1810, there were calls in Philadelphia for a "sober house" to accommodate drunkards, and a book published in Massachusetts in 1838 advocated the setting up of a network of inebriate "homes" or "retreats."[14] An abortive attempt to establish a retreat took place in Boston in 1841, and a more permanent one opened there in 1857. Others appeared in New York also in 1857, in San Francisco in 1859, in Chicago in 1863, in Philadelphia in 1872, and in parts of Canada in 1875.[15] An English surgeon and lunatic asylum proprietor, David Dalrymple, who visited several of these American institutions in 1869, initiated a campaign to have them introduced into the United Kingdom when he was elected to Parliament as a Liberal member in 1870.[16] After a number of abortive bills during the 1870s and a select committee investigation in 1872,[17] the Habitual Drunkards Act (42 & 43 Vic., c.19) was finally passed in 1879 and lasted ten years.

The Conservative government of 1874–80 enjoyed strong support from the drink industry and was therefore naturally loath to legislate contrary to industry interests.[18] However, the 1870s witnessed steeply rising alcohol consumption in both Ireland and England, public alarm at the numbers of arrests for drunkenness, and growing concern among doctors at the impact of heavy drinking on public health.[19] Given the strong feelings and powerful vested interests on both sides, the 1879 act was inevitably a compromise measure that satisfied few. Although proponents of the bill had wanted compulsory confinement in inebriate institutions at state expense, the act was in fact highly permissive. Habitual drunkards and their families had to convince magistrates of their addiction and of their willingness and ability to meet the costs of treatment. If convinced, magistrates could commit the drunkard to a licensed "retreat" for a specified period. But drunkards could not be forcibly detained in retreats against their wishes. Although the act was made permanent in 1888, by that stage its failure was glaringly obvious, for in England only seventy-three people had entered licensed retreats under its terms.[20] No retreats had been licensed in Ireland.

During the 1880s and 1890s, alcohol consumption and arrests for drunkenness declined in both Ireland and England from the levels reached in the mid-1870s. Nevertheless, there was a renewed campaign from the medical profession, supported by many newspapers, for further institutional measures to deal with chronic drunkards. The rise of eugenics as a science influenced this campaign, and much attention was focused on drinking among women. Another major inquiry took place in 1892–93;[21] an abortive bill was introduced in 1895; and, finally, a bill was passed in 1898. However, like its predecessor, the Inebriates Act was the product of a series of political compromises.

The 1898 Inebriates Act certainly went further than the 1879 Habitual Drunkards Act by authorizing the establishment of state and certified reformatories to which the courts could commit drunkards and detain them for extended periods. But significant sections of the earlier act were retained, especially those relating to retreats. The different titles of the two acts reflected changing attitudes. The term *habitual drunkard* grew out of everyday speech and implied a moral judgment because at the time, aside from the term *drunkard* being derogatory, the word *habitual* was generally associated in public discourse with the word *criminal*.[22] The term *inebriate,* however, was less familiar, Latinate, technical, and therefore more neutral. It signaled the growing medicalization of the problem of excessive drinking. As pointed out earlier, however, the 1879 act was not wholly repealed. Thus, the system instituted in 1898 was an uneasy combination of two very different approaches. One perceived the "inebriate" as sick and in need of treatment, which it was hoped would lead to rehabilitation; the other perceived the "habitual drunkard" as essentially a recidivist petty criminal, requiring punishment, which it was hoped would lead to deterrence.[23] These conflicting views were very evident in Ireland's four inebriate reformatories. Confusion as to these reformatories' basic function goes some way toward explaining their ultimate failure.

In May 1906, the Irish General Prisons Board issued a lengthy printed memorandum on the Inebriates Act, which set out in some detail the rationale behind the whole reformatory system and described its operations in Ireland since 1899. The board wanted to encourage the establishment of more certified reformatories, but it conceded that there was "a great deal of confusion" regarding some of the act's provisions. It went on to explain that the state and certified reformatories were meant to cater for two different categories of drunkard: the "tractable" and the "intractable." The Ennis reformatory, "with its stricter rules and *slightly* penal methods," was intended for the latter. However, the General Prisons Board, doubtless fostering the confusion it had sought to dispel, readily acknowledged that, "contrary to expectation," tractable cases were often the most "troublesome." Thus, the two types of reformatory operated in tandem, with "troublesome" individuals being transferred "quickly and readily" from the certified institutions to the state one, and at the same time "amenable" individuals could be sent from Ennis to a certified reformatory.[24]

In Ennis, the state wholly paid for the cost of the prison inmate, but it only contributed to the costs of the certified reformatories. The maintenance of inmates in Ennis was substantially more expensive than the cost of feeding, clothing, and accommodating prisoners in Irish jails. By 1910–11, each inmate was costing £21.19s.5d per annum, compared with only £11.10s.11d. for those serving their sentences in local or convict prisons. Staffing was also significantly more expensive because Ennis had a larger staff than was usual in a local Irish prison. Most of those employed, however—required to be total abstainers—had previously worked in the prisons. In 1910–11, in addition to a governor, there were twenty-two warders, matrons, doctors, chaplains, and servants looking after on average fifty-five inmates.[25] The governor justified this apparent overstaffing as owing to the need to blend "firmness with kindness," which threw a "heavy onus" on the staff. In addition, inmates were allowed to associate more freely than prisoners and so required greater supervision.[26]

Although the General Prisons Board was careful to refer to those committed to Ennis as "habitual drunkards" or simply as "inmates" rather than as "prisoners," the reformatory nevertheless exhibited penal features that were more than merely "slight." On admission, the reformatory's doctor took detailed medical histories of inmates, but "treatment," as defined by the governor, seems to have consisted largely of promoting physical health by means of a good diet and "moral" reform, achieved by regimentation, recreation, and religion. "No so-called specific cures of alcoholism were used." Instead, inmates were "subject to the general rules for local prisons,"[27] although these rules were mitigated by more comfortable living conditions, meant to create a "homelike" environment. During their sentences, inmates, like prisoners, progressed through three stages, each usually lasting about six months.[28] They were required to work, although for only seven rather than twelve hours a day, in order to develop "industrious and regular habits." Recreation, mainly in the form of games and reading, was encouraged so as to promote "self-control." Religious instruction was considered vital, and chaplains visited two or three times a week and conducted services on Sunday. Points were accumulated for good behavior, resulting in progression to a higher stage and the award of privileges. In the final stage of their sentence, inmates could be allowed out for walks or even to leave the reformatory for periods on parole. Punishments, which were similar to those inflicted in the prisons, largely took the form of a loss of marks, withdrawal of privileges, confinement in a special cell, wearing of a restraining jacket or muffs, or a reduced diet. At the end of their sentences, inmates, like prisoners, were released on license, under the care of a "guardian," who was obliged to report monthly to the reformatory governor.[29]

In its 1906 memorandum, the General Prisons Board extolled the successes of the institution by offering nine case histories, which included examples of "promising" inmates, including those inmates released on license who were "going on well" and some who had relapsed on release but were "not unhopeful."[30] Only three of these nine were women. This sample of cases is not therefore at all representative of the reformatory's inmates, and it is unlikely that it is representative of the reformatory's success rate, either. Another similarity between the Ennis inebriate reformatory and Irish prisons was the high number of female drunkards committed to both.[31] When Ennis opened, it had been refurbished with accommodation for equal numbers of men and woman.[32] Yet the General Prisons Board's final report on the reformatory in December 1919, just prior to the reformatory's appropriation by the British army in 1920, showed that of those discharged since 1899, 60 percent were women. In December 1919, however, only 35 percent of the general prison population was female.[33]

Not only were there far more women in Ennis proportionately than in the prisons, but the number of women sent to the reformatory did not at all reflect the number appearing before the courts charged with drunkenness. In 1899, the year Ennis opened, only 12 percent of those prosecuted in Ireland for drunkenness were women.[34] By the early 1920s, shortly after the reformatory had closed, of those the authorities prosecuted for simple drunkenness, only around 15 percent were women—although women did make up 37 percent of those accused of aggravated drunkenness. Yet of those committed to prison by the courts for all forms of drunkenness, more than half, around 55 percent, were women. After 1920, the courts were clearly far more ready to send women to prison for drunkenness than men, just as during the twenty years before 1920 they were more ready to commit women to Ennis reformatory than they were to commit men.[35]

The certified reformatories exhibited a similar pattern, for they, too, contained a majority of women. Of the three established, the ones in Belfast and Wexford were specifically for women, whereas the Waterford institution was intended solely for men. Taken together, they initially provided accommodation for eighty-one women, compared to only thirty men. Thus, it would appear that, unlike Ennis, the certified reformatories, which had to raise much of their own funding, anticipated from the outset that their clientele would be largely female.

However, in the eight years that St. Patrick's in Waterford operated before closing in March 1914, it averaged only 18.5 male admissions per annum, and St. Brigid's in Wexford, which struggled to find adequate funding and did not begin accepting inmates until March 1910, was averaging only 25.5 female admissions per annum by the end of 1914. The Belfast retreat, which was able to house 24 inmates when it moved to larger premises in Irwin Avenue in 1912, averaged 14 admissions per annum between 1903 and 1914.[36] Thus, the Belfast reformatory was expanding and generally operating up to its—admittedly very limited—capacity, which both Waterford and Wexford were clearly not doing. It is hardly surprising, therefore, that Waterford surrendered its license early in 1914, having accepted no inmates since October 1913, and that Wexford followed suit, receiving no further inmates after October 1917 and closing in May 1918.[37]

Questions remain as to why these institutions lasted for such a short time and why they largely housed women. Waterford and Wexford obviously could not fill even the small number of places that they had to offer. Belfast did expand but remained tiny and appears to have closed sometime around 1920.[38] Meanwhile, the state reformatory's numbers declined rapidly after 1910. Whereas at the end of 1910 it housed fifty-two inmates, by the end of 1914 that number was down to twenty-nine; by 1917, there were only thirteen; and two years later, shortly before closure, they had shrunk to a mere five. When Ennis was turned into a military barracks in 1920, the remaining few inmates were transferred to the large prisons for women and men in Cork city.[39]

The very unsettled political situation that prevailed in Ireland from 1912 through 1923 was obviously not advantageous to these institutions. Even before 1912, however, it had become plain that there was very little demand in Ireland for inebriate reformatories. They had originally been promoted in North America during the middle of the nineteenth century, but by the time they reached Ireland and England, it was the beginning of a new century, and attitudes to excessive drinking were changing. Thus, they were not notably successful in England, either.[40] In Ireland, local councils, nationalist politicians, the courts, the churches, and the medical profession were in the main skeptical of their value, if not openly hostile to them.

None of the new councils created under the 1898 Local Government Act (61 & 62 Vic., c.37) showed any interest in establishing a certified inebriate reformatory, which they were empowered to do under the 1898 Inebriates Act. And the registers of the Waterford and Wexford reformatories suggest that only eighteen out of the thirty-eight county and borough councils actually provided funds to help subsidize inmates from their areas sentenced to the reformatories between 1906 and 1917; and most of them put a cap on the number of inmates they were prepared to subsidize. Although the Treasury contributed 7s.0d per week, raised to 10s.6d in 1908, toward the cost of inmates, councils were expected to provide 5s.6d.[41] The drink trade was well represented on the new councils, but, in addition, councils, reflecting the views of their rate-paying electors, were reluctant to add to these electors' existing heavy financial burdens in terms of funding and managing welfare institutions.[42]

Moreover, popular attitudes to drunkenness in Ireland were fairly permissive. Public opinion, represented especially by nationalist politicians in the House of Commons and in local government, had little enthusiasm for a highly penal or punitive approach to drunkenness. Police were often reluctant to bring drunks before the courts, and magistrates and judges preferred to impose small fines or very short terms of imprisonment, even for repeat offenders, rather than a lengthy and very expensive period of confinement in a remote institution, which might deprive a family of its breadwinner and children of a parent for years.[43] Thus, in 1891, the average length of sentences imposed in Ireland for drunkenness was a mere five days. Dr. Brian O'Farrell, the certified reformatories' inspector, in his evidence to an official inquiry in 1908 singled out the courts' reluctance to use the reformatories as the main reason for the reformatories' relative lack of success in Ireland.[44] Nevertheless, as we have seen, if the courts did commit offenders to Ennis, they were much more ready to commit women than men.

The Irish churches by this period had grown decidedly skeptical of mass temperance movements, which had flourished during the 1830s and 1840s, and also of legislative sanctions, which had been actively campaigned for especially during the 1860s and 1870s. By 1900, the Catholic Church and most of the Protestant churches were focusing on promoting temperance or total abstinence among their own flocks. They had largely abandoned earlier grand schemes to rescue the drunkard and rapidly convert the whole of society to abstinence.[45] Yet all three of the small, certified reformatories established between 1903 and 1908 did have a strong denominational base.

The Belfast retreat was largely supported by middle-class Protestants and was intended for upper-working-class and middle-class Protestant women, with fees ranging from 5s.0d to £2.2s.0d per week in 1903. The "better"-class "patients" dined separately from the "working"-class ones, and whereas the latter were expected to do housework, the former were not. Dr. O'Farrell grumpily commented in 1908 that the patients were so well treated as "to make some of them unreasonable in their demands."[46] Under the 1879 act, committal was voluntary for a minimum of six months, but certification under the 1898 act meant that inmates could be held against their will if necessary.[47] However, the retreat remained very small, and its supporters struggled to raise adequate funding. The Protestant churches in Ulster certainly preached total abstinence enthusiastically, but few "respectable" families, as Dr. O'Farrell readily acknowledged, were willing to risk the public shame of committing a female member to an institution for drunkards.[48]

The Waterford and Wexford reformatories, in contrast, reflected the long-standing commitment to temperance reform that prevailed in the dioceses of Waterford-Lismore and Ferns. Yet by 1900 these dioceses were rather out of step with the approach of the Irish church generally, for the church was not especially interested in endeavors to rescue chronic drunkards. Rather, it was in the throes of launching a major and ultimately very successful crusade to enroll its most devout lay members under the banner of the Pioneer Total Abstinence Association of the Sacred Heart.[49]

Waterford had been a stronghold of temperance during the great crusade of the 1840s, and successive bishops of Ferns had been conducting their own local antidrink crusades since the 1850s.[50] But it is notable that Waterford had to turn to an English order to find a group of male religious willing to operate an inebriate institution in Ireland, and the reformatory inspector, Dr. O'Farrell, complained repeatedly of the inadequate facilities at St. Patrick's.[51] The Wexford reformatory was run by a very small female order, and, again, lack of funds was a constant problem, even delaying the institution's opening by several years. The large Irish orders, such as the Christian Brothers and the Sisters of Mercy or Charity, which played major roles in the operation of many other institutions, chose not to commit either resources or staff to this particular type of institution. Lack of strong support from the various churches was undoubtedly a major—indeed, probably a fatal— handicap for the Irish inebriate reformatories.

Thus, local councils and the churches, which could have provided essential funding for the certified reformatories, and the courts, which were supposed to supply the inmates for both the certified and the state reformatories, proved singularly uncooperative in Ireland. And even the medical profession, which could have contributed a much-needed scientific justification for such controversial institutions, was ultimately found wanting.

Members of the Irish medical profession had actively campaigned for the 1879 and 1898 acts; some doctors worked part-time in the reformatories; and the regulating bodies, the Irish General Prisons Board and the Inspectorate of Lunacy, which in the main reported favorably on the reformatories, contained significant medical representation. Yet medical opinion on how to deal with chronic drunkenness was in fact deeply divided and undergoing major shifts by 1900. Whereas many doctors were supportive of therapeutic institutionalization, many others were not. Evidence given by supposed medical experts before government inquiries often exhibited a bewildering array of contradictory opinions.[52]

The 1908 inquiry reviewing the operation of inebriate reformatories announced at the beginning of its report that "[t]here is no general consensus on the nature of inebriety." Some medical experts, the committee acknowledged, regarded inebriety as "self-indulgent drunkenness" and therefore a "vice," whereas others considered it "a disease allied to insanity." On the whole, the committee's report opted for the latter interpretation.[53] In Ireland, too, this view was being promoted. Sir Andrew Reed, an authority on the liquor-licensing laws and a former inspector general of the Royal Irish Constabulary, contributed a preface in 1908 to a book by a Belfast surgeon dealing with drunkenness and the law.[54] Reed stated that it was "well known" to the police and others who dealt with chronic drunkards that "such persons are no more morally responsible for their acts than are the inmates of a lunatic asylum."[55] Yet attempts to equate chronic drunkenness with insanity met resistance in Ireland and elsewhere.

Many were made uncomfortable by the implications of the removal of moral responsibility from the drunkard for his or her actions. Were courts then no longer to punish drunkards? In addition, viewing inebriate reformatories as comparable to lunatic asylums raised problems. By 1900, asylums in both Ireland and England were overcrowded with chronic cases, most deemed incurable. If asylums could not cure most maniacs, were reformatories, adopting similar methods, likely to be more successful with dipsomaniacs?

In order to resolve such dilemmas, some doctors attempted to reconcile conflicting approaches, viewing habitual drunkenness as sometimes the product of disease, but in other circumstances as the product of vice. Dr. H. N. Barnett, for instance, in discussing criminals, distinguished between those taking up crime as a profession and those driven to it by mental illness. The former would "sin against the light simply because they wish to sin, or in order to make money with ease"; the latter, however, "commit offences because of strong hereditary tendencies, or from a diseased brain." The former might drink heavily but were ultimately morally responsible for their actions and should be punished, whereas the latter could well have inherited from alcoholic parents a "predisposition to crime from disease," and thus imprisonment was not an appropriate response to their offenses.[56]

However, even if doctors disagreed as to whether chronic drunkenness was a disease or a vice and whether it should be managed therapeutically or punitively, they were certainly agreed on one point: chronic drunkenness in women was a far more serious problem than it was in men. There was a widespread perception in both Ireland and England during the 1890s and 1900s that drunkenness among women was on the increase. However, Irish statistics on the numbers of women prosecuted for drunkenness do not bear out this popular view. The number of prosecutions fluctuated between 1890 and 1910, but the trend was generally downward, and levels never reached those prevailing during the 1860s and 1870s.[57] But perception was all. Both the press and the medical literature portrayed drunken women as more hardened than men, as more given to reoffending, as more difficult to rehabilitate, and as far more likely to do physical and moral damage to their children and to the men with whom they consorted. Heightened fears around the turn of the century about poor public health, especially among the working class, and the dangers of the inheritance of acquired behavior focused attention on women as crucial agents in the process of racial "degeneration."[58] The supporters of the inebriate reformatories, with their largely female populations, intended them to help counter this threat.

So who were these dangerous female inebriates? Unfortunately, we know little about the 209 women who entered the Belfast retreat between 1903 and 1917; they successfully maintained the privacy that they were so obviously seeking. But the surviving reports and registers fortunately tell us more about the 151 women committed to St. Brigid's in Wexford between 1910 and 1917 and the 178 who were discharged from Ennis state reformatory between 1899 and 1919.

Dr. Patrick Considine's June 1918 report to the lord lieutenant, which was written shortly after the closure of Wexford, provides a final set of statistics on the 299 inmates of both the Wexford and the Waterford certified reformatories at this time. Most women committed to St. Brigid's were in their middle years, with 56 percent being between thirty and fifty. The inmates of Wexford and Waterford were in the main single or widowed (65 percent), and most could not read and write or only "imperfectly" so (57 percent). About 19 percent of all inmates were "troublesome" or "very troublesome." The nuns in Wexford appear, however, to have experienced more trouble than their male counterparts in Waterford. Although roughly similar proportions of women and men were transferred to lunatic asylums (2 percent) and to prisons for varying periods (13 percent), twice as many women (11 percent) as men (5 percent) were sent to Ennis.[59]

Women transferred from St. Brigid's helped boost Ennis's female population, which was already disproportionate owing to the larger number of women committed by the courts. In all, nearly two-thirds of the inmates of Ennis were women. These women came predominantly from urban areas, especially Dublin, Belfast, and Derry.[60] Like the Wexford women, most were middle-aged, but unlike them, the majority in Ennis was married. Women sent to the state reformatory had usually been before the courts on numerous occasions, and few had been convicted of simple public drunkenness, as had the women committed to Wexford. By 1906–1907, around one-third of the Ennis women had been sentenced for neglecting their children owing to habitual drunkenness; another third had committed an assault; and the final third had been sentenced for either larceny or attempted suicide. The governor reported that inmates were "drunkards of long standing" and therefore "confirmed in their ways" and not easily rehabilitated. He urged that sentences should be for the maximum of three years, but in fact most Ennis inmates were serving one to two years. Of inmates discharged before 1907, two-thirds of whom were women, only 38 percent were "going on well," compared to 43 percent who had been readmitted or had relapsed.[61] Such a statistic did not augur well for the reformatory's future success.

In his June 1918 report, Dr. Considine ascribed the closure of St. Brigid's to "the fewness of committals" and the "great advance in the cost of living," which meant that the nuns were operating the reformatory "at a financial loss, which they were not in a position to bear."[62] Prices certainly soared during the war. Thus, whereas maintaining each inmate in St. Brigid's was costing 14s.4d per week in 1915, by 1916 this amount had gone up to 17s.7d, and in 1917, when the reformatory ceased accepting new committals, it had jumped to £1.2s.4d.[63] Inflation finally spelled the end to St Brigid's, but none of the inebriate reformatories had ever prospered in Ireland. By the time they were belatedly introduced at the turn of the century, the urge to establish new institutions that had so characterized the country during the nineteenth century was on the wane. The borstal opened in Clonmel in 1906 did endure, but after 1900 it was the exception rather than the rule.

However, although it is not difficult to find factors peculiar to Ireland to explain the swift demise of the inebriate reformatories, it is important to bear in mind that they did not flourish in England either, where there was more public support for them and better funding.[64] Therefore, interpretations that focus solely on Ireland may well give a somewhat misleading impression as to the reasons why most reformatories closed within twenty years.[65] In addition, the emphasis in nearly all the Irish and English secondary literature on the reformatories' failure may not do them justice. If looked at in the short term, between 1879 or 1898 and 1914 or 1920, they can be convincingly labeled as failures in terms of their stated aims. Their supporters, especially among the medical profession, were not able to offer a compelling enough case for their effectiveness to convince impecunious local councils to supply funds or complacent magistrates to supply drunkards. But a longer-term perspective affords a rather different picture.

Later in the twentieth century, when the disease model of inebriety had come to be widely accepted under the new label *alcoholism,* dedicated institutions and programs appeared in significant numbers.[66] There is not space here to compare the earlier inebriate reformatories with the specialist alcohol units and clinics that emerged from the 1940s onward in many Western countries, but such a comparison would doubtless yield similarities as well as differences.

Perhaps the Irish inebriate reformatories were simply the victims of bad timing. They were established too late to ride the massive wave of early- and mid-nineteenth-century optimistic institutionalization, and they came too early for the mid–twentieth century's new wave of smaller, less authoritarian therapeutic institutions. They appeared during an ebb in enthusiasm for new institutional initiatives to regulate social deviants in Ireland and elsewhere, and thus they failed to thrive. However, their apparent failure may well tell us as much about contemporary attitudes and values as the apparent success of longer-lasting institutions.

7

Managing Midwifery in Dublin

Practice and Practitioners, 1700–1800

Philomena Gorey

Until the eighteenth century, childbirth and lying-in belonged exclusively within the domain of female control. The midwife oversaw labor and directed events in the birth room. The mother's friends, the so-called gossips, offered physical and emotional support to the mother throughout her labor and for her lying-in month after delivery. A woman's confinement was bound by culture, tradition, and superstition. Customs such as the enclosing and darkening of the lying-in room, the preparation of the caudle drink, and the swaddling of infants were seen as part of this ritual of childbirth.[1] Male access to this uniquely female experience was denied. Medical men were called upon only in difficult labor and then only as a last resort. Male practice, therefore, was defined by this culture. Medical men knew little of the mechanism of labor, of the anatomy of the uterus, or of the function of the placenta. When the surgeon was called, it was as an emergency, when labor was well advanced and obstructed and the delivery of a live infant remote. Then, his stock in trade was the perforation of the fetal skull, the performance of a craniotomy, and the extraction of a dead baby with the aid of crotchets and hooks.[2] As a consequence, obstetrics in this form was part of the normal practice of the seventeenth-century surgeon.[3] However, by 1730, men's scope of practice in this arena had extended beyond the delivery of a dead baby and beyond the emergency call.[4] By 1770, the prescribed norms surrounding childbirth and lying-in had been penetrated by a new breed of male practitioner, the man-midwife, who posed a threat to the livelihood of the midwife, whom tradition dictated should be married and older than thirty and should have borne children herself.[5] Because men had the opportunity and benefit of education, either through apprenticeship and, later, a university degree, midwifery was to become an empirical, clinical skill, a field of expertise where the midwife now had only a marginal role, and the birth experience would soon be dominated by institutional, scientific obstetrics.

A number of medical developments, which had their origins in Europe in the sixteenth century, accounted for this shift. First, the work of Andreas Vesalius (1514–64) illustrated the extent to which dissecting human bodies, as opposed to animal bodies, could advance anatomical knowledge and medical science.[6] During the late sixteenth century, the teaching of anatomy began to be established as part of the medical curriculum in a handful of universities—notably, Padua, Montpellier, Uppsala, and Leiden. Even though facilities were poor and opportunities to witness dissections were limited, the study of anatomy nevertheless resulted in evidence-based advances in anatomical knowledge.[7]

Second, from approximately 1640 on, men turned their attention to the pregnant female form and sought not only to discover the true mechanism of labor and the process of childbirth, but to establish themselves as necessary birth attendants, and from the mid–eighteenth century their presence in the birth room became acceptable.[8] As a consequence, the midwife saw her traditional role as birth attendant altered, her reputation as a competent practitioner challenged, and her means of livelihood eroded.[9] A very significant initiative was the invention of the midwifery forceps by a member of the Chamberlen medical dynasty, who practiced in London from around 1620 until 1730.[10] The family spanned four generations of medical practitioners and managed to keep their invention a family secret, only ever claiming to have a special expertise that enabled them to deliver live infants where previously the life of the baby would be lost.[11] Peter Chamberlen's (1601–83) daughter, Elizabeth, married Lieutenant Colonel William Walker from Tankardstown, Queen's County. Hence, a branch of the family located to Ireland.[12] Their son, Chamberlen Walker, practiced midwifery in Dublin before his death in

1731.[13] He and Johannes Van Lewen, father of Laetitia Pilkington, are the only two practitioners who can be identified as having established midwifery practices in Dublin during the 1720s.[14]

Third, the eighteenth century saw institutional midwifery established, initially for poor women, with the opening of Bartholomew Mosse's foundation, the Dublin Lying-in Hospital (later known as "the Rotunda") in George's Lane in 1745. This hospital was soon followed by the foundation of similar institutions in London, Manchester, and Edinburgh.

Finally, the old apprenticeship and guild systems of medical training gradually broke down in favor of the more scientific education awarded by the universities. Dublin surgeons had earlier disassociated themselves from the Guild of Barbers and Surgeons. They established a Society of Surgeons in 1721 in anticipation of a charter. Their efforts to place their status on a par with physicians culminated in the Society of Surgeons receiving its charter in 1784.[15] The School of Physics Act of 1800 (40. G.III c.84) gave royal imprimatur to and significantly enhanced the prestige of both branches of medicine.

By the mid–nineteenth century, midwives everywhere had assumed a secondary role and were subsequently seen as assistants to male doctors. The notion by then that childbirth was a medical event and therefore required the assistance of professional medical intervention was almost complete. Along with this notion, the benefit of long-held traditions and customs, such as the presence of the mother's closest relatives and friends with her in the lying-in room and the swaddling of the newborn infant, were called into question.[16]

This essay is intended to make some observations about the development of male midwifery in Dublin between 1700 and 1800. It considers the role of the Church of Ireland and the Counter-Reformation Irish Catholic Church in the ecclesiastical regulation of midwifery, which centered around religious orthodoxy and emergency baptism by women, in the period before 1700. It examines the emerging, if reluctant, role in regulation played by the College of Physicians from 1692, the year in which its second charter, the charter of the Kings and Queens College of Physicians of Ireland, was granted. The college was the only regulating body that granted licenses to both men and women who practiced midwifery once denominational authority withdrew. Finally, the essay traces the transition from ecclesiastical to institutional regulation in Dublin from around 1700 and examines the medical careers of three man-midwives in particular: Bartholomew Mosse, founder of the Dublin Lying-in Hospital; Fielding Ould, who is credited with discovering the mechanism of labor; and David McBride, scientist and teacher—all of whom returned to Dublin after the 1730s following their studies and observations abroad. Their careers are significant, not least because they stood directly between the demise of the apprenticeship system of medical training and the beginning of professional education and the legal requirement to be formally qualified.[17]

In Ireland, as elsewhere, the midwife was by tradition a local, married woman who had borne children herself and who may or may not have been known to the mother. Recent scholarship has contributed to a reversal of the persistent stereotyping of midwives as ignorant, incompetent, and meddlesome.[18] The writings and diary entries of contemporary practitioners reveal the work of women who were not only literate and skilled but had qualities of forbearance as well as physical and mental ability.[19] Much of the research is drawn from church licensing records, testimonials, and municipal ordinances. No such detailed research has yet been undertaken of similar Irish sources. Indeed, it is impossible to say whether such sources survive. Municipal ordinances, similar to those that began in German towns, where municipal regulation was introduced in 1452, appear to be absent in Ireland, possibly because society was predominantly rural.[20] Research already undertaken on the seventeenth-century proceedings of a number of town councils in Ireland has yielded no evidence of municipal attention to midwives. Ecclesiastical regulation and licensing by both the Catholic Church and the Church of Ireland were therefore the only extant forms of supervision in Ireland before 1692. From around 1614, both denominations had laid down guidelines for the ministering of emergency baptism by midwives and had issued decrees against the practice of witchcraft and magical healing.[21] Parish priests and churchwardens—agents of each church, respectively—were charged with the administration and surveillance of their churches' teachings.[22] The midwife's practice and activities were noted and, if necessary, included in presentments at the annual visitations of the diocesan bishop, and their numbers might be recorded sporadically in visitations and parish records. The documents and oaths were a test of the midwives' character and integrity, offering no guarantee of their professional skill. Quaker women working as midwives were not to accept offerings of money or be involved in the "sprinkling of children."[23]

Ecclesiastical regulation and licensing began to decline throughout the eighteenth century. Doreen Evenden's detailed study of seventeenth-century midwives in London traces the origins of licensing through to the decline in the church's licensing role by 1720.[24] Thomas Forbes has suggested that ecclesiastical licensing survived elsewhere in England until 1873. The latest extant license there dates from 1786. His assertion that ecclesiastical licensing faded out rather than ended abruptly does seem to be the case.[25] In Ireland, the latest extant license and oath were sworn by the midwife Mrs. Elliot to the Protestant bishop of Ossory, Charles Este, around 1740.[26] One of the latest Catholic visitations was carried out by Dr. McKenna, bishop of Cloyne, in 1785, in which the numbers of midwives in the thirty-nine parishes of the diocese were presented to the bishop, who then noted those who knew the rite of baptism and those who were "skilled."[27] Decrees continued to be issued. An 1831 decree from the archbishop of Dublin, Daniel Murray, included sections on baptism and excommunication, bearing similarities to those issued at synods two hundred years earlier.[28]

There is evidence to suggest that the arrangement between the Church of Ireland and the College of Physicians worked well for both institutions as science and religion began to converge toward the end of the seventeenth century. In 1697, Narcissus Marsh, the Protestant archbishop of Dublin, ordered Henry Phoenix to apply to the college "to be examined as to his qualifications for practicing physick." Phoenix was examined accordingly by the college's censors, and they found "that he own'd himself wholly ignorant of all ye parts of Physick except practice, and Chymestry; but on examination he was found very ignorant of ye differences, mystery and method of cure of diseases, and seemed acquainted with very few Chymical processes, or ye use of chymical remedies."[29]

The first charter for Ireland's College of Physicians, the Charter of Charles II, which was granted in 1667, makes no reference to midwives or, indeed, to midwifery. The 1692 charter gave power to the college to "examine all Middwives and to lycense and allow such as they shall find skillfull and fitt to Exercize that profession and to hinder all such as they shall finde unskillfull from practising," but because the charter's rules applied only to a radius of eight miles around Dublin, it is unlikely that regulation was implemented or extended beyond this area.[30] Only six people were admitted as licentiates between 1696 and 1742, two of whom were women. A Mrs. Cormack received a license in midwifery on of February 3, 1696 or 1697. Mrs. Catherine Banford received a similar license on January 16, 1731 or 1732.[31] Four men were awarded licenses—James Hamilton, October 1715; Matthew Carter, May 1738; Fielding Ould, August 1738; and Bartholomew Mosse, May 1742. After this date, practitioners appear to have ignored the college licentiate because the next licenses were not granted until the 1790s.[32] The declaration to be taken on admission to the college stated that licentiates should observe the college's statutes and by-laws and submit to a diploma in midwifery when the president and fellows of the college thought it was "proper to inflict."[33] Because Mrs. Cormack and Catherine Banford are the only two women whose names appear on the register, they must have been sufficiently educated to seek registration in the first place and sufficiently renowned to be accepted by the college. It is, however, likely that the physicians thought better of having women on a register of licentiates along with men. The college seems to have gotten around this problem by altering the term *license* for women to *certificate for midwifery and nurse tending*. The status of this certificate would also appear to have changed as the gulf between new knowledge among men and traditional practices by women became apparent. The college awarded these certificates until 1899, but their significance decreased when other institutions began to teach midwifery to women. The college considered that the practice of midwifery was suitable only for women and surgeons. It was seen as beneath the diagnostic abilities of physicians, not only because of its mechanical nature, but also because birth was largely seen as a natural process. In 1736, the college passed a resolution that no one would be licensed to practice "midwifery and physic" together. Anyone in breach of the regulation would have his license withdrawn and be fined ten shillings.[34]

In August 1711, the medical school at Trinity College was founded with provision for lectureships in natural philosophy, anatomy, botany, physics, and chemistry. There was no provision for the teaching of midwifery. Those under examination—such as Bartholomew Mosse, Fielding Ould, and David McBride—went abroad for their training. On their return, they found themselves confronted with a number of considerations. First, their profession was largely unregulated. For every competent practitioner there was any number of unskilled male operators who exploited the growing trend of engaging a male practitioner. Second, there were no facilities for instruction and teaching. Midwifery was quickly developing into a science. Medical men were anxious to define and name the many fetal presentations that they were encountering in the course of their practice. Most significant, they were trying to determine the physiology of labor and perfect what they knew of the second and third stages of the process of labor. They looked for the causes and treatment of obstetric emergencies and increasingly focused on the abnormalities of pregnancy and disorders associated with reproduction. Third, Mosse, Ould, and McBride were not only faced with a hostile College of Physicians—midwifery was to have an uneasy relationship with medicine until the twentieth century—but had to contend with a growing body of public opinion that believed that childbirth was best left to women and that in some cases portrayed the man-midwife as a predator of female virtue.[35] Many writers condemned the practice of midwifery by men as being indecent and immoral, appealing to the fundamental fear that any relaxation in traditional customs would break the bonds between husband and wife and eventually lead to the collapse of society.[36] Out of consideration for a woman's modesty, the male practitioner examined his patient and delivered the baby with the mother's lower body covered by a sheet.[37]

Mosse, Ould, and McBride were men of their time, not before it. They were among a small number of male practitioners in Dublin and part of a wider British and European movement that began to consider midwifery as a likely adjunct to surgery. The fact that the College of Physicians resolved to prohibit its members from the practice of midwifery in 1736 is an indication of an attempt to regulate what was already an existing trend. When these men returned to Dublin, midwives still had hegemony over normal births. The definition of "skill" in maternal and infant care simply meant the delivery of a live infant and the mother's recovery. Loss of life through obstetric emergency was an accepted part of the dangers of childbearing. All three men established practice just at a time when an emerging belief that these dangers could be dealt with by the trained male practitioner was gaining support and when labor came to be treated as a medical event rather than as a natural process.

Mosse was born in Queen's County in 1712. He was apprenticed in Dublin to the surgeon John Stone. In July 1733, the surgeon general granted Mosse a license to practice surgery.[38] Military service saw him posted to Minorca until 1738, after which time he traveled in England, Holland, and France to perfect his knowledge of surgery and midwifery. His friend Benjamin Higgins wrote that "[Mosse] became convinced of the great usefulness, if not necessity, of having a hospital for lying-in women in the city of Dublin."[39] On his return to Dublin, he obtained his license in midwifery and discontinued the practice of surgery.

Mosse opened his twelve-bed hospital for lying-in women in George's Lane in March 1745. Poor women "great with child" were admitted in labor, having been first recommended as "proper objects" by the church wardens of the neighboring parishes.[40] At first, Mosse operated the hospital on his own, with the assistance of the housekeeper and midwife Mrs. Millar. William Collum joined him as medical assistant before the hospital relocated, but the date of his appointment is not clear. The patient register for the twelve years when the hospital operated in George's Lane is detailed and complete.[41] The women who were patients there belonged to the lower orders. Their husbands were employed as artisans or tradesmen. The mother's name and age are listed, along with her husband's name and occupation, the parish from which she was recommended, her admission date, her delivery date, the sex of her child, the infant's baptismal date, her discharge date, and a column for observations. The register is significantly an indication of the length of labor—most women were delivered within forty-eight hours of admission. It is also a valuable insight into maternal and infant mortality during the early modern period and the earliest statistical table on record.[42] Of 3,975 women who delivered, 45 died; infant mortality was higher, with 4,049 live births, 372 deaths, and 138 stillborn.

By 1748, Mosse had acquired a site and negotiated a lease for the expansion of his foundation in the newly developing part of the city, Great Britain Street, the site of today's Rotunda Hospital. He identified himself so closely with the project that he oversaw every aspect of its design and construction. Funding for the hospital came from benefactions, successful petitions to Parliament, and less successful—indeed dubious—lottery schemes and activities in its pleasure gardens, where the emerging mercantile class could mingle with the aristocracy. Mosse had two ambitious plans—to succeed in obtaining a royal charter, which would secure the further development of his foundation, and to establish a school for the teaching of midwifery for "young surgeons intending to practice midwifery, as it might render it unnecessary for such to resort to France and other foreign parts for instruction; and also as a nursery to raise and transplant into several parts of the kingdom, women, who, being duly qualified, might settle in such parts as most stand in need of them."[43] He succeeded in both plans. The hospital received its royal charter on December 7, 1756, along with an initial grant of six thousand pounds.[44] Mosse unfortunately died just three years later, in February 1759, two years after his ambition was realized, having expended much of his funds on the project, but leaving his foundation as a lasting legacy of his life's work and achievements.[45]

Mosse's contemporary Fielding Ould was born in England in 1710. Following the death of his father, his mother brought him and his brother to Galway, where they were educated. At nineteen, he began his career in the anatomy house at Trinity College medical school, although he did not matriculate from there. In his *Treatise of Midwifery in Three Parts,* he states that he "spent that time which others employ in their improvement in polite Literature, in a more laborious manner; namely, in the Dissection of human Bodies."[46] He left Dublin to study midwifery in Paris. In recalling his time there, he observed, "I made the strictest Examination of every Woman, which I either delivered, or saw delivered, during my Continuance in Paris."[47] Ould returned to Dublin and in 1738 obtained his license in midwifery. He found the haphazard way in which midwifery was conducted in the city intolerable, in particular the manner in which any quack or empiric could set up in practice and pose as a competent practitioner. Both the College of Physicians and the Society of Surgeons turned a blind eye to the necessity of establishing a standard of practice or regulation for men entering the profession. Notwithstanding this lack of standards, because it was becoming fashionable to engage men-midwives, the expertise of men such as Ould and the more competent professionals reflected well on all male practitioners. As he expressed the problem, "[T]here is no Method of hindering such Impostors, from committing these outrageous Villanies on the Public."[48]

By 1742, Ould had completed the only work he ever published, *A Treatise in Midwifery in Three Parts,* dedicating it to the president, censors, and fellows of the College of Physicians and submitting it to them for their approval, which they duly gave it. In his *Treatise,* he accurately describes the internal rotation of the fetal skull during labor. He had observed that the fetus's head was always directed toward the shoulder as it descended into the pelvis. It was previously thought that this presentation of the fetal skull was abnormal. His *Treatise* met with some opposition, particularly from an older contemporary, Thomas Southwell, who charged him with inaccuracies in both anatomy and physiology.[49] Nevertheless, his observation is acknowledged as being the first step toward an understanding of the mechanism of labor.

In 1756, having established a large private practice, Fielding Ould applied to the College of Physicians to be examined for a license in physic. The college refused, citing their by-law the prohibited the practice of midwifery and physic together. Dissatisfied with this response, he applied to Trinity College for permission to be examined for a bachelor of medicine. The university refused on the grounds that Ould's request was "judged inconvenient at this time, and likely to occasion much uneasiness in the College of Physicians."[50] Ould persisted, and in 1759, the year he succeeded Mosse as master of the Dublin Lying-in Hospital, he was granted a liceat by Trinity College, which he presented to the College of Physicians. The physicians refused to pursue his application, whereupon the university agreed to examine him and granted an MB to him in January 1761. The College of Physicians immediately withdrew its support of the university by refusing to examine candidates for medical degrees, and the connection between the two bodies was severed and not reestablished until 1785, when Ould was eventually awarded his license in medicine.

David McBride was born in Ballymoney, County Antrim, in 1726. After he was apprenticed locally, he entered the Royal Navy as a surgeon and remained in that capacity until 1748. Following this service, he studied anatomy in Edinburgh under Alexander Munro and midwifery in London under William Smellie.[51] He came to Dublin in 1751, where for some time he combined his midwifery practice with a pursuit in scientific experiments. He was a founding member of the Medico-Philosophical Society, which was established in 1756. The society at first consisted of approximately seven to ten members, who met fortnightly to present their experimental findings and to discuss their scientific observations. Among the many experiments McBride conducted, he discovered a cure for scurvy and a method for accelerating the process of tanning leather, for which he petitioned the Irish House of Commons for a patent, although nothing seems to have come of it. In 1764, the University of Glasgow conferred a degree of doctor of physic on him in recognition of his work.[52]

Between the years 1749 and 1760, McBride kept a journal of his midwifery practice in which he recorded 149 detailed accounts of deliveries he attended.[53] Although the entries are haphazard—some years he recorded only a few deliveries—the journal offers clinical descriptions of complications and his efforts to treat them. As a source, it gives a unique insight into the manner in which male practitioners conducted their practice and promoted the development of man-midwifery in Dublin in the mid-1700s. McBride either refers to the woman by name, which suggests familiarity or that his attendance was prebooked, or as a "poor" woman—for example, "Poor woman in Francis St., April 1756"—which confirms the evidence that men-midwives attended poor women not only as charity cases, but to gain obstetric experience as well. A pattern of repeat business emerges. Several women were delivered of between five and six children each, at intervals of around eighteen months, and he attended a number of "poor women" from Loftus Lane, which suggests some of his practice came by word of mouth. His practice extended geographically from Bolton Street and King Street north of the Liffey and from Dolphin's Barn to Dame Street south of the river.

Of the 149 births he attended, 85 were normal, and many involved delivery by a midwife. For the remaining 64, a number of the obstetrical emergencies and abnormal presentations that we know today are described in detail, except of course without the modern medical terms. Placenta praevia was presented as "violent flooding in the end of the seventh month . . . the placenta was growing to the lower part of the uterus," and prolapsed cord occurred when he "found upon breaking of the membranes the cord to come down."[54] Eclampsia is described in harrowing detail in case no. 147, when McBride attends a young woman—Mrs. Bryan's daughter—who was "seized with violent convulsions which were preceded by an almost total loss of sight and violent pain in the head." These "fits" occurred on and off for six weeks before he was called. McBride attempted to deliver her child, even though his description presents a picture of a woman who must have been close to death. Her delivery failed, her uterus ruptured, and she died shortly thereafter. It is clear that nothing could have been done to save his patient, yet McBride is obviously upset with the outcome. He concludes: "I was immensely shocked that I should have interfered, and not rather have left her to the pains, which I certainly should have done, as there was at the time I saw her, no urgent necessity for delivering her. But I thought her delivery was the luckiest thing that could have happened to her and so it certainly would have proved if she had either been left to nature, or it could have been done without injury. Every labor and abortion should be trusted to the natural pains, unless something very urgent requires the assistant of the hand."[55] The journal illustrates a typical mid-eighteenth-century practice—a mix of booked and emergency calls, the use of forceps in difficult labor or a crotchet when the infant was found to have died in utero, references to abnormal presentations that the practitioner had read about and was now encountering himself for the first time, and, finally, the satisfaction of a live birth when it seemed certain that the child was already lost.[56] It also makes clear the extent to which "natural pains" were seen as part of the birth process.

McBride established a private medical school at his house in Cavendish Row, now Mountjoy Square, while his midwifery practice grew throughout the 1760s. From a memorandum in his fee book, it appears that he attended 1,065 midwifery cases from 1767 to 1777.[57] He was appointed teacher of midwifery at the Rotunda Hospital in 1774, after the course of lectures was established there. However, he died unexpectedly of pneumonia in December 1778 at the age of fifty-two. McBride had intended to publish the results of his scientific experiments, to include them in one body of work, but this volume was never completed, so his research—in particular, his treatment of scurvy—was never recognized. His midwifery journal in the *Miscellanea Medica* is a very significant legacy because it is the only extant account of obstetric practices in Dublin during the mid–eighteenth century.

Each of these men—Mosse with his charity foundation, Ould in his pursuit of regulation and standards of practice, and McBride as scientist and teacher—were dedicated in the pursuit of their efforts. As a city, Dublin was a perfect location in which to realize their ambitions. It was on the periphery yet not outside the dynamic changes in the economic and political structures of eighteenth-century Europe. It was large enough to attract medical men whose attitudes reflected the medical enlightenment that was taking place, yet small enough to allow their endeavors to succeed without the competition they might face in larger centers. Finally, poverty in Georgian Dublin offered a steady supply of "poor lying-in women" whose labors could be used for practice and teaching.[58] Ould and McBride's achievements might not be seen to compare with the great medical discoveries on the nineteenth century, but they must be placed within the context of eighteenth-century medicine, which relied so heavily on patronage.[59] Mosse and Ould sat in on the meetings of the Dublin Lying-in Hospital Board of Governors, but rarely contributed. The minutes of the meetings in the earlier years, which allow a fascinating insight into the hospital's social and architectural history, are of little obstetric value to the researcher. Those masters who followed—William Collum (1766–73), Frederick Jebb (1773–80), and Henry Rock (1780–86, died in office)—did not write obstetrical works, so it is impossible to account for obstetrical procedures or practices at the hospital for those years. It was not until Joseph Clarke's tenure, from 1786, that we learn of initiatives to treat puerperal fever, even though outbreaks had been recurring since 1767. By then, infant mortality was also recognized as a threat, and Clarke wrote extensively on it.[60] When Mosse, Ould, and McBride returned to Dublin, they all had benefited from having received the best teaching or practical experience that was available at the time and continued to be in touch with trends abroad after their return. Through their zeal, initiative, and considerable achievements, they paved the way for the next generation of practitioners, who had the benefit of university degrees, among them William Dease, who was to become the first president of the Royal College of Surgeons, and the aforementioned Joseph Clarke, who pioneered the response to puerperal fever at the Rotunda in the 1780s and 1790s.[61]

The formal teaching of midwifery did much to advance the role of men in midwifery and gradually assisted in challenging the esteem in which female practitioners had been held. This decline in the office of midwife began at around the time teaching was initiated by William Smellie in London in the 1740s. Instruction was established at the Rotunda Hospital in 1774 amid controversial circumstances, chiefly on grounds of propriety. The debate was publicly played out between the incumbent master, William Collum, and his assistant, Frederick Jebb. Collum was against instruction on midwifery, especially to women, whereas Jebb was for it, and both anonymously published pamphlets setting out their reasons for their very differing points of view.[62] Women were eventually instructed "by themselves" and attended until they were "sufficiently well qualified for practice." Whereas both men and women learned the anatomical structure of the female pelvis, knowledge of surgery and physics was deemed unnecessary for the female practitioner. Her practice was limited to an ability to know the difference between a normal and complicated labor so that she could call the male practitioner if necessary and to the care of the mother and baby after delivery. The basis of instruction for women was to teach them "how far they can act on their own responsibility . . . but points out to them the line beyond which they cannot safely venture."[63] The lecture demonstration offered a new field of study and proved that the best way to teach science to those with little or no basic knowledge of it was to show how it worked.[64] Each scientific discipline used models for demonstration purposes. Midwifery used the mechanical doll to demonstrate labor. Those who established private schools advertised lecture courses in the press and made much of the acquisition and importation of such "machines," expounding on their representation of "real women and children."[65] David McBride and others used Smellie's model of instruction in private medical schools from the 1760s. Teaching by these radical practitioners challenged the wisdom of the traditional rules and customs governing childbirth. Men as midwives would succeed only if the female practitioner could be shown to be not only deficient in her knowledge, but a danger to the mother and her child.

By 1800, the involvement of men in midwifery was very evident. Traditional methods of assistance in labor were gradually giving way to new surgical techniques, although there is little evidence to suggest that the midwifery forceps were widely used in Dublin throughout the century. Given the limited educational opportunities for women, men's involvement was inevitable, particularly because sepsis, the recognition and treatment of puerperal psychosis, and the management of pain in labor were to dominate nineteenth-century midwifery. However, it must be stressed that mothers themselves, in particular those who could afford it, were decisively opting to engage the male practitioner in favor of the midwife, believing that in the interest of their own safety and that of their infants the merits of an increasingly male-dominated profession outweighed attendance by a perhaps skilled but less educated midwife.[66]

8

Lady Dudley's District Nursing Scheme and the Congested Districts Board, 1903–1923

Ciara Breathnach

This chapter outlines the attempts the Lady Dudley scheme made in tandem with the Congested Districts Board (CDB) to organize domiciliary medical care and to improve public health and sanitation in the West of Ireland from 1903 to 1923.[1] In the absence of egodocuments from officials or the native population, this chapter relies heavily on the scheme's and CDB's annual reports.[2] Although repetitious in nature, both sources—observations by nurses and CDB officials—provide us with an indication of medical, cultural, social, and economic circumstances in the West during this timeframe. The Dudley scheme's annual reports are of particular use because they incorporate detailed case notes and some interesting photographs of nurses interacting with patients.[3] This essay also attempts to tease out the relationship between medical care, the nurses, and the people.[4] Poverty and associated problems such as malnutrition and poor living conditions were a great challenge to practitioners of modern medicine during the period under review.

Lady Rachel Dudley (1876–1920, née Gurney) was the wife of William Humble Ward, third earl of Dudley, who was appointed lord lieutenant of Ireland in 1902.[5] The Dudleys had a holiday home in Connemara, an area of Galway whose inhabitants had endured particular distress throughout the nineteenth century. Although evidence of distress was still visible at the turn of the century, people were no longer at "risk of starvation." However, Lady Dudley was particularly perturbed that in remote areas of the West no provision was made for nursing the sick poor in their own homes. In fact, outside of dispensaries and union (workhouse) hospitals, only four district nurses were working in the West, and they were maintained by external funding.[6] Two were supported by special funds (a Manchester Fund and the West of Ireland Association); the *Irish Homestead*[7] newspaper funded the third; and Queen Victoria's Jubilee Institute for Nurses (QVJIN) provided the other one, in Achill.[8]

To fully appreciate the role of the district nurse and the value of public health care in the West, it is necessary to give a brief overview of the Irish health-care system in the latter half of the nineteenth century.[9] Under the 1851 Medical Charities Act (14 and 15 Vic., c.68), Ireland was divided into 723 dispensary units. Each unit was managed by a committee composed of guardians and rate payers until the 1898 Local Government Act (61 and 62 Vic., c.37); after that, guardians were given sole authority).[10] Under this regime, the appointment of medical officers was unaccountable; it was done by election on an annual basis by poor-law guardians who more often than not served their own political agendas. This flaw in the system did not go unnoticed; a letter to the *Irish Times* in December 1903 criticized the election process and suggested that for the sick poor to be served more efficiently, appointments should be made by open competition.[11] Indeed, Ruth Barrington argues that the extent to which doctors (who from 1874 had the additional task of being medical officers for health) engaged in extracurricular activities was "to the detriment of their medical duties." She also highlights that local authorities were loath to increase tax rates, meaning the amount spent on health care for the poor remained the same year after year.[12] Further, local taxation was not an option in the West, where there were few "resident gentry or well-to-do inhabitants of the middle classes" to shoulder the burden, and without the wealthier classes it was impossible to raise voluntary contributions.[13] Several witnesses to local board government inquiries mooted ideas to locate "efficient nurses" in remote areas, but without serious consideration or funding, nothing came of the suggestions.[14]

There was an eclectic mix of unqualified and traditional medical practitioners in the West, most notably "handy women," who acted as midwives, or "wise women," who advised on all ailments from ulcers to abscesses. In urban areas, chemists were prescribing for all matters and acting as dentists. According to official reports to Parliament, bonesetters, cancer curers, and individuals who were described as "spectacle quacks" were also in operation.[15] Regardless of the three medical officers in the Dunfanaghy Union in 1909, it was found that the local shopkeeper prescribed and sold drugs and recommended various acids for dermatological conditions, "often to the disfigurement of the patient."[16] By 1900, people who resorted to formal medical health-care institutional options were limited to district hospitals and union hospitals, but the former were considered an adjunct to the "poor house," and this stigma meant that the majority of sick poor "preferred to die at home rather than enter an institution."[17] Generally speaking, medical care was inextricably linked to the poor-law system, which in the popular mindset was a euphemism for the "workhouse," an institution that aspiring smallholders despised. A sick person could avail himself or herself of treatment at dispensaries, smaller units manned by a medical officer, if a person held a black ticket or in the home if he or she held a red ticket; both types of tickets were obtained from the local poor-law guardian. Barrington also notes the dispensary system was notoriously corrupt in that guardians doled out tickets to rich and poor alike in exchange for votes.[18] This corruption did little to inspire confidence. From a professional perspective, Nurse Bridget N. Hedderman noted the people of Aran perceived the dispensary "as a kind of guillotine or deathtrap."[19] In a report to Dublin Castle in April 1889 on the "alleged distress in Donegal," William Lawson Micks,[20] in his capacity as a local government board inspector, also noted the reluctance to engage with formal systems of poor relief. He cites relatively low indoor and outdoor relief statistics, stating that the "tenacity with which country people cling to their homes is so well known that nothing short of the most acute suffering and utter despair will compel families to run the risk of abandoning their houses even temporarily and to become inmates of the workhouse."[21]

In addition to the medical system's apparent shortcomings and the people's unwillingness to engage in it, not all areas had the benefit of a medical officer. Some congested districts—those districts with living conditions so poor that they could not support the people who lived in them—were so remote that the delay in obtaining medical assistance cost lives; this was especially true in the case of the islands. Nurse Hedderman wrote how her appointment to Aran located her nine miles away from the nearest doctor, "a situation not without risk as there was no special concession for me: laws that applied to nurses on the mainland were equally applicable here."[22] That the people were slow to engage with official medical care meant that the real delay in seeking medical assistance was much longer than normal, so patients were usually on death's door by the time doctors and nurses intervened. Monsignor Walker of Burtonport wrote how it was "impossible for the dispensary doctor to reach the island [either Arranmore, Rutland, or Inisfree] in stormy weather, and consequently the sick are left to the mercy of the winds and waves; and the sad cases of deaths which occurred in such circumstances have been the source of the greatest pain and anxiety to myself and the resident priest on the Island for a long time."[23] Many congested-district residents were very impoverished and could not afford the doctor's fee. For the majority, when they were ill, it was a case of "trusting to chance," and as a result many people died, especially women in childbirth.[24] Midwifery services were not prioritized. Laurence Geary notes that in 1851 there were no midwives in Munster or Connaught and only three in Leinster and four in Ulster, and the situation did not improve until nursing and midwifery and its training were formalized in 1919 with a registration act.[25] Distinctions between "trained" and "qualified" were crucial to the debate on nursing as a profession or vocation. Union hospitals were not fully exploited as maternity services in the West, and therefore union hospital nurses' ability to aid the birthing process in a meaningful way was questioned.[26] Lady Dudley noticed that where the boards of guardians could not provide maternity nurses, situations were pitiful; instead, "the people assist each other," and the poor supported the destitute. These areas could not afford to raise the monies necessary to employ a nurse, so external funding was of the utmost importance in the provision of domiciliary health care.[27]

Inspired by the high level of social inequity, Lady Dudley wrote a series of letters that appeared in Irish newspapers throughout 1902 and 1903, highlighting the lack of proper health care in the West, and from this attention a subscription fund evolved. This money was used to start the "Dudley scheme for the establishment of district nurses in the poorest parts of Ireland" in 1903. A few areas were selected for a pilot medical scheme to start "cottage" dispensaries in the more remote parts of the West or those areas farthest away from existing health-care provision. Lady Dudley's actions were not unusual and must be viewed in the wider context of philanthropy and social consciousness of the time.[28] To ensure that the nurses were trained in medicine, surgery, and midwifery, the Dudley scheme liaised closely with bodies associated with the QVJIN. This institute emanated from a public fund that was collected in 1897 in honor of Queen Victoria's Golden Jubilee and was subsequently used to fund training as well as district nursing schemes.[29] There were two affiliated training institutions in Ireland: Catholic nurses were trained at St. Laurence's, and Protestant nurses were trained at St. Patrick's Training House, both in Dublin.[30] It was envisaged that the Dudley nurses would be stationed on their own; to this end, supplementary district training was given.

Meanwhile, the CDB had been operating in eighty-four districts along the western seaboard in the counties of Donegal, Leitrim, Sligo, Roscommon, Mayo, Galway, Kerry, and West Cork since 1891.[31] Although the board was relatively well funded, health care did not fall under its remit; the board was expected to improve living standards in the designated districts through the development of agriculture, fisheries, existing cottage-based industries, and the creation of markets. It was not directly responsible for people's health issues, but it could not ignore the appalling living conditions. One nurse commented how a house she visited "was a most wretched one, with practically nothing in it. The patient was lying on a bit of grass on the floor, with no covering except an old skirt and jacket she had on. There was no under-clothing, bed or bedclothing. . . . It was the most pitiable state of affairs that anyone could imagine, and I shall not forget my experience of that day for some time."[32] The board's first systematic attempt to deal with health fell under the rubric of sanitation issues; for this, the Parish Committee Scheme was founded in 1897.[33] In short, the board delegated authority to local committees to fund and supervise improvement works on houses. The Parish Scheme's initial aim was to remove animals out of the family dwelling and to move the cesspool from immediately outside the door to an allotted twenty feet away from the house. That same year the CDB agreed to pay the wages of a Jubilee nurse stationed at Achill Island, County Mayo.[34] Strictly speaking, the board was not permitted to spend its money employing a nurse, but it continued to do so until 1 May 1899; after that, the costs were paid out of the Achill Disaster Fund.[35]

Once the initial expenses of furnishing a house and equipping the nurse with a bicycle and the necessary medical stores (which amounted to £55) were paid, the Dudley committee, which was established to support district nurses, estimated that it cost between £108 and £112 per annum to place a nurse in a rural area.[36] Where suitably furnished houses were available, the initial outlay was reduced to between £90 and £100 per annum, but accommodation suitable for a trained nurse was usually unavailable in the selected poor districts.[37] In October 1904, the committee approached the CDB for help in finding accommodation in the congested districts of Ballycroy, County Mayo; Glengariff, County Cork; and Arranmore Island, County Donegal. The board agreed either to purchase or to build cottages at the specified locations on the condition that the committee paid the interest on the capital sum.[38] In 1906, the board provided cottages for nurses at Annagry, County Donegal; Dooks and Caherdaniel, County Kerry; and Bealadangan, County Galway.[39] It was not difficult to convince the CDB to get involved because it had always been concerned with people's health but had been curtailed by legislation. Aside from home-improvement schemes, the board had been running small coffee stalls for fishermen at Teelin and Malinbeg since 1894, and in later years similar stalls were opened at Downings Bay and Kincasslagh. These stalls were designed to combat what the CDB felt was excessive alcohol consumption among fishermen and employed women at six shillings a week to sell coffee at a penny per cup.[40] Because the board was separate from any particular political ministry, people accepted its help a little more readily than they would help from government agencies, so an affiliation to the board served the Dudley committee well. Indeed, the Dudley committee admitted that without CDB support it would not have been able to operate in the congested districts and "would have been compelled most reluctantly to move the nurses, who were doing excellent work, elsewhere."[41] The accounts of the Dudley committee, in table 8.1, make clear the extent to which the committee was financially dependent on the CDB.

Once established, the Dudley committee was overwhelmed with appeals for nurses from both overworked doctors and local clergy, who were frustrated by the lack of facilities, but one of the stipulations for

Table 8.1
Location and Year in Which the CDB Houses Were Built

Location of CDB House	County	Year
Geesala, Ballycroy	Mayo	1904
Glengariff	Cork	1904
Arranmore	Donegal	1904
Anagry	Donegal	1906
Caherdaniel	Kerry	1906
Dooks	Kerry	1906
Spiddal	Galway	1908
West Cove	Kerry	1908
Derrybeg	Donegal	1909
Achill	Mayo	1909
Pulathomas	Mayo	1908
Bealadangan	Galway	1909
Roundstone	Galway	1911
Kiltimagh	Mayo	1911
*Tory Is	Donegal	1911

* Temporary residence.

Sources: CDB, Seventeenth Annual Report (Dublin: CDB, 1908), 34; CDB, Eighteenth Annual Report (Dublin: CDB, 1909), 25; Lady Dudley's Scheme, Third Annual Report (Dublin: n.p., 1906), 11–12; CDB, Twentieth Annual Report (Dublin: CDB, 1912), 31.

establishing a district nurse was that the area needed to collect as many subscriptions (donations) as possible.[42] In this regard, the people were granted active agency in the care of their communities. Following this subscription process, the committee provided the deficit funds for the maintenance of the nurse. There were a few exceptions to this rule; for example, in Roscommon a local committee had enough funds to maintain its own Jubilee nurse.[43] In Lissadell, County Sligo, Sir Josslyn Gore Booth guaranteed the costs from 1912 until 1921.[44] The *Irish Homestead* newspaper provided funding for two nurses from 1901 in Foxford and later at Pulathomas until 1907, when it approached the Dudley committee to take over.[45] When the CDB bought Tory Island in 1903, conditions were very primitive; there was a population of "355 persons, separated by 8 miles of sea from the nearest doctor." The board negotiated with other bodies, such as the Commissioners of Irish Lights and the Guardians of Dunfanaghy Poor Law Union, to maintain a nurse on Tory Island, and even the impoverished islanders made subscriptions voluntarily in support of the service.[46] In this instance, the board agreed to pay £12 a year toward the cost of providing a qualified nurse.[47]

Funding was an issue that required careful consideration because the expense involved in supplying a nurse was substantial. Table 8.2 shows the cost of providing nineteen nurses in 1909–10. As the table highlights, salary payment was the largest expense, but accommodation costs would have been much higher were it not for the CDB, which provided fifteen of the nineteen nurses' homes by 1912.[48] Despite the fact that most of the nurses used bicycles, traveling costs remained higher than rents and taxes owing to some patients' remote location. The committee relied heavily on subscriptions, and although Lady Dudley moved to Australia in September 1908, she continued to support the Irish initiative from there.[49] She arranged for Sir Ernest Shackleton, who had sojourned at her home in Australia, to give a lecture in Dublin on his return from the *Nimrod* Antarctic expedition, and it raised £315 for the scheme.[50] That year the CDB gave £50 to the Dudley scheme and continued this grant in aid of the scheme until the board's dissolution in 1923.[51]

The district nurse was theoretically supposed to work alongside and under the direction of the local dispensary doctor, but the Dudley

Table 8.2
Budget, Lady Dudley's Scheme, 1910

Receipts	Pounds (£)	Shillings (s)	Pence (d)	Expenditure	Pounds (£)	Shilling (s)	Pence (d)
Cash at Bank of Ireland	781	8	10	Nurses Salaries	1,806	6	11
Deposit	502	0	2	Rents and taxes	119	4	11
Cash in secretary's hands	3	18	6	Furnishings and repairs	113	6	2
Donations	190	14	3	Medical appliances, stores, and nourishments	77	19	8
Subscriptions*	1,688	19	5	Traveling expenses	232	8	7
Dividends and income tax refunds	363	3	7	Sundries	105	1	9
Collecting boxes	10	11	5	Management salaries	125	0	0
Annagry Christmas tree	1	1	0	Printing and stationery	57	9	8
Leyden fund	24	0	0	Sundry expenses, including postage	48	13	1
Spiddal fund		10	0	Traveling and inspection	32	1	0
Nurse's stoves	8	11	0	Annagry Christmas tree	1	1	0
Emergency cases	13	9	8	Leyden fund	32	10	9
Interest on deposit account	8	19	1	Nurse's stoves	8	11	0
Shackleton lecture	315	12	6	Emergency cases	9	13	1
				Investments	509	9	0
				Balance in bank	645	3	9
Total	3,944	0	4		3,944	0	4

* Including interest on Irish Women's Memorial Fund given by the QVJFN.
Source: Lady Dudley's Scheme, Seventh Annual Report (Dublin: n.p., 1910), 22–23.

nurses worked mainly on their own initiative. More often than not, nurses were called because the doctor was unavailable; Nurse Brady, based in Annagry, County Donegal, commented after one case that "[t]he doctor had not yet arrived. . . . I thought at the time I should certainly lose him [the patient]. I do not know what these poor things would have done without the nurse's services[;] several times this month it has been impossible to get a doctor, the latter having so much to do."[52] The absence of a doctor was a regular occurrence. In a letter to the Dudley fund, Father Anthony Timlin wrote, "Short a time as your nurse has been here, she has been the means of saving the life of a poor woman. The doctor was from home when sent for, and were it not for the nurse it is generally believed the poor woman would have been lost to her weak little family."[53] In areas where nurses, unlike doctors, were accepted unequivocally, they had a twofold position, that of health-care provider and educator; one priest noted how "she [the nurse] acts the part of instructress in matters of hygiene, cookery and cleanliness; and as the poor are apt and anxious to learn, we expect great after good as the result of her services."[54] Nurses were nearly always female; they were perceived as maternal figures, and the remit of those engaged in the public health-care setting was broadly defined. On entering a household, a nurse was expected to conduct domestic duties, such as cooking and cleaning as well as caring for children.

As a result of CDB initiatives, many significant improvements occurred in living standards (through the parish committee schemes), but the CDB was a self-help agency, and it did not receive a unanimous response from the people. As a consequence, many substandard, unsanitary dwellings remained in use in parts of the West. When Nurse De Largy was relocated to Foxford (following a four-year stint in Dooks, County Kerry), she was deeply upset by the level of destitution there; she remarked how her first case "was rather a shock. Half the room was little more than a dung heap. At the other side was a big turf fire pouring smoke into the room (for there was no chimney) and round it were a man and woman, five children, a dog, a calf, a donkey and four or five fowls."[55] In this instance, the patient was a baby with chronic pneumonia, and, according to De Largy, the pneumonia was caused directly by the poor living conditions. The very design of this type of cabin was not conducive to good health, being damp and poorly venti- lated and lacking a chimney. These conditions led to a high number of respiratory diseases, and the risk factor was exacerbated by cohabita- tion with animals. Poor housing stock and families living in clusters also aided the spread of fever and disease.[56]

Despite the high levels of training, Dudley nurses had much to reconcile given the poor reputation that assistant nurses had in work- houses.[57] An obvious social and cultural gulf existed between the two classes—the educated nurses and the poor local people—and the resi- dent population initially challenged the authority of female health-care providers. That the nurses lived in sturdy houses, wore uniforms, and used bicycles and on occasions motorcars meant that they were visibly a different class from the resident women, and a reluctance to engage was apparent particularly among the women of the congested districts. Hedderman found that "the men's conversion to modern methods is much more pronounced than the women's. . . . The women cling to their ancient beliefs with a tenacity which is hard to credit."[58] Unsur- prisingly, perhaps the biggest obstacles to advancing better practice were the extent to which folk medicine was used and the power held by local handy women and bonesetters. Nurse Hedderman noted on the Aran Islands, "Until recently our islanders knew nothing of modern nursing. . . . [T]hey adopted ways as old-world and quackish as they were unscientific."[59] The prevalence of ethnomedicinal practice, faith healing, and other less expensive forms of self-medication using patent medicines also worked against proponents of scientific medicine.[60] Mrs. Hazell of Cashel House, County Galway, remarked how the people were "most ignorant and allow sick people to eat and do most unheard of things. It is against ignorance of this sort the nurses have to fight and they will no doubt bring wisdom and cleanliness to many homes."[61] When Nurse Rosina Hayes attended a maternity case in Carna, she found that the only reason she was called was that the local "handy woman" was drunk and was unable to deliver the child. The expectant mother explained that she had not called for medical assistance in the first instance because the neighboring women said the handy woman was "lucky."[62] In another instance, Nurse Brannagan found it difficult to convince the women of Derrybeg to follow her instructions regarding "measley children," and they continued to fill them with "horrid whiskey" and "piled dirty clothes" on them.[63] An anonymous account in 1908, five years after the induction of the Dudley scheme, noted a case of a young boy who had broken his leg, and his parents sent for a bonesetter. The child was in severe pain, and only after the priest's intervention would they allow the nurse to tend to him. Under no circumstances would they allow the child to see the doctor, despite the nurse's repeated efforts to get them to do so. In this instance, the nurse was perceived as the bridge between the people, the clergy, and the doctor. More accounts highlight how the people were happy to adopt a hybrid approach to medical health care that embraced modern medical practice but did not abandon traditional remedies. The following story illustrates this point:

> Had been attending a case of ulcerated leg for some days. I called unexpectedly one evening and found the patient had been treating her leg in an extraordinary manner. I discovered a large piece of moss, with earth attached to it, laced on the open sore, with the earthen side next it. I naturally felt quite irate and asked why my treatment had been abandoned. I received a long explanation of the virtues attached to the moss cure, and was told an old woman prescribed it. . . . [S]uperstition was, of course, at the back of all this. I merely relate this as an instance of some of the difficulties a nurse has to meet in dealing with patients of this class.[64]

Among the nurses, there was little tolerance of ethnomedical practices; its persistence reminded them of the social gulf that existed between them and their patients. Ethnocentric tones were probably inadvertent, but the discourses on the body that can be gleaned from these reports are almost that of redemption, sanitation, and reclamation from all that was ill about rural western society.

It took a while before the nurses won their localities' trust and respect; with it, they began to have a profound impact on health care and on raising levels of cleanliness. In stark contrast, the lesser-trained nurses in union hospitals were not viewed in the same favorable light; one Limerick child described them as not being "right nurses," but "oul wans wud dirty necks an yallah sthrings to their caps."[65] Maria Luddy cites cases whereby lay women carried out work in lieu of maintenance in institutions, but more significantly she highlights that from the 1860s the religious orders, such as the Sisters of Mercy, were making efforts to take control of union hospitals, and they subsequently supported and perpetuated "the existence of a cheap welfare system."[66]

On the strength of the Dudley scheme's success, the Vice Regal Commission on Poor Law Reform in Ireland recommended more "cottage hospitals" for remote districts of the Northwest, to be "attended by the dispensary doctor and with a fully trained Nurse of the Jubilee class."[67] A party of Parliament members who visited the West in 1906 reported how "deeply impressed" they were "with the value of the work of Lady Dudley's nurses in these districts. They say that the elevating and refining influences of such devoted women cannot be overstated, and they are rewarded by the gratitude and affection of the people to whom they minister."[68] In August 1907, the report of the Vice Regal Commission on Poor Law Reform described the scheme as "a remarkable and unquestionable success." In 1909, the commission proposed that a complete overhaul of the system be made, that doctors be paid out of parliamentary funds, and "that the hospitals should be taken completely out of the Poor Law." This proposal was rejected in favor of a "transfer of all infirmaries and hospitals to the County Public Assistance Authority, which would co-ordinate the medical institutions of their area, and organize an outdoor service, including the Medical Dispensary Service and the appointment of nurses for nursing in the homes of the necessitous."[69] But this proposal did not go into effect, nor did it entice the government to invest directly in district nursing schemes.

Before long, it became obvious to the Dudley committee that working in the congested districts was very physically demanding for the Jubilee nurses. Travel to patients often included cycling, hiking over hills, traversing fields, sometimes paddling in boats— often in darkness. Nurses were expected to conduct all medical and educational duties; they were exposed to infectious disease and, because of the abject poverty they witnessed, psychologically disturbing situations. On arrival, nurses had to deal with issues of health, malnutrition, and sanitation; in every respect, the nurses were overworked. It was also found that the nurses' diligence was expended often to their detriment, and that in most cases for ethical and moral reasons they willingly risked life and limb. Both Nurse De Largy, stationed in Dooks from 1907, and Nurse Ellen Donald, who was in Derrybeg in 1909, contracted typhus while performing their duties.[70] Nurse Hedderman, who was stationed on Aran, later recounted "the hardships connected with maternity work, in one of the loneliest and most isolated districts in the West of Ireland."[71] Like many other Victorian institutions, the committee in charge of the Dudley scheme was patriarchal and felt "responsible for their [the nurses'] appointment and regard the wellbeing [sic] of their nurses as a sacred trust."[72] Two nurses (Leyden and Trinham) were "forced to resign on account of ill-health" because of "the hard and trying conditions of their lives with constant exposure to weather[,] long hours of work and incessant anxiety and responsibility."[73] By 1910, the committee had recognized the "arduous nature of their duties," and in 1913 it was decided to put a maximum limit of three years on the amount of time nurses could spend in the congested districts.[74]

From 1913 to 1923, the Dudley committee operated smoothly but did not expand because from the outset efforts were hampered by financial problems. Following the implementation of the 1911 National Insurance Act, costs increased, and that year the QVJIN decreed that each of the affiliated societies should pay £40 toward the training of each nurse.[75] During the Second World War, financial limitations meant a drain on funds and left a mere twenty-three nurses in twenty-one districts.[76] In 1916, the committee even scaled its annual report down to a one-page document to cut back on printing costs.[77] The situation improved slightly after Lady Dudley's tragic drowning while she was on holiday in Connemara in 1920. Lady Mayo collected £40,000 in the United States as a memorial.[78] This money was used to sustain the current number of nurses, though the Dudley scheme failed to expand; its optimum number of nurses was twenty-one, a relatively small number considering the fact that there were eighty-four congested districts.

Although this low number was in part owing to the lack of funds, the few women applying to the Jubilee nursing schemes was a more pressing issue. It was most difficult to entice Catholic women into the scheme, despite its scope for upward mobility.[79] Nationalist and sectarian issues also prevented Catholic women from entering the Jubilee training institutes because the latter were perceived as Anglophile institutions (despite the fact that the Catholic nurses were trained at St. Laurence's separately from Protestant Jubilee nurses). The fallout was that some areas lost their nurses; for example, in 1914 the position in Pulathomas was vacant for more than a year.[80] In addition, the lack of participation of Irish-speaking women posed communication problems, and the committee later introduced remunerative incentives for nurses to become proficient in the Irish language.[81] As Barrington remarks, "[T]he service was uneven and depended entirely on local initiative," and in the grander scheme only 21 of Ireland's 174 district nurses in 1917 were employed under the Dudley scheme.[82] Although Barrington is very critical of the scheme, she is careful to note how invaluable the service was to the sick poor living in remote districts. Albeit a small-scale operation, the relationship between the CDB and the Dudley committee was a very practical and productive one. At the last CDB meeting held on 29 May 1923, it was decided that all CDB property would be presented as gifts to the respective communities. In other words, the Dudley committee and the district nursing scheme had the benefit of the houses free.[83] The Dudley scheme subsequently enjoyed good relations with the Irish government, and it continued until 1974, after which the respective health boards reemployed the Dudley nurses.[84]

The long tradition of local authorities using local clergy, benevolent landlords' charities, and programs such as the Dudley scheme as a panacea for its own shortfalls in the provision of health care and sanitation in remote rural districts was difficult to redress, and this situation did not change in independent Ireland. In the 1927, the *Report of the Commission on the Relief of the Sick and Destitute Poor Including the Insane Poor,* the existence and "extraordinarily good work" of the Jubilee nurses were acknowledged, but no alternative system proposed. Indeed, the report took the continuance of the scheme for granted.[85]

Although the provision of privately funded schemes alleviated local authorities' huge burden of responsibility, it also allowed them the bad habit of not budgeting sufficiently for health care in general, not to mention domiciliary health care. In this political climate, where local authorities effectively ignored their responsibilities regarding health-care provision, voluntary initiatives such as the Dudley scheme were absolute necessities.

9

"The Wages of Sin Is Death"

Lock Hospitals, Venereal Disease, and Gender in Prefamine Ireland

Laurence M. Geary

> Mary Shortall that was in the lock with the pox.
> —James Joyce, *Ulysses*

> The relief this hospital affords is compleatly [*sic*] secured to the destitute and the friendless, as all persons afflicted with the venereal disease are admitted and extern patients receive advice and medicine, thereby in a great measure preventing the more general dissemination of this dreadful malady.
> —Statement by the governors of the Westmoreland Lock Hospital, 25 September 1819

P rostitution has been designated the second-oldest profession, a premise that confers a certain antiquity on venereal disease, if, indeed, it does not make this disease the oldest human infection. Prostitution and venereal disease historically were intimately related, and nineteenth-century society blamed women for the prevalence of both. In Ireland, prostitution was never a crime, but the practice met with widespread social disapproval, much of it based on sanctimony, self-righteousness, and hypocrisy. Some perceived prostitution as a social nuisance, an offense against public decency; others objected on moral or public-health grounds. Despite society's concerns and objections, little attempt was made to regulate prostitution or control venereal disease in Ireland until the passage of the Contagious Diseases Acts of 1864 (CDAs, 27 and 28 Vic., c.85).[1]

The CDAs were introduced in specified garrison and port towns in the United Kingdom of Great Britain and Ireland, including Curragh, Cork, and Queenstown (Cobh) in Ireland, to redress the alarming levels of sexually transmitted diseases in the army and navy. The acts allowed for the compulsory inspection of suspected prostitutes for venereal disease and for their detention and treatment if infected. As Carmel Quinlan has noted, the CDAs and the subsequent clamor for their repeal sharpened debate in Ireland and Britain on prostitution and on the existing sexual and moral double standard that arose from society's perception that men and women's sexuality differed. Male sexual desire was seen as active, female as passive and receptive. The prevailing social standard afforded men a sexual license that was withheld from women. Society demanded continence of women, but not of men; sexual activity in the latter was condoned as normal behavior, a sign of masculinity, but condemned in women as abnormal or aberrant.[2]

The debates surrounding the introduction of the CDAs, the import of the acts, the fierce opposition they aroused, and the subsequent repeal of the legislation in the 1880s have received considerable attention from historians.[3] The focus of this chapter is not the CDAs themselves or the legislative response to prostitution and sexually transmitted diseases, but the institutional treatment of venereal disease in Ireland prior to the introduction of the CDAs. From early in the nineteenth century, the institutional response was marked by the same sexual and moral double standard that was to prove so controversial half a century later when evolving social forces brought such concerns more into the public gaze.

In 1755, surgeon George Doyle opened a hospital in Rainsford Street, Dublin, for the treatment of women and children suffering from venereal disease. The hospital relocated on a number of occasions, including a fourteen-year sojourn in suburban Donnybrook, before settling permanently in Townsend Street in the center of Dublin.[4] The hospital opened on its new site on 20 November 1792 "for the indiscriminate admission, without recommendation, of indigent persons affected with the venereal disease" and was renamed the Westmoreland Lock Hospital after the lord lieutenant.[5] According to "Erinensis," the *Lancet*'s Irish correspondent, "[V]enereal disease and poverty [were] the cheap prices of admission."[6]

Unlike Dublin's other hospitals, which were voluntarily or philanthropically funded and managed, the Westmoreland Lock Hospital was a state institution; it was entirely funded by Parliament and was managed by government appointees. Paternalism, pragmatism, and prudery were imbued in the managerial and operational philosophy; there was little evidence of charity or compassion, except perhaps for vulnerable, potentially reformable young women, in particular rape victims who found themselves diseased through no fault of their own.

Two other institutions treated venereal disease in the prefamine period in Ireland: St. John's Fever and Lock Hospital, Limerick, and the South Charitable Infirmary, Cork. St. John's opened in 1773 primarily as a fever hospital, but one ward was set aside for the treatment of women suffering from venereal disease, these "unfortunate victims of seduction and its consequent miseries having no other hospital available to them."[7] Of the 2,999 patients who were admitted to the lock ward in the years 1820–36 inclusive, 31 died, and the remainder were discharged.[8]

By 1820, the eight-bed venereal ward for the treatment of female patients in the South Charitable Infirmary was under financial pressure and threatened with closure. The trustees appealed successfully to the lord lieutenant for an annual government grant of £200, which, they said, would enable them to maintain two lock wards, each containing eight beds. They contended that "an ample lock establishment for females" was essential to cut off "the source of infection." The Cork trustees stressed "the melancholy prospect" facing the city's population of upwards of ninety thousand if the government ignored their appeal, stating that there was no other refuge for women "who may have been seduced into the paths of infamy" or who had become infected as a result of the dissolute habits of profligate husbands.[9]

The initial patient intake at the Westmoreland Lock Hospital was 128; in November 1793, 42 beds were added, and another 80 in May 1796, making a total of 250. The original admissions register noted the numbers of patients presenting at the hospital but did not specify gender, age, occupation, or place of residence.[10] Between 20 November 1792 and 31 December 1818, 39,558 individuals were admitted to the hospital, and another 99,982 attended as out-patients. In the decade 1809–18, after improvements in admission procedures, the registers recorded the ratio of male to female patients as seven to ten and of Protestants to Catholics as one to six.[11]

A major cause of managerial concern was the failure of significant numbers of patients to complete their treatment, thereby contributing to the continued dissemination of venereal disease.[12] For instance, in the three-year period to January 1808, 255 patients "eloped" from the hospital, and another 114 were discharged for irregular conduct.[13] A military guard had been posted in the hospital earlier to prevent patients from leaving without permission. However, the contiguity of the guard room to the female wards had entirely predictable consequences, "an intercourse prejudicial to the patients and to the soldiers themselves."[14]

The regulations governing patient behavior and the patients' relationship with the hospital, staff, and other inmates were bureaucratic and restrictive, dictated by the prevailing moral climate and laced with a strong eighteenth-century autocratic flavor. Patients were forbidden to "swear, use profane, abusive or obscene language"; to gamble, smoke, quarrel, or make "any offensive noise" in the hospital; to spit on the walls or floors; to soil the bedclothes; or to pilfer or damage property or clothing. They were to behave respectfully to the nurses and all officers of the hospital and with "decency and regularity during divine service." Patients were confined to their own wards and expressly forbidden to visit those of the opposite sex. Spouses were not allowed to sleep in the hospital. Patients in the married women's ward who misbehaved could be expelled. Anyone who violated the regulations could be confined in a lock-up ward and placed on reduced diet. Flagrant offenders faced summary expulsion.[15] Such a regime was the norm at the time and was not specific to either the Westmoreland Lock Hospital or the other lock institutions in Ireland.

On 31 August 1808, the lord lieutenant, Charles Richmond, appointed a three-man committee—John David La Touche, a member of the well-known banking family; social activist William Disney; and prominent medical practitioner George Renny—to inspect and report on the hospital and a number of other Dublin charities that received regular government funding. The committee claimed that venereal disease was increasing throughout the country, which they attributed to the expansion of the military and naval services, noting that troops were permanently quartered in every village and town in Ireland. Furthermore, the committee detected "an increased profligacy of manner amongst the lower order of females," owing, they claimed, to the influence and ubiquity of the armed forces.[16]

In November 1808, Westmoreland Lock Hospital housed 163 female and 90 male inmates, and such was the demand for places that the committee proposed that female applicants should be given priority. "The policy of this arrangement in checking the farther propagation of the disease is abundantly evident," they argued. The implication of the statement—that women were largely or wholly responsible for spreading venereal disease—was equally apparent. According to the committee, female applicants had "a stronger claim to compassionate attention" because they were "more destitute and helpless" than males afflicted with the disease, a claim that could be realized by excluding men entirely from the Westmoreland Lock Hospital and by treating them in the existing Dublin hospitals, which, it was argued, should be provided with an additional one hundred venereal beds at government expense.[17]

In November 1819, the government, concerned once again about the use of public funds, instructed Renny and Philip Crampton, the surgeon-general, to conduct another inquiry into the Lock Hospital. In their report, they claimed that the government had established the institution to relieve "a great mass of human suffering" and to reduce the incidence of venereal disease, but the hospital had not fulfilled these "humane intentions." Among the reasons given for this failure was the difficulty of preventing "an intercourse between male and female patients in any building within the same roof" without substantially increasing supervision, which, in turn, meant increased costs. In addition, no attempt had ever been made to provide for the moral and religious instruction of the younger inmates or to teach them industrious habits. There was no system of classifying patients in the hospital, no attempt to separate the young from the old, the reformable from the incorrigible. Visitors until the time of this report had had unrestricted access to patients on certain days of the week, an opportunity that some used to recruit "the younger and best looking females for the supply of the brothels in town." This practice was facilitated by "the persuasions and misrepresentations of the numerous confirmed prostitutes" in the hospital and with the connivance of some of the nurses.[18]

Crampton and Renny argued that the maintenance of wards for men in the Lock Hospital, offering both a private retreat during the course of the illness and the possibility of a cure, had stripped venereal disease of much of its terror. They claimed that men had become indifferent to acquiring or communicating infection. The apprentice or mechanic who was disposed "to spend a few weeks in absolute idleness, in the most profligate society," and in comfortable circumstances could do so "at a price no higher than acquiring a venereal disease."[19] From this general premise, Renny and Crampton concluded that the Westmoreland Lock Hospital—and, by extension, similar institutions—encouraged idleness and vice, with inevitable consequences for the incidence of venereal disease in society.

Furthermore, Renny and Crampton argued, infected males did not deserve the same degree of compassion as females, nor did they have the same claims on public relief. Men were "often seducers of innocence" and contracted venereal disease by indulging their "vicious propensities." They were "stimulated to expose themselves to it by their depraved appetites alone." In contrast, women were "too often the melancholy victims of seduction" and, abandoned by parents and friends, were forced into prostitution in order to survive.

Crampton and Renny recommended the closure of the wards for men and the conversion of the hospital into one for "the cure and reformation of 160 diseased females." In a classic exposition of the double standard of morality, they claimed that the continued institutional treatment of female venereal patients was dictated "by imperious necessity and real benevolence, as every diseased woman is not only in herself the centre of a circle of infection, whose radius is indefinite, but an object of

peculiar compassion, in every view that can be taken of her truly destitute and unhappy condition."

Crampton and Renny's arguments were of course entirely specious,
and their extraordinary recommendation to exclude infected males
from the Westmoreland Lock Hospital was both ill conceived and without any scientific basis. Their faulty analysis and dangerous proposals
were prompted by the nineteenth-century social standard that indulged
men sexually while criticizing, patronizing, and attempting to cocoon
women.

Crampton and Renny suggested that the supervision of this all-
female institution should be entrusted to "a few benevolent governors
and governesses," individuals who were willing to devote their time to
"the gratuitous and faithful discharge of such a duty." They observed
that it was implicit in the philosophical fabric of such an institution that
the cure of disease without a corresponding moral reformation was of
little benefit to the individual or to society. To this end, they advocated
a fivefold classification system in the hospital, with a matron to oversee
each of the five groups:

1. Patients who were under twenty years of age
2. Older patients
3. Married women
4. Patients who had suffered relapses while recuperating in asylums or
    penitentiaries
5. "Refractory patients or very abandoned females"

Crampton and Renny recommended a restriction on visitors, a
reduction in the medical staff, the nonadmission of medical students
under any circumstances, presumably on moral grounds, and, finally,
the closure of the out-patient dispensary and the transfer of its functions to the House of Industry, a quasi-workhouse. They claimed that
such a facility was inappropriate in an institution reserved exclusively
for females. There were other objections to treating venereal disease
in dispensaries, including the possibility of mercury poisoning arising
from injudicious and irregular usage and the difficulty of persuading

"patients of the lower order" to persevere with a course of treatment after the primary symptoms had disappeared. Those who thought they were cured were mistaken because there was no conclusive remedy for syphilis or gonorrhea in the nineteenth century and would not be until the availability of penicillin from the 1940s on. However, the belief that they were cured prompted some to resume their old way of life, thereby spreading venereal disease.

The moral climate that surrounded the treatment of female venereal patients in general hospitals may have influenced the decision to convert the Westmoreland Lock Hospital into an institution exclusively for women. Several Dublin doctors testified that there were "great objections" to the practice of treating women for such diseases, and women suffering from venereal complaints were generally excluded from these institutions.[20] Female venereal patients were also admissible to the Richmond Hospital, one of three government-funded hospitals attached to the Dublin House of Industry, but the governors were reluctant to accept them because these individuals were regarded as debased and diseased, and there were objections to associating "women of virtuous character and women of bad character together." Dr. Hamilton, one of the surgeons to the Richmond Hospital in the mid–nineteenth century, had on several occasions admitted "women of the town," as he termed them, to his wards in the hospital, prompted by the women's entreaties, their diseased appearance, their assurances of proper conduct, and their exclusion from the other Dublin hospitals. He was aware of the general objection to mixing them with "innocent women," but he trusted in their promises to behave. As it transpired, the problem did not lie with the venereal patients, but with the general workhouse hospital inmates who treated the infected women with such contempt that "a fierce spirit of resistance was excited in them," resulting in "violent and abusive language" and the general disruption of the hospital. Thereafter, female venereal patients were almost entirely excluded from the House of Industry hospitals.[21]

The decision to convert the Westmoreland Lock Hospital into an institution for women created an acute shortage of hospital beds in Dublin for diseased men. The government responded by supporting thirty beds in Dr. Steevens' Hospital from 1820[22] and a number of others in the Richmond Hospital. However, these initiatives did little to stifle the many complaints from medical practitioners about the inadequate facilities for treating sexually transmitted infections in men.[23]

Crampton and Renny's recommendations in relation to the Westmoreland Lock Hospital took effect 4 March 1820. After the closure of the men's wards, a new board of governors applied itself to redressing the perceived abuses in the institution, including the nursing staff's drunken and neglectful habits. Petty and demeaning regulations governing admission and patient behavior were added to the existing ones. Any woman who refused to have her hair cut or who did not bring with her "at least one decent suit of female clothing" was refused admission. Inmates were expressly admonished, on grounds of decency and personal health, not "to expose themselves by looking out of the windows."[24]

The governors claimed that it took several years of commitment and effort on their part to convert the institution into "a place of sobriety, order, and zealous attention to duty" and "to render the superior officers efficient, and persons of exemplary lives." The result, according to the governors in 1838, was that "every justice" was now afforded to "the unhappy inmates."[25] It may have been the governors' complacency and pomposity that led "Erinensis," the *Lancet*'s man in Dublin, to dismiss them contemptuously as the "tinkers of the broken chinaware of female virtue" and to reject their reforms as a great blow to medical education in the city.[26]

On 13 August 1829, the lord lieutenant appointed another commission to inquire into several institutions in Dublin, including the Westmoreland Lock Hospital, which received government funding, his action prompted by ongoing concerns about the use to which public monies were put. The six-man commission, which included Crampton and Renny, noted that the classification system recommended by the 1819 inquiry had been adopted and that great care was now taken "to separate the novice in crime from the hardened offender, and the married woman who is the victim of her husband's profligacy from those whose disease has proceeded from their own personal misconduct."

The commissioners added that they would give every possible assistance to any woman who was remorseful and anxious to alter her lifestyle.[27]

The primary function of the Westmoreland Lock Hospital and of all such institutions was a public-health one: to control the spread of venereal disease. In addition, the governors believed they had an implicit moral obligation to address the broader question of prostitution in society and to dissuade the vulnerable and the young from a life on the streets. According to the governors, many of their young patients had been seduced—often forcibly and against their will—and their families had disowned them on discovering that they were infected with venereal disease. The Lock Hospital afforded such victims an opportunity to escape from a life of prostitution. It was accordingly essential to segregate "the hardened profligate" from "the recent victim of seduction" and to steer away young, potentially reformable girls from "a vicious course of life." This could best be achieved, the governors believed, by restoring these girls to their families or by admitting them to penitent asylums or reformatories.[28]

There were four such institutions in Dublin at the time, the most important being the Lock Penitentiary, which was established in 1794 on Dorset Street "for the reception, accommodation and employment in useful industry of unhappy females, who, after their cure has been completed, are desirous to relinquish a vicious life and to follow better courses."[29] The raison d'être of this and similar refuges was piously captured in the following quatrain:

Ye, alas, who long have been
Willing slaves of death and sin,
Now from bliss no longer rove,
Stop, and taste redeeming love.[30]

The 1829 commission argued that the Lock Hospital's role in promoting the "moral improvement" of such individuals entitled it to continued financial support from the government.[31] Lock hospitals differed from all other institutions for the relief of the sick poor, a difference that arose from their "peculiar nature," to quote an 1842 government committee of inquiry into Dublin charities.[32] Venereal disease was seen as self-inflicted, the consequence of passion and vice, and its victims, other than the innocent ones depicted earlier, were deemed undeserving of charity. As a result, institutions for the relief of venereal disease found it almost impossible to attract voluntary financial support, which meant that either the state became involved, or such institutions ceased to function.[33] In the early 1850s, Thomas Byrne, surgeon to the Westmoreland Lock Hospital, ascribed the institution's lack of popular support to the fact that venereal disease was "too delicate a subject to bring before the public," and he dismissed as "perfectly utopian" the notion that an institution whose inmates had "brought the disease on themselves by their own guilt would be supported by ladies going round begging for it."[34]

The Westmoreland Lock Hospital was funded entirely by Parliament, an involvement that sat uneasily with current economic thinking. Government concern over this usage of public funds was reflected in the appointment of inquiries in 1808, 1819, 1829, 1842, 1854, and 1855 to consider whether government funding of the hospital and a number of Dublin charitable institutions should be continued, modified, or terminated. In June 1829, the Select Committee on Irish Miscellaneous Estimates suggested that such public support should be based on four criteria: (1) "the proved utility of the charity"; (2) "the improbability of its maintenance by private aid only"; (3) "the contribution of funds locally raised by subscription or taxation"; and (4) "the strictest economy in salaries and all other expenses."[35]

The half-century after the Act of Union witnessed the gradual erosion of the Westmoreland Lock Hospital's financial base, which, of course, had implications for the service provided. Table 9.1 shows the level of public funding for the institution between 1801 and 1827. After that, Parliament voted for a sum of £3,490 in 1828 and of £3,060 in the following year.[36] From 1828 to 1838, the average annual parliamentary grant was £2,813. In 1838, the grant was reduced to £2,500 and remained at that amount until 1848. Thereafter, it was reduced by 10 percent per year. The projected grant for 1855 was £1,000.[37]

Table 9.1

Level of Public Funding for the Westmoreland Lock Hospital, 1801–1827

Period	Annual Average (£)
1801–1803	5,932
1804–1806	7,111
1807–1809	9,019
1810–12	7,386
1813–15	7,813
1816–18	8,314
1819–21	5,133
1822–24	2,606
1825–27	3,412

Source: Westmoreland Lock Hospital annual reports, Royal College of Physicians archives, Dublin.

On 23 December 1837, the Treasury reminded the lord lieutenant that the Westmoreland Lock Hospital was in constant breach of one of the four criteria for public funding laid down by the 1829 Select Committee on Irish Miscellaneous Estimates and that unless private subscriptions were raised in aid of the hospital, it could not guarantee a continuation of government support. The governors responded with a lengthy memorial to the lord lieutenant in which they stressed the hospital's success "in effecting the object for which it was instituted" and in conferring "important moral benefits" on the unfortunate inmates. They argued that it was essential to establish and adequately fund "national lock hospitals for female patients," claiming that the annexation of venereal wards to general hospitals was insufficient. The governors contended that many infected women were driven by necessity into "this unhappy course of life," and others were "innocent sufferers through the medium of vicious husbands." The governors viewed the Westmoreland Lock Hospital as a national institution devoted to curbing the incidence and virulence of venereal disease. The rigid exclusion of "women affected by the venereal" from every other hospital in Dublin meant that if the Lock Hospital were closed, these "wretched objects" would "be cast in helpless misery on the world, not alone to certain death, but as long as life continues, to the diffusion of unrepressed pestilence."

The governors sketched an alarming picture of the ravages that syphilis would wreak on "the lower classes of society" in the event of the hospital's closure, a sketch that was grossly inflated for obvious, money-generating reasons. "The worst forms of phagedaena (hospital gangrene) would undoubtedly prevail to a desolating extent," and new types of infectious diseases might be generated that would expose society to "such a pestilence of lues (syphilis) as once carried death and terror on its wings." The governors argued that lock hospitals offered the only safeguard against this possibility, the only means of suppressing venereal disease among the poor. These institutions' inability to secure voluntary contributions placed the onus on government to support them and to protect society from "the consequences of national infirmities."[38]

The governors' submission was infused with social classification and stereotyping. Their concern for the moral and physical welfare of the women involved and for the general community was undoubtedly genuine, but the impression given is that profligate carnality and its consequences applied exclusively to the lower orders, who were perceived to have less physical and moral control than the higher social classes. As a consequence, the latter were paternalistically obliged to protect their social inferiors from their own passions.

The 1854 Select Committee on Dublin Hospitals introduced a new element to the venereal equation: concern for the health and well-being of the armed forces, a concern sharpened by the military demands of the Crimea. "It appears that in large garrison towns the establishment of a lock hospital for females is the best mode of preventing venereal disease among the soldiery." The committee recommended continued public support for the Westmoreland Lock Hospital on the grounds that "venereal disease constantly incapacitates and even causes the discharge of the soldier at the very age that he is most serviceable to the country."[39]

In the following year, a similar committee recommended an annual parliamentary grant of £2,600 to the hospital and the restoration of bed capacity to 150.[40] Since 1 April 1854, the number of beds had fallen to 40, and all attempts at classification had been abandoned. "The old and the young, the hardened and the comparatively inexperienced in vice were associated in the same wards." The committee stressed the evil effects of such a system in an institution whose function should be to prevent "the spread of the moral contagion no less than that of the physical disease." It proposed a threefold classification to remedy this "great evil":

1. General patients
2. Patients admitted with special recommendations
3. Patients from these two wards who were anxious to amend their ways and penitents in asylums or penitentiaries who had suffered a relapse

The committee claimed that the adoption of this classification system would also address the perceived deficiencies in religious instruction and training in the institution.[41]

The pious moralizing and religious sentiment that permeated the management of the hospital, the different inquiries into the institution in the first half of the nineteenth century, and the annual reports of the Board of Superintendence of Dublin Hospitals, a body that came into existence in the wake of the 1855 inquiry, were reflected in the dreary, depressing, and deteriorating physical fabric of the institution itself.[42] The essence of the Westmoreland Lock Hospital, from the time it opened on Townsend Street in 1792 until it was demolished in 1955, was captured in the gloomy inscription, printed in large red letters, over the chapel door: "The wages of sin is death."[43]

Sexual activity—premarital, conjugal, illicit, or deviant—may indeed have proved fatal to participants who were unfortunate enough to contract venereal disease before the discovery of penicillin. Not all cases of syphilis progressed to the tertiary or fatal stage, but for those that did, the experience for the victims was distressing, painful, and irreversible. In the eighteenth and nineteenth centuries, therefore, lock hospitals could not cure venereal disease, but by isolating the afflicted, they may have lessened the incidence and virulence of the infection. These institutions, in conjunction with penitent asylums or reformatories, may also have discouraged some women from engaging in prostitution. However, the ensuing moral and epidemiological impact was blunted by society's acceptance that the male biological imperative excused men's sexual activity and that women alone were the sites of venereal infection.

10

"Sickness," Gender, and National Health Insurance in Ireland, 1920s to 1940s

Mel Cousins

This chapter looks at the administration of the Irish national health insurance system in the years after the establishment of the Irish Free State in 1922. It examines, in particular, gender-related issues in the administration and reform of the national health insurance system. The implications of this assessment for broader debates about whether data on illness in national health insurance systems can be interpreted as evidence of morbidity or simply as absence from work are also considered. The chapter first outlines the background of the national health insurance system in Ireland and then moves on to discuss concerns that emerged, particularly in the 1930s, in relation to women's (in particular married women's) perceived high claim rate under the national health insurance scheme. In addition, it looks at whether these concerns can be explained by higher female morbidity. Finally, it discusses the broader debates about the meaning of national health insurance records.

The UK national health insurance system of 1911 also applied to Ireland. Unlike the rest of the United Kingdom, however, the medical benefit scheme under the National Insurance Act of 1911 (1 and 2 Geo. V, c.55), which provided for access to general practitioner care) did not apply to Ireland, and national health insurance in Ireland provided entitlement primarily to weekly benefits during sickness and disablement.[1] The act insured all employed persons older than sixteen who were manual workers and nonmanual workers with earnings of up to £250 per annum. The national health insurance scheme was premised on different treatment of men and women. The scheme paid a maximum rate of 15 shillings per week for men and 12 shillings per week for women for up to twenty-six weeks, and disablement benefit was payable after the expiry of sickness benefit at a flat rate of seven shillings and sixpence.[2] Sickness and disablement benefit were payable where a person was incapable of work by reason of some specific disease or bodily or mental disablement.[3] However, a woman was not entitled to sickness or disablement benefit for four weeks after confinement unless her husband was suffering from a disease or disablement not connected (directly or indirectly) to her confinement.[4] The insured person and his or her employer paid their contributions at a weekly rate of 8 shillings for men and 7 shillings for women and, to each contribution, the state provided 0.44 shilling.

The state did not directly administer Ireland's national health insurance. Because of the existence in Britain of a network of industrial and friendly societies, Prime Minister David Lloyd George provided that such societies administered these benefits. Government-appointed insurance commissioners approved and supervised them. The act established separate Irish insurance commissioners. However, in Ireland, there was a much weaker network of friendly societies, and thus in many cases they had to be created for the purpose of administering national health insurance. Prior to Irish independence, many Irish persons were insured with British societies, and Irish societies could have non-Irish members. However, following independence, the national health insurance system was nationalized, and persons insurable in the Irish Free State were required to be insured with Irish-approved societies.

As a result of the island's having a largely agricultural and self-employed workforce, and because self-employed persons were not insured under national health insurance, the national health insurance system had a different impact in Ireland. In 1923, only about 420,000 persons out of a total workforce of about 1 million were insured under the act; of those insured, 124,600 (29 percent) were women.[5]

Under the original provisions of the 1911 act, upon marriage a woman was suspended from receiving benefits unless she could prove that she would continue to be employed after marriage. In 1924, the Irish government established a Committee of Inquiry into the national health insurance scheme.[6] In its interim report in 1925, the committee recommended that women's membership in an approved society should terminate on marriage and that such women should be compensated by the payment of a marriage grant. The 1929 act implemented this proposal without any serious opposition.[7]

The Irish national health insurance scheme was not a pay-as-you-go system but rather based, at least notionally, on an actuarial and funded approach.[8] National health insurance was accordingly to be actuarially valued by the UK government actuary every three years because the actuary acted on behalf of the Irish Department of Local Government and Public Health after independence. This meant that an assessment was made of the national health insurance scheme's financial viability on a regular basis, looking at both income and expenditure.

A 1928 assessment showed that some societies were in danger of bankruptcy; and as a result, in 1932, the new Fianna Fáil government decided to amalgamate and abolish the approved societies. The new National Health Insurance Society (NHIS, Cumann an Arachais Náisiúnta ár Shláinte) replaced the previous scheme. Thus, instead of being insured with one of sixty-five approved societies, each insured person was now insured by the NHIS. Although the amalgamation does not appear to have had any direct impact from the gender perspective, it did centralize the records of all insured persons. The proactive NHIS quickly began analyzing the claim records.

The NHIS immediately expressed concerns about women's claim rates.[9] In 1923, approximately 30 percent of persons insured under national health insurance were women, and during that year women made 30 percent of all claims for sickness benefit. Over the period 1927–28, the proportion of women insured under national health insurance did not increase (fig. 10.1). However, by 1928, the proportion of sickness benefit claims made by women increased significantly to 38.5

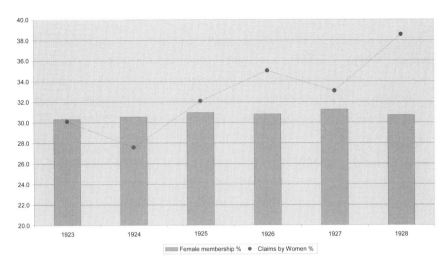

10.1. NHIS membership and claims by gender, 1923–28. *Source:* National Health Insurance Commission, *Administration of the National Health Insurance* (Dublin: National Health Insurance Commission, 1929). Membership data for 1928 compiled from *Sláinte* (1936).

percent. The NHIS carried out a third periodic valuation of the finances of national health insurance on 31 December 1928. This report showed a marked deterioration in the NHIS's financial position compared to the previous valuation in 1923. It attributed the deterioration to "the heavy expenditure in disablement benefit which far exceeded anticipation, particularly in respect of women members."[10] Figure 10.1 shows membership data for 1928.[11]

In the period 1928 to 1935, the average benefits claimed by men fell significantly, driven particularly by a fall in the claim level for sickness benefits (fig. 10.2).[12] In contrast, the average benefit paid to women saw minor increases but included a significant rise in claims for disablement benefit. Contemporary analysis made these numbers look somewhat worse because officials underestimated the level of growth in membership, thereby overestimating the per capita benefit levels paid per member.

For the period prior to the Irish government's 1932 amalgamation of friendly societies, only aggregate-level data are available. However,

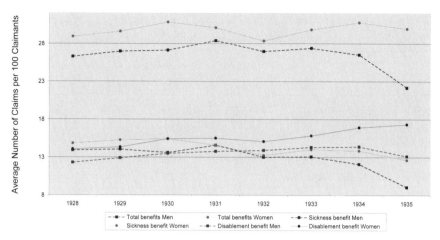

10.2. Claims for health insurance benefits by gender, 1928–35. *Source:* Data compiled from Women's National Health Association, *Sláinte* (1936). Data are adjusted to take account of actual membership figures as set out in Department of Social Welfare, *Social Security* (Dublin: Department of Social Welfare, 1949), as opposed to the estimated figures used in *Sláinte*. It should be noted that the original calculation underestimated membership growth, thereby overestimating per capita expenditure.

the unification of the societies in one NHIS allows a much more detailed examination of these statistics. In 1938, Ruairi Ó Brolcháin presented a paper to the Statistical and Social Inquiry Society that examined the claim record in some detail (assessing the data for the first full year of the NHIS's operation in 1935).[13] This paper provided a breakdown of the claim record for 1935 by sex, marital status (of women only, revealingly), illness, county, age, occupation, number of claims, and duration of incapacity. The vast majority of members (70 percent) were men, and the bulk of the remainder consisted of single women or widows. Only 3 percent of total membership consisted of married women. Domestic servants composed more than 50 percent of all insurable single women.

As set out in table 10.1, the average duration of claims from men and single women was similar. However, the average duration of claims from married women was significantly higher. In addition, the average number of claims per member was significantly higher for single women

Table 10.1

Claim Rates and Duration by Gender, Ireland, 1935

| | Men | Women | | Both Sexes |
		Single	Married	
NHIS Membership Total	335,400	137,100	3,400	486,00
Average Duration of Claim (in weeks)	14.54	14.16	20.71	14.81
Average Claims per Member	0.18	0.23	0.44	0.20
Duration of Claim per Member (in weeks)	2.58	3.24	9.16	2.95

Source: Data compiled from Ruairi Ó Brolcháin, "Examination of the Sickness Experience for the Year 1935 of Persons Insured under the National Health Insurance Acts," *Journal of the Statistical and Social Inquiry Society of Ireland* 16 (1938–40): 53–72.

and even greater for married women. This meant that the total duration of claims per member was somewhat higher for single women and dramatically so for married women.

As can be seen from table 10.2, the average age of married women members was more than six years older than that of men, which may have contributed to some extent to the higher claims level.

Claims rose steadily with age for men and women. However, as shown in figure 10.3, married women's claim level was significantly higher at each age bracket, so that age alone cannot explain the higher claim rates.

Ó Brolcháin's study also examined the illness recorded as affecting each of the different groups. However, as emphasized in the study itself, some caution needs to be attached to these data. First, the examination focused on inability to work rather than on the detailed medical reasons for that incapacity. A more complex medical condition might accordingly be recorded under one heading only. In addition, the reason for the initial incapacity might change over time, but this change might not be reflected in the medical certificate. Further, Ó Brolcháin argued that "there is no doubt that such illnesses as tuberculosis, venereal disease and cancer are not always correctly certified because of the passive or active objection of those incapacitated."[14]

Table 10.2

Average Age of Insured Persons by Gender, Ireland, 1935

Insured Persons	Average Age
Men	36.25
Single Women	28.06
Married Women	42.68
Both Sexes	34.18

Source: Data compiled from Ó Brolcháin, "Examination of the Sickness Experience."

With these qualifications in mind, the main illnesses affecting men were rheumatism, microbic fevers, and respiratory diseases. Rheumatism and microbic fevers also affected single women, followed by diseases of the blood (in particular anemia). In the case of married women, the main illnesses recorded were rheumatism, pregnancy, and "diseases of women." It is clear that, to some extent, pregnancy and diseases particular to women did contribute to married women's higher claim rate. However, these conditions accounted for only 15 percent of total sickness and disablement claims and were generally of a reasonably short duration. They accordingly can also go only a small way toward explaining the significant differences in claim rates.[15]

In the following year (1938), an official study was carried out looking at the claim experience under the Irish national health insurance scheme. Taking advantage of the unification of societies, the Department of Local Government and Public Health commissioned the UK actuary's office to carry out a special investigation of the claim record in comparison with the UK experience. This investigation was to be the first detailed comparison of the actual experience of claims with the assumptions upon which the scheme had been based.[16] The Irish standard[17] was based on the UK standard adopted in 1912 and somewhat modified for women in 1918. However, as the UK actuary pointed out, the UK standard never purported to be a standard applicable to Irish conditions. Given this qualification, the report also compared the Irish experience with the recently revised British standard based on its own claim experience. As shown in figure 10.4, the study revealed that

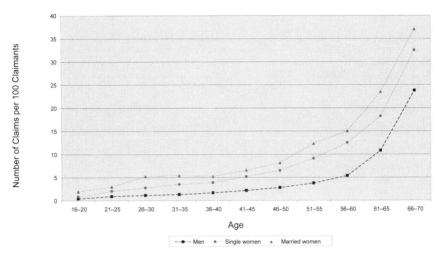

10.3. Average duration of receipt of benefits by gender, 1935. *Source:* Data compiled from Women's National Health Association, *Sláinte* (1936).

women's claim experience for both of sickness and disablement benefit was significantly higher than men's.

Perhaps more important, the analysis showed that, with the exception of men's sickness benefit claims, the claims experience significantly exceeded the standards. Although the Irish standard was "admittedly inappropriate," the British provision was based on actual recent data, including married women's "heavy claims experience" in Great Britain (see fig. 10.5).

Age was found to be a "significant factor" in the claims experience. In the case of men and single women, there was a steady rise in the period spent on sickness benefit by age. However, this increase was insignificant compared to the much more dramatic age-related increase in claims for disablement benefit. Older workers tended to exhaust their entitlement to sickness benefit and then move on to the long-term disablement payment. Married women had a significantly higher claims experience for sickness benefit in the younger age group, which actuaries believed was associated with pregnancy. However, married women also had a significantly higher disablement benefit claims experience.

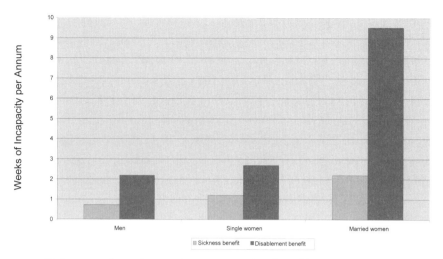

10.4. Claim experience by gender, 1935–37 (weeks of incapacity per annum). *Source:* Data compiled from *Report on the Investigation of the Sickness Claims Experience of the Unified Society* (1935–37), Department of Social Welfare File IA91/53, National Archives of Ireland, Dublin. The report was not published but was laid before the Oireachtas (Parliament).

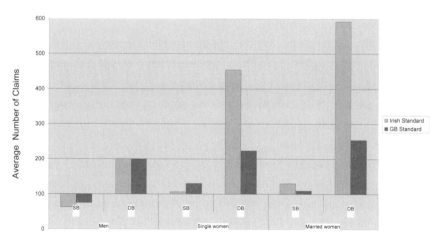

10.5. Claims experience as ratio of Irish and Great Britain standards, 1935–37. *Source:* Data compiled from *Report on the Investigation of the Sickness Claims Experience of the Unified Society* (1935–37), Department of Social Welfare File IA91/53, National Archives of Ireland, Dublin. The report was not published but was laid before the Oireachtas (Parliament).

The actuaries reported that there was no significant difference in age distribution by gender that would explain the different rates of claim.

The review concluded that married women's claims "appear[ed] notably excessive." It suggested that the certification system might lead to an increase in claims and to a prolongation of claims. In addition, the review pointed out that the rate of sickness benefit for men and single women was the same in Ireland as in Great Britain, but that the rate of disablement benefit was in fact higher for men and single women in Ireland. The rates for married women were higher in all cases because the reductions that had been made in the United Kingdom in 1932 "to preserve the financial equilibrium of the scheme" had not been replicated in Ireland.[18] As the review pointed out, wages were lower in Ireland, and it went on to argue that "here without doubt, is to be found one explanation of the higher level of claims, and especially for the prolongation of claims."[19] The review summarized that the sickness benefit experience was broadly acceptable but that claims for disablement benefit appeared excessive and required appropriate investigation of the genuineness, frequency, certification, and supervision of claims to determine if the existing experience was normal.

Following submission of the report to the Department of Local Government and Public Health, a representative of the UK actuary's office visited Dublin to discuss certification and assessment of claims. However, although the archives are incomplete, it would appear that there was little enthusiasm in the department for significant change in this area.

A further actuarial report on the NHIS's overall financial position was completed in 1941.[20] This report again reviewed the experience of sickness claims, updating the data to 1938. As can be seen in figure 10.6, women's claims remained significantly higher than men's, and married women, in particular those in the younger age ranges, had significantly higher claim rates than single women.

Compared to the UK experience (fig. 10.7), Irish men's claim rate was overall somewhat higher, and both single and married Irish women were significantly more likely to claim benefits than their UK counterparts.

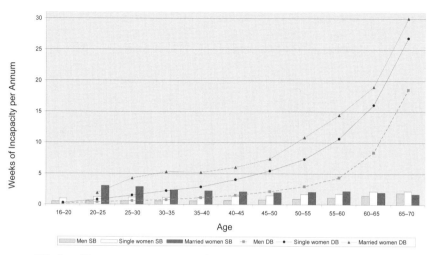

10.6. Weeks of incapacity per annum by age and gender, 1935–37. *Source:* Data compiled from *Actuarial Report on the Financial Position of the National Health Insurance System,* File S.12457, National Archives of Ireland, Dublin.

The actuarial report concluded that "drastic revision" of the existing approach to claims would be necessary to change this position but believed that it was "doubtful . . . whether a material and sustained improvement in the position can be secured" as long as the existing procedure for medical certification continued (see fig. 10.7).[21]

In 1942, Seán MacEntee, the newly appointed minister for the Department of Local Government and Public Health, asked his officials to identify measures to improve the checking of claims and medical certification "with a view to the eradication of the claim habit."[22] Although the files indicate that a separate report was being prepared in relation to the problem of high sickness experience, there is no indication of any significant action in this regard.[23] The primary focus of the Department of Local Government and Public Health—indeed, the main purpose of the actuarial review—was the reform of the system of funding of national health insurance in order to allow the use of accumulated resources for additional benefits.[24] It would appear that this issue and, of course, the wide range of issues raised by the Second World War took

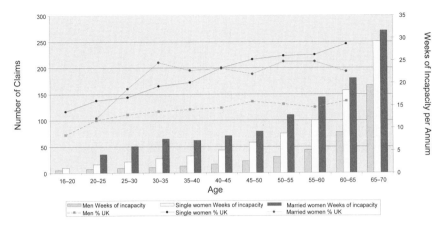

10.7. Weeks of incapacity per annum by age and gender in comparison with the United Kingdom, 1936–38. *Source:* Data compiled from *Actuarial Report on the Financial Position of the National Health Insurance System,* File S.12457, National Archives of Ireland, Dublin.

key policymakers' attention away from the issue of claims experience. In any case, having risen in the period to 1940, claims for and expenditure on health insurance benefits stabilized or fell (particularly for women) in subsequent years (before rising significantly in the postwar period; see table 10.3).

Can the differential claim rates for national health insurance benefits be explained by higher morbidity among women? "Morbidity" can be understood as the incidence of sickness or disease for a specific population. There is unfortunately an absence of any comprehensive data on morbidity among Irish persons in the relevant period.[25] Data are available on the incidence of certain diseases, as are administrative data on the use of, for example, certain hospital services. However, these data are of little assistance in establishing morbidity levels for insured workers both because the data available are far from comprehensive and because insured workers make up a specific subgroup of the population as a whole.[26]

One piece of relevant evidence relates to the claim record for "additional benefits" provided under the national health insurance scheme (see table 10.4). Such benefits were provided primarily in relation to

Table 10.3

Claims and Expenditure on Sickness Benefits by Gender, Ireland, 1939–1949

	Sickness Benefit				
	New Claims		Payments (£)		
Year	Men	Women	Men	Single Women	Married Women
1939	44,595	24,031	159,988	74,776	12,466
1940	46,948	26,034	158,610	79,130	11,877
1941	42,367	24,518	153,594	78,484	11,138
1942	39,936	23,707	136,580	76,729	10,259
1943	—	—	145,841	74,626	10,849
1944	44,480	24,294	149,419	72,227	9,907
1945	46,357	24,761	151,274	71,955	9,803
1946	52,329	24,966	161,439	70,144	9,423
1947	55,625	25,054	232,525	93,181	15,822
1948	51,347	24,619	265,189	111,980	20,761
1949	55,878	27,603	293,885	123,041	23,895

	Disablement Benefit				
	New Claims		Payments (£)		
Year	Men	Women	Men	Single Women	Married Women
1939	5,599	3,750	219,900	112,919	38,428
1940	5,403	3,745	221,130	115,866	38,937
1941	5,089	3,727	216,597	119,741	38,038
1942	4,430	3,237	204,209	120,265	36,913
1943	—	—	194,292	118,278	35,876
1944	4,874	3,151	185,081	117,616	33,943
1945	4,747	3,199	184,834	118,814	33,174
1946	4,913	2,995	189,500	119,720	32,340
1947	5,704	3,030	327,636	180,643	50,238
1948	6,382	3,581	406,772	215,861	60,462
1949	7,488	4,228	455,793	234,063	65,881

Source: Annual reports of the NHIS secretary, 1939 to 1949 (1943 missing), Department of Social and Family Affairs Library, Dublin.

dental, hospital, and optical care (representing more than 95 percent of total expenditure on such benefits). These benefits represented payments toward the cost (in full or in part) of medical treatment and were payable whether the person was in employment. Thus, there was no issue concerning work disincentives for such benefits. Insured women claimed hospital benefits in proportion to their membership in the scheme. But analysis carried out by the NHIS indicates that women's claims for dental and optical benefit were significantly higher than would be expected based on the ratio of their membership to men's membership.[27]

Thus, this evidence is largely inconclusive, indicating that, on the one hand, women were no more likely to avail themselves of hospital services than men, but that, on the other, they were more likely to avail themselves of dental and optical benefits.

Detailed data *are* available in relation to mortality rates. Tony Fahey has examined the issues concerning women's mortality rates in early-twentieth-century Ireland. Although Fahey's emphasis is somewhat different from that of this study, his paper does offer relevant insights. His study asserts that Ireland in the early twentieth century was an exception to general demographic patterns in that Irish women had almost no life-expectancy advantage at birth over Irish men and that their death rates were higher than men's over a wide range of ages. He points out

Table 10.4
Claims for Additional Benefits by Gender, Ireland, 1944

Additional Claim	Benefit Difference	Men	Expected Women[1]	Actual Women
Dental	17,100	7,600	15,800	+8,200
Hospital	5,200	2,300	2,200	−100
Optical	9,000	4,000	7,000	+3,000
Other	4,000	1,500	2,200	+700
Total	35,400	15,700	27,800	+12,000

Source: Data compiled from Cumann an Arachais Náisiúnta ár Shláinte (National Health Insurance Society), *Secretary's Report Year 1944* (Dublin: Department of Social and Family Affairs, 1944).

that "female mortality disadvantage was very much a characteristic of rural Ireland," whereas in urban areas women's life expectancy showed the normal pattern and exceeded men's expectancy by the two- to three-year margin, as was common in Europe.[28]

Possible explanations for this pattern include male dominance, maternal mortality, and health-selective emigration. Fahey rejects these explanations on the basis that although it might be assumed that "males were dominant in rural Irish society," there is no evidence that this dominance produced an impact on mortality rates; maternal mortality was "far from being a major cause of death in the 1920s in Ireland or elsewhere," and the Irish level did not appear to vary significantly from the rates in other European countries.[29] Emigration was in fact more likely to have raised the health profile of those who remained behind rather than to have lowered it.

In seeking an alternative explanation, Fahey highlights a number of points that are relevant to this study. First, he argues that "being single had health advantages for both women and men, operating primarily through their lack of children and the consequent reduced risk of overcrowding in housing (and possibly other forms of impaired living standards) compared to married people with families." Second, such advantages worked to the particular benefit of men because there were far more single men in the national population than single women. In addition, "there were sharp divergences between urban and rural areas in the distribution of single men and women and the consequent distribution of mortality advantage."[30] Single men were heavily overconcentrated in rural areas, whereas single women were overrepresented in urban areas.

Interestingly for this study, Fahey highlights the special position of female domestic servants. This group was based largely in urban areas and constituted up to 20 percent of the female population in Dublin in 1926. Domestic servants were in an unusual position because, despite the low status of their work, they normally had exceptionally good housing conditions (in comparative terms) and unusually low mortality rates. Roy C. Geary's calculation of the standardized mortality rates by occupation for the period 1901–1910 indicated that domestic servants had the lowest mortality rate of any major occupational group in Ireland.[31] As will be recalled, domestic servants constituted more than 50 percent of the single women group in the data for this study.

Unfortunately, it is difficult to compare directly the issues discussed in Fahey's study with those raised in this chapter. One cannot necessarily expect that the incidence of mortality and morbidity would be the same for particular occupational groups—although one might expect some correlation. In addition, the fact that data for men are not broken down by marital status makes it more difficult to compare the sickness rates of single women with those of men. However, the evidence presented by the national health insurance data is not inconsistent with Fahey's argument. Single women (of whom more than 50 percent were domestic servants) do not show a very high level of sickness absence (although perhaps higher than one might expect given their apparently low mortality rate).[32] Married women, by contrast, as Fahey would predict, do have very high rates of sickness absence.

There was clearly a belief among policymakers, as echoed in the actuarial review, that women's benefit claims were influenced by factors such as the proportion of previous earnings replaced by the sickness insurance payment, which were not directly linked to incapacity to work. At this point, it is almost impossible to decide conclusively whether this view is "correct" or whether Irish women's morbidity was significantly higher than men's (and British women's). However, the extent to which married women's claims exceeded those of men and single women as well as the extent to which women's claims for disablement benefit exceeded the standard set in Great Britain (where women's claims were already perceived to be high) suggest that factors other than morbidity were at play in Irish women's decision to claim national health insurance benefits.

These findings again raise the question as to whether, in fact, sickness absence can be equated with morbidity. Focusing primarily on the nineteenth-century records of friendly societies, James Riley has argued that these records indicate that morbidity increased at the same time as mortality declined.[33] John Murray, in contrast, has suggested that such records cannot reliably be interpreted as indicators of morbidity and that, instead, they should be seen simply as indicators of sickness absence. Murray argues that sickness rates cannot be inferred directly from insurance claim rates and that "insurance claims should not be equated with evidence of sickness, although in many cases there is a strong relationship between the two."[34] The NHIS's experience in early-twentieth-century Ireland would appear to support the latter view. Although, given the absence of independent evidence of morbidity among the insured population, it is impossible to establish comparative morbidity levels conclusively, the evidence would seem to suggest that a broader range of features influenced the claim records of married women under the NHIS. In the vast majority of cases, there clearly was a strong relationship between sickness absence and sickness. The NHIS was of the view that "real malingering," in which there was absolutely nothing wrong with the person, was "not as common as is generally supposed."[35] However, even making allowance for the older age of married women and for pregnancy as well as diseases common among women, it remains difficult to explain the extent of married women's higher claim level on health grounds alone.[36]

Economic incentives provided an obvious alternative rationale for the high claim rate. In the Ireland of the 1930s, unemployment and underemployment remained relatively high. The general tendency of public policy was to discourage married women from pursuing paid work. However, the state provided few financial incentives for women to do so. Although unemployed married women were entitled to unemployment insurance, in the 1930s this insurance was payable only for a maximum of thirteen weeks in each year. Once entitlement to the insurance-based payment was exhausted, married women, unlike men, were generally not entitled to the means-tested unemployment assistance.[37] There accordingly was a considerable incentive for married women to claim the open-ended incapacity benefits. The rate of benefit was not high in comparative terms, but the maximum rate of sickness benefit did represent 50 percent of the average weekly earnings of a female worker in industries producing transportable goods in 1938, and it was not affected by any other income in the household (such as the husband's earnings).[38]

This chapter has discussed the administration of national health insurance in Ireland in the early twentieth century, focusing on gender differences in claims for benefits. It has shown that contemporary assessment found that women—in particular, married women—had a much higher rate of claim than men and that Irish women had a much higher rate of claim than would have been expected based on British norms. It is suggested that although some of this higher claim rate may have been owing to poorer health and more frequent pregnancy among Irish women, it is difficult to explain this differential purely on health grounds. It seems likely that married women took account of broader social issues, including the limited availability of alternative income sources such as unemployment assistance. This finding emphasizes the extent to which social security schemes are negotiated in their implementation by the claimants as well as by the policymakers and administrators. It also contributes to the debate in the literature on health insurance. The real question is whether records should be seen as an indicator of morbidity or simply of sickness absence. This chapter supports the latter interpretation.

Two further points arise. First, given the concerns about the level of claims by married women, why was nothing or very little done about such a level? I suggest that this lack of action was largely owing to the structure of the scheme, which was administered by an independent body, the NHIS, and funded largely by employer and employee contributions. The Exchequer contribution was limited, and the concern of civil servants and politicians was primarily with the viability of the scheme rather than its detailed operation. Action would have been forthcoming only if women's claim level had threatened the underlying financial viability of the national health insurance scheme. Despite the concerns, the relatively small number of women, in particular married women, insured under the scheme limited their financial impact.[39] In addition, the particular conjuncture favored inaction. The focus of both Department of Local Government and Public Health officials and the NHIS in the late 1930s and 1940s was on altering the scheme's financial basis so as to provide additional benefits. Furthermore, the Second World War raised a range of broader concerns and led to the stabilization or fall in women's claims.

Second, it is important to note that the story does not end in the 1940s. This account finishes in the 1940s largely for data reasons. The advent of the Second World War put an end to the production of detailed studies of the impact of national health insurance.[40] But concerns continued to be reflected in the 1949 White Paper on social security.[41] The White Paper proposed the unification of the existing unemployment and sickness insurance schemes (renamed disability benefit). It recommended that no distinction should be made between single persons of the two sexes on the basis that their needs were the same. However, it also set out specific concerns about employed married women, who, it suggested, presented "some special features":

> Married women normally look to their husbands for maintenance, and those of them who engage in employment do so, generally speaking, in order to augment the family income. The sickness experience of this class has been exceptionally heavy, and if the higher benefit rates became applicable to them, it is to be feared that the degree of malingering would be even worse than it has been. It will hardly be considered unreasonable if, in order to reduce the very serious and obvious danger of malingering, the husband—who is legally obliged to support her—should be asked to make some financial sacrifice for his wife if she should become ill and it is, accordingly, proposed that a somewhat lower sickness benefit rate be granted to married women, except in cases where their husbands have deserted them or been legally separated from them.[42]

These proposals were implemented in the Social Welfare Act of 1952 (1952/11) and a lower rate of disability benefit for married women continued to be paid until the 1980s, when the law was changed as a result of European Union legislation.

It may well be that similar issues arose in the largely undocumented intervening decades.[43] In the 1980s and 1990s, concerns again surfaced about women's overclaiming, this time leading to specific measures to tie access to disability benefit more closely to participation in the labor force.[44] Richard O'Leary's study of women on disability benefit (prior to the introduction of such measures) suggests that factors relevant to women's staying on disability benefit included issues related to incapacity such as age and the type of incapacity, but also broader issues such as prior unemployment and unemployment levels. He believes that the entry of women into long-term receipt of disability benefit was related "not just to health status but to other factors affecting their relationship with the labor market," such as the presence of children, prior unemployment, and the rate of local female unemployment.[45] But despite these measures, gender differences among claim rates of disability benefits remained significant.

This study highlights the importance of not assuming that issues such as national health insurance claim records or morbidity rates are unproblematic concepts. It would be foolish, as Noel Whiteside points out, to take "administrative classifications at face value and assume they reflect some sort of social reality."[46] In looking at insurance claims experience and at morbidity, this chapter has attempted to establish the relationship between one rather subjective factor for which good data are available and another rather subjective factor for which no comprehensive data exist. National health insurance data clearly do not simply reflect some underlying social reality of morbidity. Rather, the existence of national health insurance constructs a new social reality: being a national health insurance pensioner is just as much a reality as being sick. And it seems likely that although morbidity obviously influences national health insurance claims, the existence of national health insurance may also affect the manner in which people construct the social reality of morbidity.

11

"A Perpetual Nightmare"

*Women, Fertility Control, the Irish State,
and the 1935 Ban on Contraceptives*

Sandra McAvoy

States permit or restrict access to fertility control for a range of reasons, including concerns about demographics, health, and culture.
Their decisions may also say much about contemporary attitudes to
women. The Irish 1935 Criminal Law Amendment Act (1935/6) crimi-
nalized the importation and sale of contraceptives. It was a measure
that brought the law into line with the teaching of the dominant Roman
Catholic Church and marked a break with a neighboring British culture
in which contraception was increasingly accepted. No special provision was made in the 1935 legislation for women for whom pregnancy
involved a threat to life or health. Archive evidence indicates, however,
that these women's needs were understood by at least some of those
involved in drafting it and that the original proposals involved restricting access to contraceptives while permitting doctors to prescribe them.[1]
This chapter looks at evidence on access to birth control information
and literature in the period following Irish independence in 1922 and
at how key political decision makers, who were determined to impose a
Roman Catholic morality on the state, brought about the ban.

There is no reliable quantitative evidence on the import, sale, or use
of contraceptives in Ireland before or after independence from Britain in
1922. A 1934 response from the Revenue Commissioners' Office to an
inquiry about this issue merely reflected the variety of preparations and

goods manufactured as contraceptives in this period, which included rubber sheaths (condoms), diaphragms, sponges, cervical caps, cocoa butter quinine spermicidal pessaries, spermicidal creams and jellies, and materials used in douching.[2] It explained that contraceptives were

> not invoiced as such nor described as such in official Customs documents. The rubber variety would appear in our documents and records as "Rubber manufactures, other sorts not elsewhere specified or included."
>
> The soluble materials used to effect the like purpose might be "medical preparations, dutiable or non-dutiable" or even "preparations of oil, butter etc. etc. not medical."
>
> The invoices usually cover the former by the term "rubber goods" the latter by "preparations" . . . (according to the ingredient).

The commissioners saw no reason for special classification, as the memo further explained: "Our original consideration of these articles sprang [?] from our administration of the prohibition against the import of 'indecent and obscene articles' and we decided that the articles in question above were not within the prohibition."[3]

The fact that by 1934 the customs authorities did not consider contraceptives to be covered by measures prohibiting "indecent and obscene" articles might imply a recent change of attitude. In 1926, although the Department of Posts and Telegraphs indicated that there was little scrutiny of the packet post, it was still returning to senders birth control advertising or contraceptives occasionally identified in the postal system and threatening to prosecute them. The department was, however, conscious that it was overstretching its powers and that the legislation it drew on, the British Post Office Protection Act of 1884, had ceased to be applied in Britain in 1908 (also the year of the last Irish prosecutions for sending contraceptives through the post) because "of the reluctance of the British courts to give a decision as to whether such articles are indecent."[4]

What evidence is there of the use of contraceptives in Ireland? One source of information is a 1921 contribution to the letters pages of the

British Medical Journal by obstetrician Gibbon FitzGibbon, then master of Dublin's Rotunda maternity hospital. Responding to suggestions by British anti–birth controller Dr. Halliday Sutherland that Ireland was a birth-control-free zone, in which large families lived happily and infant welfare clinics and societies for the prevention of cruelty to children were unnecessary, FitzGibbon addressed a number of issues. In the process, he provided interesting material on knowledge of birth control in Ireland. He wrote that, in his experience, although most married couples "did not avoid the first or second infants," once incomes were stretched, the possibility of a further pregnancy became "a perpetual nightmare." His impression was that many of his middle-class patients spaced or limited the numbers of their children without suffering the mental or physical health problems anti–birth controllers attributed to the practice of family limitation.[5] In another letter, he commented,

> In my experience birth control has no ill effects, and does not promote either nervous disorders or sterility. Many of my patients restrict their families to the dimensions of their incomes and when the latter has become capable of the greater burden have voluntarily increased the former. They are, in my opinion, the better and happier for doing so. It is far better for parents to have two or three children and to be able to bring them up well fed and well educated than to have an unlimited number which means constant deprivation. That appears to me to be the chief difference between the working classes and the middle classes.[6]

FitzGibbon's observations support suggestions based on demographic evidence that although there were regional variations, by the early twentieth century, particularly within professional and managerial groups and among Protestants, some Irish couples attempted to plan their families by spacing and restricting numbers of pregnancies.[7] Given the unreliability of many methods of birth control used at the time, commercial as well as home made, it is unlikely that demographic statistics reflect the scale of attempts at family planning.[8]

FitzGibbon did not describe the methods used by his patients. If practice in Ireland reflected that in Britain, it is likely that some relied on withdrawal, abstention, or abortion, but a number of statements in his letter and article touched on key issues in contemporary debates and implied that he was talking about contraception. His suggestion that the medical profession must decide whether doctors should provide "sound" family-planning advice or leave patients prey to "deleterious advertisements" referred to an important aspect of the birth control movement. Until the 1920s, the medical profession in the British Isles was slow to involve itself with the issue. Without that involvement, during the late nineteenth and early twentieth centuries the provision of contraceptives developed as an unregulated commercial activity. Users bought information booklets and contraceptives directly from commercial outlets or by post through newspaper and magazine advertising. It is difficult to quantify the extent to which Ireland shared aspects of a British culture in which, following the First World War, birth control was increasingly accepted. As late as 1920, a Dublin chemist was prosecuted under the 1857 Obscene Publications Act (20 and 21 Vic., c.41) and 1842 Dublin Police Act (5 and 6 Vic., c.27) for displaying poster advertisements for contraceptives and books containing contraceptive information. The size of his stock of birth control literature, 240 books, that the authorities seized and burned may suggest there was a healthy market for such material in Dublin.[9]

FitzGibbon was clearly speaking of either home-made or commercial contraceptives when he alluded to the potential of methods used by women to change the balance of power within marital relationships. Rejecting the concerns of anti–birth controllers that removing fear of pregnancy "prostituted the wife" and led to "undue indulgence," he argued that sexual desire was normal in a "healthy clean-minded woman," and on the question of women who wished to control their fertility, but whose husbands refused to cooperate, he asked: "Why not give the power to the wife? She probably cannot resist him otherwise."[10]

FitzGibbon did not address women's health concerns, possibly because he did not conceive of any argument against contraception in such circumstances. He did refer to the social and economic consequences of failure to restrict family size, using the example of the deprivation endured by the dependents of small farmers. He argued that their children were "reared weaklings," that mothers were constantly nursing, and that older children, denied parental care and education, became "drudges for the younger." He also provided an interesting perspective on the issue of sex outside marriage, though these comments may have been related to the wider British debate. Attributing late marriage to an awareness among young people that uncontrolled childbearing brought misery, he expressed the view that delaying marriage did not necessarily mean accepting celibacy and that the resulting problems included both the spread of venereal disease (which might not be recognized until after a late marriage) and girls who "go wrong in what may be called an amateurish way" after "having their affections trifled with without any prospect of security of tenure." FitzGibbon suggested that knowledge of birth control might encourage early marriage and reduce these health and social problems and that closer child–parent relationships in small families would have sociomoral benefits—in particular, that tighter parental control might impact on "the moral laxity of late years." With reference to that "moral laxity," FitzGibbon reported that contraceptive information was readily available in certain circles: "[I]f a girl wants to find out about preventative methods there are plenty of people ready to give her all the information. It is not to the medical profession or decent married people she will go for the information."[11]

The points made by FitzGibbon suggested that by 1921 many Irish couples understood from personal experience the benefits of birth control and practiced it, probably using a range of means that may have included commercial contraceptives. Some possibly tried the more makeshift methods Dáil deputy Dr. Robert Rowlette referred to in 1934 when he suggested that attempts to ban contraceptives would be ineffectual because it was "common knowledge that contraceptive apparatus is manufactured with the greatest ease from the ordinary contents of any household."[12]

Although FitzGibbon saw fertility control in a positive light, it was an issue on which the medical profession was divided. In 1923, for example, Henry Corby, professor of obstetrics and gynecology at University College, Cork, published a paper in a special birth control edition of the British medical journal *The Practitioner*. Perhaps representing an older generation of doctors,[13] one that found the subject distasteful, Corby was "thoroughly convinced that the use of contracepts [sic] of any kind is distinctly dangerous to health." Believing that an exchange of body fluids during sexual intercourse was essential for the well-being of both partners, he condemned the use of chemical spermicides, coitus interruptus, and condoms, equating the use of the latter with masturbation, a practice that he believed damaged the nervous system and led to impotence in men and loss of "natural feeling" in women. Corby also rejected social and economic arguments for family limitation but indicated that he had recommended safe-period fertility control when the woman's health was at risk. Because the approximate dates of the safe period were not confirmed in medical literature until 1930, it is not surprising that in the case he quoted as an example, the woman became pregnant.[14]

In 1924, the Catholic Church's position on birth control was laid out in an article by anti–birth controller Reverend Vincent McNabb published in the *Catholic Medical Guardian*. It made it clear that women's health considerations were irrelevant to church policy and warned that doctors who advised women that they "ought" to avoid pregnancy because of a danger to themselves or their unborn child breached Catholic medical ethics. McNabb emphasized that in the church's view the primary purpose of sexual intercourse was procreation, and the only permissible methods of birth control involved "conjugal and virginal chastity."[15]

Opponents of birth control scored a success when they influenced the report of the 1926 Evil Literature Committee and the subsequent 1929 Censorship of Publications Act (1929/21). The committee was a state inquiry established because Ireland had signed the 1923 International Convention for the Suppression of the Circulation and Traffic in Obscene Publications. This convention required signatories to examine the need for national legislation on "obscene publications" and to define which printed matter would come within the scope of new laws.[16] Delegates from the Catholic Truth Society of Ireland and a number of witnesses organized by Catholic social movement activist and Jesuit priest Father Richard Devane, implied that imported British birth control "propaganda" in the form of books, pamphlets, advertising material, newspaper, and magazine articles was widely available, at least in Dublin. They suggested that literature explaining the use of contraceptives was obscene and that knowledge of contraception encouraged sexual activity outside marriage. Effective use of contraceptives required sex education, and one passage, marked for the committee's attention, illustrated how candidly such pamphlets purveyed sexual knowledge:

> This fertilization is brought about by the insertion of the penis into the vagina of the female. The excitement of sexual intercourse causes the penis to grow stiff and rigid, enabling it to be worked up and down the vagina, and when the height of sexual excitement is reached, the semen is shot from the penis into the vagina, from whence it may penetrate to the womb, and if it comes into contact with any active female germs, fertilization is certain to take place, resulting ultimately in the birth of a child.[17]

The committee's report perhaps inevitably stated that aspects of birth control literature provoked "the strongest repugnance" and that it opened "the way to sensual indulgence for those who desire to avoid the responsibilities of the married state." It noted that Ireland's inherited British law on the dissemination of information on contraception was "laxer" than that in British dominions and many European states. The report acknowledged the evidence of Protestant witnesses, however, that "the growing opinion in Great Britain in support of the propaganda is beginning to exist in the Saorstát, and the practices recommended to be followed by a limited number of persons." Separating concerns about birth control literature and the use of contraceptives, and despite recommending strict control of the former, the report also acknowledged Protestants' view that attempting to prohibit contraceptive use "would be an unwarranted interference with individual liberty." It recommended "[t]hat the sale and circulation, except to authorised persons, of books, magazines and pamphlets that advocate the unnatural prevention of conception should be made illegal, and be punishable by adequate penalties." The committee did not define who the "authorised persons" might be, but it acknowledged the view of Protestant witnesses that the medical profession might be considered an appropriate channel through which to direct information about birth control.[18] When the birth control sections of the censorship bill that followed from the committee's report were discussed in the Dáil and Senate, there was general acceptance that censorship of birth control information was necessary, and although Protestant senator Sir John Keane argued the case of women with medical reasons for avoiding pregnancy and those living in poverty for whom childbearing could be the "last straw," he accepted that information on contraception might be misused.[19] The resulting sections of the 1929 Censorship of Publications Act defined the advertising of contraceptive drugs and appliances as "indecent and obscene" and made it an offense to publish or sell publications advocating contraception or abortion. This step may have marked a return to Victorian understandings of "obscenity," but the legislation applied only to printed matter. Contraceptives remained legal, and material in state files indicates that advertising and information trickled into the country in the early 1930s.[20]

Although there was acknowledgment in 1926 that a pro–birth control strand of public opinion existed in Ireland, the official position not only of the Roman Catholic Church but of all the major Christian churches was that the use of contraceptives was unacceptable. A willingness to take account of women's experiences and health needs influenced the 1930 Lambeth Conference of the Anglican Church, of which the Protestant Church of Ireland was a part, when it accepted that the practice of contraception might be justified where "a birth would involve grave danger to the health, even to the life of the mother, or would inflict upon the child to be born a life of suffering; or where the mother would be prematurely exhausted, and additional children would render her incapable of carrying out her duties to the existing family." The conference also accepted that women and men should be perceived as equal partners, that sexual relations within marriage were not solely for the purpose of procreation but had a spiritual dimension, and that this 'sex-life . . . is a primary part of the process of soul-education."[21] Thirteen Church of Ireland bishops attended the conference, and the bishops of Cork and Derry, the Right Reverend C. B. Dowse and Right

Reverend J. I. Peacock, were members of the committee that drew up the birth control resolution. Prominent clergyman and church scholar Canon James Blennerhassett Leslie, responding to the Lambeth decision in a September 1930 article in the *Church of Ireland Gazette,* suggested that any other conclusion would have "run counter to biological and medical science," which the bishops had on another occasion declared was "a Revelation of God."[22]

Canon Leslie's article was one of the few containing positive references to birth control published in Ireland in the 1930s. In part, this lack of a positive response may have been owing to the increasing effectiveness of the 1929 censorship legislation, but it was probably also owing to a series of developments that demonstrated the increasing political power of the Catholic Church and inhibited opposition. A key step was Pope Pius XI's encyclical letter *Casti Connubii,* issued on the last day of December 1930. It reaffirmed the Roman Catholic position, condemning contraception, sterilization, and abortion as "criminal abuse" of marriage and dismissing arguments about family limitation on women's health grounds as "false and exaggerated."[23] For sincere Catholics, this papal pronouncement must have been hugely important. It provided ammunition for a Catholic anti–birth control lobby that had begun to ask questions about Protestant medical ethics in the light of the Lambeth Conference decision. In a published February 1931 Lenten Pastoral, the Catholic archbishop of Tuam, Dr. Thomas Gilmartin, raised objections to the appointment of Protestant doctors to state dispensary posts.[24] In the same month, the *Catholic Bulletin* published an anonymous article attacking the Protestant ethos of the Trinity College, Dublin, medical school and calling for Catholic resistance in the face of the Lambeth decision. This resistance, in effect, would associate opposition to birth control with Irish nationalism.[25] In July 1931, when discussing a draft pharmacy act, anti–birth controllers within the Pharmaceutical Society of Ireland forced the society's council to accept a clause condemning the sale and supply of contraceptives or abortifacients as unethical.[26]

In mid-February 1931, Archbishop John Harty of Cashel privately made it clear to the government that he would denounce the appointment of any Protestant dispensary doctor within his diocese. The Cumann na nGaedheal government of conservative Catholic W. T. Cosgrave might have been expected to sympathize with the hierarchy's position, and, indeed, a memorandum of the period notes: "Government prepared to meet the wishes of the Bishops, and to make the sale of contraceptives illegal, as far as the law is competent to do so."[27] This option was not acted on. With Protestants' employment rights protected by the 1923 Constitution, Cosgrave warned the bishops that to publicly disagree with the government would undermine both its authority and church–state relations.[28]

Though the crisis died down, the medical profession felt the repercussions of this highlighting of ethical differences between Catholic and Protestant doctors. Tony Farmar has pointed out that Protestant doctors saw their incomes from private practice fall and that in July 1931 the archbishop of Dublin, Dr. Edward Byrne, as chairman of the board of the National Maternity Hospital, made it clear that he would block the election of a Trinity College graduate to the post of master of the hospital.[29] There were fears, too, that the birth control matter might affect the job prospects of Catholic National University of Ireland graduates who hoped to work in Britain.[30] This issue became even more sensitive from July 1930, when the British Ministry of Health formally recognized the relationship between birth control and women's health and authorized local authority clinics to provide contraceptive advice to married women whose health might be threatened by pregnancy.

Considerations around their employment as much as the 1929 Censorship Act may have silenced many pro- and anti–birth controllers within the medical profession, but some must have seen the effects on women of too frequent childbearing. In 1933, Bethel Solomons, the Jewish master of the Rotunda Hospital, Dublin, addressed the issue of contraception only indirectly when he wrote on the potentially tragic consequences of some health problems during pregnancy in a paper published in the *Irish Journal of Medical Science*. He warned that "women with nephritis should not become pregnant; so long as they do there will be deaths," and that those suffering "decompensated cardiac disease should not marry, and if they do, they should not become pregnant or they will surely die."[31] In a 1934 *Lancet* paper, "The Dangerous

Multipara," Solomons listed the complications associated with multiple pregnancies, including rupture of the uterus, kidney damage, eclampsia and other forms of toxemia, hemorrhage, contracted pelvis resulting in disproportion or malpresentation, placenta praevia, and morbidly adherent placenta. He argued that risks to the health and life of women increased steadily after the fifth pregnancy and that the maternal death rate among those bearing a tenth child was five times that of all women in pregnancy. The article's message was that family limitation was essential to the reduction of maternal morbidity and mortality rates, but even in a British publication Solomons did not risk explicitly advocating contraception, something that by the 1930s might have impacted his career in Ireland.[32]

If censorship was intended to route information on contraception through the medical profession and had apparently inhibited advocacy of birth control, why was it found necessary to introduce a prohibition on contraceptives? A recommendation on restricting access to contraceptives was made in the 1931 report of the six-member Committee on the Criminal Law Amendment Acts (1880–85) and Juvenile Prostitution (the Carrigan Committee).[33] Established in 1930 to review existing legislation on sexual crime, contraception was a secondary issue for the committee, but, like the Evil Literature Committee, it associated access to contraceptives with sexual promiscuity. A decade after FitzGibbon made his observations on family limitation, this committee's impression was that contraceptive use was "extremely prevalent, not only in the cities and larger towns, but also in villages and remote parts of the South and West of the country. . . . [S]o common in some places were [such] articles in use that there was no attempt to conceal the sale of them, and places were mentioned to which the supply of such articles comes regularly by post to recognised vendors."[34] Although one member, Jesuit priest Reverend John Hannon, called for a prohibition on contraceptives, the committee recommended that access should be restricted through legislation similar to the 1920 Dangerous Drugs Act (10 and 11 Geo V, c.66)—that is, in certain cases at least, doctors might prescribe contraceptives, and authorized stockists might supply them.[35] The Carrigan report was judged too controversial for publication, but a small all-party committee of Dáil deputies (the Geoghegan Committee), chaired by Minister for Justice James Geoghegan, was established in 1932 to consider the Carrigan recommendations and agree which measures would be included in a Criminal Law Amendment bill.[36]

Although Geoghegan had been one of the Catholic Truth Society of Ireland delegates to the Evil Literature Committee, the committee did not recommend a ban. A November 1933 Department of Justice memorandum indicated that the committee members considered that the implications of banning contraceptive drugs had been inadequately researched and that they should not be included in a prohibition. On contraceptive appliances, the Geoghegan Committee accepted that "it would be unduly severe on persons who did not regard the use of such appliances as improper, and who were advised by their Doctors to employ them, to prohibit completely the importation and sale of such appliances."[37] The outline for legislation drafted by the committee in 1933 allowed that "qualified medical practitioners should have power to prescribe and to supply such appliances to their patients." They would, however, be required to keep registers of supplies received and "full particulars of the persons to whom such appliances were supplied."[38]

How, then, was this intention translated into a prohibition? Sean T. O'Kelly, Fianna Fáil minister for the Department of Local Government and Public Health, appears to have been one of those responsible for that change. At an early stage in the drafting of legislation, he declared himself "unable to concur in the instruction . . . so far as it empowers qualified medical practitioners to prescribe and supply the appliances in question to their patients."[39] O'Kelly's position on the women's health issue—presumably that of the government, of which he was vice president—was made clear when he addressed a September 1933 League of Nations meeting in Geneva: "The practice of contraception for any purpose was abhorrent to the people of many countries, including Ireland. The association of such recommendations with measures taken for maternal welfare would be calculated to bring health centres into disrepute in the minds of the faithful and to nullify the efforts made by the governments in the sphere of public health."[40]

Three months later, when the proposed legislation was discussed at an Executive Council (cabinet) meeting on 8 December 1933, O'Kelly was delegated to obtain "authoritative advice" on the matter.[41] It is not clear whether the advice was to be legal or theological—it was probably both—but the result was communicated to the Geoghegan Committee: "[A]ll appliances and substances for contraception are to be definitely prohibited and no exceptions whatever are to be made."[42] One committee member, the Protestant Trinity College TD, Professor W. E. Thrift, objected and insisted that "a doctor should be allowed to import and distribute such articles without being guilty even of a technical offence."[43] It was clear, however, that the Executive Council had no intention of making allowances for non-Catholic thinking on contraception.

Since the political parties had agreed to accept the Criminal Law Amendment bill without debate in the Dáil, and censorship meant it would be difficult to ignite public discussion, the possibility of a challenge to the contraception section already seemed remote. The only Dáil deputy to make a stand against the prohibition was Dr. Robert Rowlette, professor of materia medica and pharmacy at Trinity College, who had experience of the problems faced by the parents of large working-class families through his work in the Charitable Infirmary in Jervis Street, Mercer's, and Sir Patrick Dun's hospitals. Rowlette warned that a prohibition would have "very grave effects on the health of respectable and virtuous married women" whose medical history meant that pregnancy could be a health or life-threatening condition and argued that "a considerable number of people both in this and in other countries" did not object to the use of contraception in such circumstances.[44] A number of senators made similar statements. Sir John Bagwell, for example, argued that contraceptives were "justifiable when it means the prevention of disease, the avoidance of injury to health, and possibly danger to life. That is a view held by quite respectable, good living citizens. . . . It is a very frequent thing to have contraceptives used by women under medical advice, responsible medical advice."[45]

Protestors were in the minority, however, and the legislation passed. In August 1935, a consignment of quinine pessaries ordered by Henry

Bell Ltd., a Waterford chemist's shop, was confiscated and destroyed. Charged under the new legislation, Bell Ltd. argued that it was "bound to keep in stock every species of drug which might alleviate suffering" and that the pessaries could be used for purposes other than contraception.[46] The Probation Act was applied in this case. By contrast, in 1936 a Fownes Street, Dublin, store owner received a sentence of six months with hard labor, reduced on appeal to the maximum £50 fine, for stocking fifty skin condoms and an unspecified quantity of rubber condoms.[47] The message was driven home–the Irish Free State was a Catholic state—and a statement of distance between British and Irish cultures had been made.

What were the effects of the introduction of the prohibition? Beneath the churchmen and politicians' rhetoric lay the untold stories of women who suffered health problems and for whom pregnancy was a death sentence. For such women and their partners and for those on limited incomes, the "perpetual nightmare" identified by FitzGibbon must have been deepened by the reduction in access to both information and increasingly reliable options. Many, presumably the majority, accepted Catholic teaching on birth control. Some with knowledge and experience of contraceptives imported them in plain packets or smuggled them from Northern Ireland or Britain. There remained the less reliable alternative of withdrawal and the methods acceptable to the Catholic Church, abstention and the safe period.[48] In the decades following the ban, however, Dr. Michael Solomons (son of Bethel Solomons) had patients who, when advised to control their fertility, confided that "abstinence from sex during an 'unsafe period' required a degree of self-control unknown to their husbands."[49] Caitriona Clear has pointed out that by the 1950s Irish doctors were world experts on the "grand multipara."[50] It is arguable that the ban delayed the emancipation of Irish women—not least by subordinating their rights to life and health to their reproductive functions.[51]

12

"A Probable Source of Infection"

The Limitations of Venereal Disease Policy, 1943–1951

Susannah Riordan

O n 4 July 1951, Ireland's Department of Health inspector Dr. P. R. Fanning noted that "it is very doubtful if it is politic or possible to establish a VD [venereal disease] service that could be described as wholly satisfactory."[1] This remark, written in the immediate aftermath of the "mother-and-child scheme" controversy, might be taken as a speculative comment on the likely response of religious and medical opinion to such a service. In part it was, but it was also an epitaph to eight years of futile efforts to address Ireland's venereal disease problem in the Department of Local Government and Public Health and its later version the Department of Health. And although the Catholic Church and the medical profession had played some part in the failure, the main responsibility lay with the politicians and administrators. Successive attempts had fallen victim to internal politics, abrupt policy changes, political dogmatism, and poor drafting. Throughout the period, only two factors remained constant: an unwillingness to challenge the climate of secrecy surrounding these diseases and an adherence to gendered behavioral stereotypes that was politically useful but administratively counterproductive. These factors were interrelated. One of the victims of the department's policy of discretion was its own capacity to reach informed decisions.

A scheme for the diagnosis and treatment of venereal disease in Ireland had been established in 1917. Following the recommendations of the Royal Commission on Venereal Diseases, which reported in 1916, local authorities were empowered to establish free clinics with 75 percent of the cost reimbursed by central government. By 1922, schemes were functioning only in Dublin City Borough and in Dublin, Kildare, Wicklow, and Monaghan counties, all served in practice by clinics in Dr. Steevens' and Sir Patrick Dun's hospitals in Dublin.[2] In 1919, concerns about the treatment of former servicemen led to the provision of free supplies of Salvarsan (the specific remedy for syphilis made available by Paul Erlich in 1910) or its substitutes to qualified general practitioners in counties without a venereal disease scheme.[3]

In 1924, prompted by the army's concerns about its rates of venereal infection, an interdepartmental committee of inquiry was established by the Departments of Defence, Justice, and Local Government and Public Health. By the time the committee reported in March 1926, the army had addressed its problem through the adoption of disinfection stations.[4] However, the report, based on military statistics, countered the prevalent view that venereal disease was primarily spread by prostitutes and argued that it represented a significant public-health problem among the civilian population. The report recommended that venereal diseases should become notifiable (anonymously in the first instance, but by name if the patient refused or discontinued treatment). It further recommended a range of measures designed to improve the education of medical professionals and the Local Government and Public Health minister's powers to compel local authorities to establish treatment schemes.[5]

The Department of Local Government and Public Health dismissed the report on the grounds that it had not proved that venereal disease was a significant problem in the civilian population, that recommendations dealing with prostitution, prisoners, and inmates of public institutions were the responsibility of other departments, and that the proposed scheme of notification ran counter to the existing principle of confidentiality.[6] The department also opposed publication of the report, against the will of its signatories and the cabinet, but after consultation with the Catholic archbishop of Dublin the report was suppressed.[7]

Between 1926 and 1951, venereal disease schemes were established in the Cork, Limerick, and Waterford county broughs and in all counties except Cork, Donegal, Dublin, Kilkenny, Mayo, Meath, Sligo, the North Riding of Tipperary, and Waterford.[8] The preparations available free to general practitioners were extended in 1948 to cover a range of therapeutic substances, including penicillin.[9] However, despite its "innovating tradition" in the period,[10] the Department of Local Government and Public Health proved remarkably resistant to change in the treatment of venereal disease. None of the legislative or educational recommendations of the 1926 report was implemented.[11] No significant developments occurred between 1922 and 1942, and the annual reference to venereal disease in the department's report was little more than a complacent footnote. Indicating that the schemes were succeeding in reaching patients where and when treatment was most required, it acclaimed the generally downward trend in the number of cases treated at the Steevens and Dun hospitals (the only statistics available between 1924 and 1944) (see fig. 12.1), and the hospitals described fluctuations in either the total figure or the ratio of in-patients to out-patients.[12]

The single file that contains the department's general correspondence on venereal disease between 1930 and 1953 bears witness to its zeal in avoiding unnecessary expenditure but otherwise suggests a lack of enthusiasm and even of expertise. In May 1932, for example, a woman from Sligo was informed that although no free scheme was available in her county, her medical practitioner could apply for free supplies of Salvarsan—information that would have proved of little value to her given that she was suffering from gonorrhea, not syphilis.[13]

From 1940, the venereal disease rates began to rise (as figure 12.1 shows). The early years of the decade were marked by a new level of concern among medical professionals, welfare organizations, and public representatives, although there was no consensus on the causes or appropriate response. The annual reports by county medical officers of health (CMOs) occasionally prompted local venereal panics.[14] Reports from the army and turf camps indicated rising levels among recruits.[15] Some blamed returned emigrants for the rise. In April 1944, an anonymous letter reported that one such man, now working at Drumlish

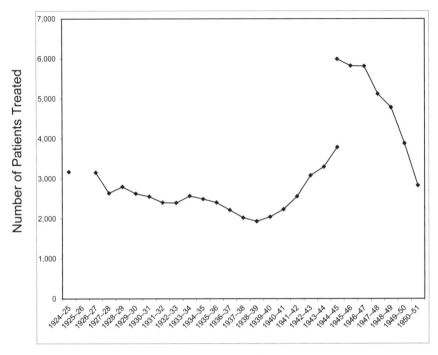

12.1. Patients treated under venereal disease schemes, 1924–51. Between 1924–25 and 1944–45, the only published figures were those from Dr. Steevens' and Sir Patrick Dun's hospitals. In 1951, estimated figures from all schemes dating back to 1944–45 were published for the first time. *Source:* Data compiled from Department of Local Government and Public Health reports for the years 1925–45 and Department of Health, *Report* (Dublin: Department of Health, 1950–51).

creamery, was "all swarmed with clap or that dirty disease that is contracted by bad living,"[16] and questions were asked in the Oireachtas (Parliament) as to what measures were being taken to examine and quarantine people entering the country.[17]

Two new studies drew attention to worrying patterns. In March 1942, it was reported that Wassermann reaction tests (antibody tests for syphilis) conducted on all women attending the Rotunda Hospital's antenatal clinic had led to a positive result in 4 percent of cases. The hospital's usual policy of testing "suspected individuals" traditionally produced positive results of 1.0 to 1.5 percent. The implication was that syphilis went undetected in 75 percent of women's cases.[18]

The second study, of patients attending Dr. Steevens' Hospital, was published by a surgeon at that hospital, J. C. Cherry, in June 1943. Cherry identified three key problems: that women tended not to present for treatment (the present increase being almost totally accounted for by male cases); that the rate of defaulting, or failure to complete treatment, among male patients was higher than 50 percent for syphilis and 75 percent for gonorrhea; and that patients who presented late did so as a result of lack of information about treatment facilities. He argued that patients were also deterred by inconvenient clinic times, long delays, and a lack of privacy. But Cherry's main argument was that non- and late presentation and defaulting could best be addressed by the provision of information, and he warned against the social consequences of thousands of infected soldiers and workers returning to Ireland, "where everything militates, both materially and morally, against helping them to continue treatment."[19]

Public discussion of venereal disease was becoming increasingly acceptable. This change may reflect an awareness of the groundbreaking publicity campaign launched by the British Ministry of Health in 1942,[20] but the most direct impetus was the May 1944 request by the Catholic archbishop of Dublin, John Charles McQuaid, that Jervis St. hospital should establish a venereal disease clinic.[21] This initiative prompted the *Irish Times* to report on the enthusiasm of a group of "prominent Dublin doctors" for a publicity campaign among other measures.[22] The *Journal of the Medical Association of Éire* more cautiously emphasized the moral aspects of disease and recommended that consultation should take place between civil servants, medical professionals, and the church as to the benefits of such a campaign.[23] On 20 June 1944, Minister for Local Government and Public Health Seán MacEntee was asked in the Dáil whether his department had taken any steps to cope with the spread of venereal disease. The *Irish Times* regarded his reply—a simple "yes"—as a significant policy u-turn.[24] In fact, it was typically both correct and misleading.

Since April 1943, the Department of Local Government and Public Health had been giving new attention to venereal disease, and consideration was given to consulting religious leaders about a publicity campaign.[25] MacEntee and his colleagues surveyed general practitioners as to incidences of privately treated cases, and the results, completed in April 1944, indicated a substantial increase—from 1,940 cases in 1938 to 2,938 in 1943. It was believed that the results yielded an underestimate because only 104 of 960 Dublin practitioners responded.[26] Private practitioners' reluctance to supply information would continue to prove significant.

The department also began to consider the possibility of developing a uniform scheme of local-authority clinics. Between January and September 1944, the department's Public Health and Public Assistance sections debated whether county homes or county hospitals were more suited to the purpose. The debate centered around which institution offered greater anonymity but reflected the Public Assistance Section's fears that a uniform scheme would transfer responsibility for venereal disease from the Public Health Section to it.[27] The discussion was suspended when the two sections agreed that the majority of existing local schemes were adequate and halted in November by newly appointed chief medical adviser Dr. James Deeny pending research into the treatment implications of penicillin.[28] Although officials continued to give periodic attention to schemes for improving the existing facilities for diagnosis and treatment, these schemes were overtaken by alternative proposals devised by Deeny and, ultimately more successfully, by the parliamentary secretary with responsibility for public health, Dr. Con Ward.

In his contribution to the debate, medical inspector Dr. C. E. Lysaght argued that "if any of us who have written in this file had the misfortune to contract V.D.," this person would consult his general practitioner, and most sufferers would take this course. Public clinics were of limited value because they were likely to be attended by "only the most degraded and poorest type of persons."[29] The belief—unsupported by empirical evidence—that venereal disease sufferers who were not treated privately were inclined to avoid treatment or to default was at the heart of Deeny's and Ward's proposals. Both sought to address the epidemiological aspects of venereal disease, emphasizing the control as well as the treatment of disease, and both sought to give CMOs the responsibility for case finding and case holding.

Deeny proposed to make venereal diseases anonymously notifiable.[30] In addition to providing accurate statistics, it was hoped that this measure would give CMOs insight into the geography of infection and permit them to investigate contacts. This approach had been recommended by the 1926 report and had recently become favored by elements of public opinion, perhaps reflecting further British developments in the form of Defence Regulation 33B. This regulation, issued in November 1942, compelled anyone named as the source of infection by two or more patients to undergo examination and treatment.[31] Both the British and Irish initiatives were posited on the importance of vectors of disease, sources of multiple infections (presumably prostitutes) who could be dealt with without threatening the anonymity of those who reported them.

Deeny also proposed to involve private practitioners in case finding and case holding. He proposed that in addition to free therapeutic material and their normal fees, such practitioners should be paid 10s for every notified case of gonorrhea treated until cured and 6s for each intravenous injection and 3s.6d for each nonintravenous injection administered in a case of syphilis.[32]

The secretary of the Department of Local Government and Public Health, James Hurson, was opposed to the scheme.[33] The Department of Finance was also initially hostile. Local Government and Public Health offered no evidence that the proposal would induce patients who would otherwise not seek treatment to do so and admitted that its estimate of the cost, £3,500, was a guess.[34] Finance Secretary M. A. Kiely unearthed a copy of the 1926 report—with such difficulty that she was convinced that no one in Local Government and Public Health was aware of its existence—and discovered that none of the report's recommendations on medical education had been effected. She argued that Local Government and Public Health had contributed to the medical profession's unwillingness to address venereal disease and that "the suggestion that doctors should be bribed to attend V.D. patients is, I think, most objectionable in principle and the fact that the bribe suggested is probably inadequate does not make things any better."[35]

Nonetheless, the scheme was approved on a trial basis by Finance Assistant Principal Louis Fitzgerald after "a very full discussion" by telephone with Deeny.[36] This decision is intriguing, and still more so is Local Government and Public Health's refusal to entertain Finance's suggestion that publication of the details of the public schemes would be more advantageous. In formal submissions, it was merely stated that publicity was not thought advisable.[37] Finance officials were informally told that there was clerical opposition to such a move.[38] There is no record of such opposition in the Local Government and Public Health's venereal disease files, in the minutes of the meetings of the Catholic hierarchy in the 1940s, or in the correspondence between Archbishop McQuaid and the Department of Local Government and Public Health. Perhaps soundings of clerical opinion had been taken, but it is curious that such a key decision should be taken in an apparently casual manner. It suggests that the department's interest in publicity was at best half-hearted.[39]

Deeny's scheme was developed until September 1946, when it was suddenly abandoned in favor of the venereal disease provisions contained in Dr. Con Ward's public health bill of 1945, which later found expression in the Health Act of 1947 (1947/28) sponsored by minister for health Dr. Jim Ryan.[40]

The infectious diseases provisions of the 1945 bill that were intended to apply to venereal diseases were enacted almost without alteration under the 1947 act and became operative under the Infectious Disease Regulations of 1948 (SI No. 99/1948).[41] Although section 38 of the 1947 act included additional safeguards, it retained the power proposed to be given to CMOs under the controversial section 29 of the 1945 bill to order the compulsory detention of a person who was "a probable source of infection with an infectious disease" until satisfied that "such person is no longer a probable source of infection."[42]

Responsibility for this new emphasis on compulsion lies primarily with Ward, who had indicated from the time he entered the Dáil in the that he shared the view that venereal disease sufferers either went to private practitioners or remained untreated. Instead of the government's wasting money on free schemes, he had stated in 1928, "people suffering from this disease should be isolated until they are certified to be cured."[43] They were irresponsible and dangerous, he had commented a year later: "[T]he people who contract this disease are people who will spread it. . . . It is very often spread innocently through lavatories, towels, drinking utensils, etc. I say in all seriousness that the public should be adequately and completely protected from contracting these contagions in that innocent way."[44]

To the Dáil's surprise, Ward repeated his insistence that venereal diseases were frequently spread by nonsexual means almost twenty years later during the debates on the 1945 bill.[45] However, his failure to apply those sections of the bill dealing with the movement of persons, the disposal of furnishings and utensils, and the sale or letting of dwellings to venereal diseases suggests a possible dichotomy between his medical understanding and his political understanding of venereal infection.[46] Fear—and fear that could be openly admitted—was a useful ally.

Minister Jim Ryan did not refer to "innocent" infection, but he took pains to associate compulsory measures with venereal disease and with prostitution: "I now say that one of the first and most important conditions which these provisions are intended to counter is the spread of venereal disease contracted from prostitutes soliciting in the streets."[47] He argued later that "there is no chance, I am afraid, of cleaning up that disease except we get the prostitutes into some institution where they can be treated and that can only be dealt with under this section."[48]

This association disarmed criticism of compulsory measures, which in fact applied to a wide range of infectious diseases and all sufferers. Section 38 featured prominently in the Catholic hierarchy's protest against the infectious disease provisions of the 1947 act.[49] It is possible that this focus was deflected not only by concerns about the "mother-and-child" provisions, but also by uncertainty about the state's rights where prostitutes were concerned. Archbishop McQuaid would later agree with his adviser John A. Horgan that although "the moral theologians seem to have steered clear of these modern problems, or to offer no definite treatment," the state had a right to detain prostitutes. McQuaid added,

"[W]e are in a quite different region when we treat of ordinary persons, who are not prostitutes, male or female. In such cases the State ought not to intervene or enclose with compulsion."[50] Whether McQuaid was aware of it or not, Ryan's suggestion that the provisions of section 38 would be utilized only in the case of prostitutes led McQuaid into an uncharacteristic position of theological uncertainty.

The concerns about venereal disease voiced in 1952 by the Catholic hierarchy subcommittee established to examine the 1947 act were formulated mainly by Bishop Michael Browne of Galway and were ephemeral and ineffective. They included the suggestion that if the "reasonable precautions" that persons suffering from infectious disease were obliged to take against infecting others included the avoidance of marriage, the matter of state interference with the sacrament of marriage might arise.[51]

The lack of sustained criticism of compulsory detention is reflected in historian Ruth Barrington's suggestion that although the measure was severe, the Department of Local Government and Health could argue that it was necessary: "Many prostitutes refused to accept treatment for venereal disease and continued to spread infection. The powers of arrest and detention in the Bill were primarily aimed at such women and at tinkers, who were suspected of being primary sources of typhus infection."[52] It is certainly the case that the measure was aimed at prostitutes and travelers, persons whose civil rights had few champions. However, the argument that the compulsory detention of prostitutes was either a necessary or a valuable means of halting the spread of venereal disease was anecdotal. General Richard Mulcahy pointed out that Ward had provided information neither about the prevalence of syphilis and gonorrhea nor whether there had been any difficulty in persuading sufferers to seek treatment voluntarily, but he was a lone voice.[53] In general, deputies agreed that in the case of venereal disease "provisions that are considered drastic must . . . be considered necessary."[54] Assumptions about the source of venereal infection and the behavior of sufferers made venereal disease a special case. Even Mulcahy withdrew his objection to the provision that blood samples might be taken from patients by force in the light of Ryan's explanation that "we had some hope that . . . we might be able to deal with some of those people who are spreading venereal disease. Such people are rather intractable and rather uncooperative when they are taken into hospital." "I cannot see," Mulcahy said, "that a doctor will have to rely on that particular subparagraph in any particular case apart from that but I do think that it might be necessary in such a case."[55] The opposition was prepared to grant extraordinary powers to the state on the mere suggestion that they would be used only against venereal disease sufferers.

There was no informed debate on compulsion either among civil servants or public representatives, and the transparent weaknesses of the measure went unremarked. First, the state had no powers to compel treatment other than continued detention.[56] Second, it could not be guaranteed that someone being treated for syphilis was not infectious and likely to remain so for between two and three years. For how long were sufferers to be detained? More significant, the Department of Health (the new name of the Department of Local Government and Public Health) failed to recognize that it had already reason to doubt whether such detention was possible in the first instance.

The power to detain a person who was "a probable source of infection" derived from Emergency Powers (No. 46) Order of 1940, which had been issued following an outbreak of typhus associated with a group of travelers.[57] Under the order, warrants were issued in thirty-eight cases, none of which was venereal.[58] On two occasions prior to the introduction of the 1945 bill, requests had been made to issue such warrants, and a third case arose in October 1946.

Earlier, in April 1943, just as officials had begun to review the treatment facilities, Templemore gardai requested a warrant to detain two named women alleged to be responsible for the increased rate of gonorrhea in the Tenth Infantry Battalion.[59] And in January 1944, a corporal in the army named a woman as the source of infection for himself and two others.[60] The first request was denied.[61] The second case was referred to the Attorney General's Office, where it was argued that without a medical examination, which the minister of local government and public health had no power to compel, there was no evidence that the woman was suffering from venereal disease. Furthermore, even if she was infected, it could not be categorically stated that she was "a probable source of infection."[62] In general, it was virtually impossible to define someone as "a probable source of infection" without a blood test indicating that she or he was suffering from a venereal disease at an infectious stage and without evidence (despite Ward's views) that she or he was likely to engage in promiscuous sex.

This final point regarding the behavior of a person suspected of having a venereal disease was made starkly when the third request to issue a warrant was made in October 1946 by the Louth CMO in the case of a twenty-two-year-old woman described as a "tramp." She had been diagnosed with syphilis at an infectious stage and had declined to continue treatment.[63] Opinions were canvassed within the department. Deeny believed that the case met the criteria for detention, but that it would be impolitic in the climate surrounding the public-health bill.[64] Others had doubts, and John Garvin, principal officer of the department's Public Assistance Section, raised the point that decided the minister's course of action: "[I]n this case there is evidence of infection but not that the patient is in the habit of infecting others."[65] The gardai were instructed to report on whether the young woman's "known habits" could provide evidence that she was a "probable source of infection." The investigation resulted in a pathetic description: "While in Dundalk the girl was not known to be soliciting or importuning for immoral purposes and no complaint was made to the Garda to that effect. She sang on the streets occasionally. We have no evidence that her habits give rise to a probable source of infection, except the rumour had it she was a depraved character and the fact that she was suffering from a venereal disease."[66]

Although these cases may have encouraged Ward and Ryan's concentration on female vectors of disease, these men remained unwilling to recognize the flaws inherent in their policy of compulsory detention. This unwillingness suggests either that each was pursuing his own agenda independently of his officials or that the lines of communication in the Department of Health were ineffective or that both were manipulating public fears about venereal disease to achieve controversial means of controlling other diseases. It also highlights the department's continued failure to develop expertise in venereal disease control.

Interparty minister for the Department of Health Dr. Noël Browne added to these difficulties by attempting to marry compulsion with his department's long-term aims of expanding the facilities for treatment and making CMOs responsible for case finding and case holding.[67] The Infectious Disease Regulations of 1948 not only gave effect to the infectious disease provisions of the 1947 act but also introduced anonymous notification. Medical practitioners were now obliged to notify the CMO of each case of venereal disease they diagnosed and three months later to indicate whether the case was being adequately treated. Browne expressed the hope that such statistics would "enable us to form a better picture of the prevalence of the disease and to make arrangements for its treatment accordingly."[68]

In addition, section 13 (1) of the regulations, which applied to all infectious diseases, directed a CMO, "on becoming aware, whether from a notification under these Regulations or otherwise, of a case or an suspected case of an infectious disease or of a probable source of infection with an infectious disease in his district[,] . . . [to] make such inquiries and take such steps as are necessary or desirable for investigating the nature and source of the infection, for preventing the spread of infection and for removing conditions favourable for infection." Unlike the schemes devised by Deeny, the regulations made no direct provision to address defaulting on continued treatment—which several commentators saw as a particular problem among male patients.

In May 1949, P. Raymond Oliver claimed in the *Journal of the Medical Association of Éire* that as many as 80 percent of male patients in Dublin defaulted, compared with 20 percent in London. He attributed the problem to two main causes: lack of information and lack of follow-up care.[69] The article inspired a four-part series on venereal disease in the *Irish Times* in July that was in the main sensational, anecdotal, and inconclusive, but that provoked a lively correspondence.[70]

Browne's willingness to provide detailed answers to the *Irish Times*'s questions compared favorably with medical professionals' reluctance to go on the record. His replies were published in full and unchallenged, and he and his department emerged relatively unscathed. Between the time he was first approached for comment by the *Irish Times* investigator and the publication of the series, Browne announced in the Dáil that "a revised scheme for dealing with venereal disease is under consideration at present and will be communicated to health authorities as soon as some difficulties have been cleared up."[71]

The positive impression created by this announcement and by Browne's promotion of the 1948 regulations bore little relation to the fact that the latter were predictably proving unworkable in the case of venereal disease. This outcome had become apparent when in May 1949 two cases were brought to the department's attention. In the first instance, it had emerged during a court case that the plaintiff, a woman who traded in fruit and vegetables, was suffering from syphilis. The judge alerted the gardai to CMOs' powers to prevent persons identified as probable sources of infection from working with food. The second instance was that of a male syphilis sufferer who was known to have discontinued treatment. In both cases, a positive diagnosis had been made, but of syphilis in a noninfectious stage, and Department of Health inspector Dr. P. R. Fanning gave his opinion that no powers existed unless this diagnosis could be *proved* to the contrary.[72] A second round of debate took place as to whether any powers existed even where a diagnosis of venereal disease at an infectious stage had been made.

Financial officer E. MacArdle, whose initial reluctance to believe that the regulations were intended to apply to venereal disease bears further witness to the lack of continuity in venereal disease policy, argued that in all circumstances "a person could only be described as a potential rather than a probable source of infection."[73] Her colleague, Brendan Hensey, believed that the intention behind the 1947 and 1948 measures was to regard "anybody with VD in the infectious state [as] a probable source of infection if he is physically capable of infecting another even though he may claim that he intends not to take actions which would infect another." However, he was not convinced that the intention had been achieved as drafted, and so he recommended that legal opinion be sought.[74]

The matter was never resolved because the Department of Health's legal advisers became aware that it was irrelevant. The only circumstances in which prima facie evidence of venereal disease in an infectious stage appeared sufficient to empower CMOs to detain venereal disease sufferers or compel them to seek or continue treatment was when formal notification was received from the attending physician. However, such notification was strictly anonymous. The CMO could not officially become aware of the patient's identity. Thus, although he had the power to act, he would not have the ability to do so.[75] A decision was taken: compulsory powers ought not ordinarily to be used in cases of venereal disease, and the minister of health's express permission should be sought before using these powers in exceptional cases.[76] By June 1951, even this avenue had been closed: because the minister had been given an appellate function in cases of compulsory detention under the act, it was deemed impossible for him to give any advice whatsoever on this matter to CMOs.[77]

Although the situation in which the Department of Health found itself has elements of farce, it had a human cost. Not only had the regulations failed in practice, but they had been drawn up under the influence of behavioral stereotypes that bore little relationship to the social factors that left venereal disease untreated or inadequately treated. One such factor was parents or guardians' refusal to permit the treatment of infants. Fanning reported in July 1951 that he had been approached by CMOs in two such cases. The minister's appellate function prohibited comment, but in any case the CMOs had no power to compel treatment: "[T]he denial of adequate treatment to these infants was almost certainly calamitous."[78]

However ineffective the CMOs' powers, their formal obligations under the regulations led ironically to a further impasse when many general practitioners declined to operate the system of notification so long as the Department of Health had the power to investigate cases. In April 1950, the *Irish Times* reported that the minister of health was at odds with the medical profession over three issues: the deregulation of streptomycin, the notification of venereal disease, and the mother-and-child scheme. It was suggested that what was necessary was the "pouring of oil over troubled doctors."[79] Browne's efforts in this regard were no more successful in the case of venereal disease notification than in the other matters.

Browne's announcement that his department was considering a revised treatment scheme was accurate insofar as officials had been giving sporadic attention to this project since 1943. The *Irish Times'* renewed interest had prompted a hasty review of progress, but little else. Serious attention to the venereal disease scheme began in June 1951 following Browne's resignation. Thomas O'Sullivan, an assistant principal in the Public Health Section who had begun to take a keen interest in the subject, told Kiely of the Department of Finance that "there is still a great deal of pressure from various sources to get 'something done' about v.d. and that advantage is being taken of the present lull in the Dept. to get a move on."[80]

There was considerable reason for optimism. The official figures were falling (see fig. 12.2), and the majority of counties now had a scheme for the diagnosis and treatment of venereal disease either locally or by arrangement with an urban center. The counties that had no scheme were known to make arrangements for patients.[81] Responding to a circular issued in September 1951, the majority of CMOs claimed to be content with the existing arrangements and saw no need for the provision of local treatment centers.[82]

In a sense, the debate had come full circle. Given the failure of the notification scheme, the available statistics were no more reliable than they had been at any point over the previous thirty years, and it was impossible to judge whether the CMOs' views reflected a satisfactory venereal disease service or mere complacency.[83] Every initiative devised within the Department of Health over the previous eight years of planning either had been abandoned or had failed to work in practice, and it was unlikely that the situation could be altered. O'Sullivan spelled out the opposition that he foresaw as attending any attempt to introduce what he called a "comprehensive plan for ensuring the accuracy of statistics, the tracing of all cases and the treatment until cure of all cases."

This opposition could be based on many reasonable and unreasonable objections e.g. legitimacy of securing specimens for test by subterfuge—laboratory tests for V.D. are not extremely reliable—the disease is not infectious at all stages—infectious cases are not necessarily

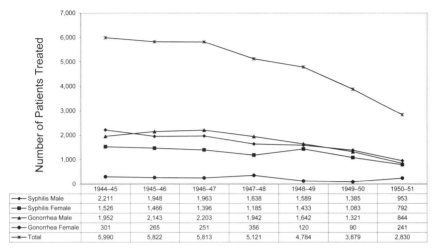

	1944–45	1945–46	1946–47	1947–48	1948–49	1949–50	1950–51
Syphilis Male	2,211	1,948	1,963	1,638	1,589	1,385	953
Syphilis Female	1,526	1,466	1,396	1,185	1,433	1,083	792
Gonorrhea Male	1,952	2,143	2,203	1,942	1,642	1,321	844
Gonorrhea Female	301	265	251	356	120	90	241
Total	5,990	5,822	5,813	5,121	4,784	3,879	2,830

12.2. Estimated numbers of patients treated under venereal disease schemes, 1944–51. *Source:* Department of Health, *Report* (Dublin: Department of Health, 1950–51).

a public danger—the liberty of the individual not alone as regards isolation and treatment but also as regards freedom from the unwelcome attention of public health staffs which can prove a source of embarrassment as regards employment, family and home life—breach of medical confidence—undue interference in what is reputed to be a lucrative portion of private practice in the case of medical practitioners who treat this disease—morality—bureaucracy, etc.[84]

It was this memorandum that elicited the remark from Fanning, one of the few officials who had contributed to every stage of the debate, that a satisfactory scheme was neither politic nor possible.

O'Sullivan, who was newer to the game, suggested that although it was unwise to fly in the face of public opinion, the department might take steps toward the formation of an "enlightened public opinion" through a discreet publicity campaign.[85] His recommendation was not accepted.

Between 1943 and 1951, considerable advances were made in the treatment of venereal disease. Penicillin was introduced; health authorities were obliged to make provision for diagnosis and cure (under the

Infectious Disease Regulations of 1948); and the network of free clinics was extended. The official figures had returned to a trend of continuous decline after the exceptional short-term increase in cases during the emergency. The crisis was over. Yet the mood within the Department of Health was clearly one of unease and suspicion that untreated venereal disease represented a significant hidden threat to the public health. There was no reason to believe that the picture that Dr. J. C. Cherry had painted in June 1943—of women who were unaware of their condition, of men who were given every incentive to discontinue treatment, and of a population of sufferers who had not the slightest idea where to go for treatment—had changed. Irish public opinion had been considered sufficiently robust to tolerate discussion of the incarceration of prostitutes, but not of symptoms or of the addresses of clinics. Ward, Ryan, and Browne had arguably focused on the pressure "to get something done" rather than on venereal disease. Officials' efforts had been marked by brief phases of enthusiasm followed by long periods either of neglecting the situation or of confronting the dilemmas posed by the most recent initiative. Despite the very real constraints described by O'Sullivan, the record of the Department of Local Government and Public Health and then the Department of Health in this regard is an undistinguished one. The social cost can only be imagined.

13

Prophylactics and Prejudice

Venereal Diseases in Northern Ireland during the Second World War

Leanne McCormick

Recent years have seen an awakening of interest in the history of venereal diseases (VD) in Ireland. The focus, however, has been largely on the southern counties and the activities of the Irish Free State.[1] As with so many areas of social and medical history, the situation in Northern Ireland has been neglected. This chapter aims to help redress this imbalance by tackling the overlooked issue of VD in Northern Ireland, focusing in particular on the Second World War years. Although research on the history of VD has often focused on decisions made at central government level, some recent studies have considered the enforcement and impact of VD legislation at a local and regional level.[2] It is apparent from this work that central governmental strategies and proclamations often differed from the reality at a local or regional level.[3] As Roger Davidson has contended, "[T]he social response to VD was heavily determined by the interaction of issues of public health, public order and public morality at a local level."[4] As the most politically divided, socially conservative, and economically disadvantaged part of the United Kingdom, Northern Ireland provides a valuable case study considering how VD legislation was implemented at a local level and how local attitudes and beliefs influenced the situation.[5] This chapter considers the years of the Second World War because they saw increased governmental attention concerning VD with the presence of large numbers of British and foreign troops, in particular Americans, which added a new perspective to VD prevention and control.

The Government of Ireland Act of 1920 (10 and 11 Geo 5, c.67) partitioned Ireland, setting up two governments and two parliaments, one for the six counties that were to form Northern Ireland and another for the twenty-six southern counties that became the Irish Free State (then Éire in 1937). The new state of Northern Ireland was faced with a situation wherein one-third of the population, Catholic nationalists, was hostile to its existence and wanted a united Ireland. The Northern Irish Parliament was dominated by Unionists who were intent on maintaining links with Britain and not relinquishing any power to Nationalists. Nationalists elected to the Northern Ireland House of Commons refused to take their seats until 1927.[6] Northern Ireland was therefore in a complicated political situation—part of the United Kingdom yet physically separated from it, politically separate from the Irish Free State yet sharing a land mass. This peculiar situation was most starkly evident during the Second World War, when Northern Ireland was at war on the side of the Allies, whereas Eire remained neutral, leaving one-quarter of the island under blackout conditions even while the other three-quarters were "lit up."

However, both North and South of the island were united in the belief that VD was largely unknown in Ireland and by their reluctance to engage in major preventative or treatment schemes. The Royal Commission on Venereal Diseases (RCVD), which was established in London in 1913 to investigate the prevalence of VD, recommended in its 1916 report that free treatment centers were set up across the United Kingdom. In Ireland, North and South, the establishment of these centers was problematic and met with resistance. There was a general opinion among local councils who were to draw up treatment schemes that this approach was not something they should be involved in, that VD not widespread, and that those infected would be better treated at a central location and not in the community.[7] In several counties in Northern Ireland, reluctance to establish treatment centers led to many having to travel to Belfast to be treated. Londonderry[8] County and County Borough demonstrated the most determined resistance, and no VD treatment scheme was implemented until 1943, when, forced by the war emergency, the government demanded treatment centers be established. Wrangling over staffing and finance issues, however, ensured that it would be several more years before the centers were eventually established.[9] The turbulent political situation of the early 1920s and the creation of new health structures on both sides of the border also hindered the implementation of treatment schemes.[10] In comparison with other parts of the United Kingdom, there was little publicity about prevention and treatment of VD in the interwar period, and it was not until the outbreak of the Second World War and in particular the arrival of US troops in Northern Ireland in 1942 that the situation began to change.

War has traditionally been associated with an increase vigilance regarding venereal infection, and it was concern about the health of the military that in the past had prompted government legislation concerning VD.[11] The Contagious Diseases Acts (CDAs) of 1864 (27 and 28 Vic., c.85), for example, were introduced in response to the high levels of VD among troops and the resultant loss of manpower.[12] During the Great War, the British government, under pressure from its allies, had introduced the Defence of the Realm Act 40d (4 and 5 Geo V, c.29), which made it an offense for any woman suffering from VD to have sexual intercourse with a soldier or to solicit a member of the military to have sex with her. Any woman suspected of doing so could be detained for examination and treatment and possibly imprisoned. This act was regarded as a return to the CDAs of the 1860s and provoked similar condemnation and campaigning from women's organizations concerning the injustice of the legislation, the condoning of a sexual double standard, and the unfair treatment of women. Although facing similar pressure from its allies during the Second World War to legislate concerning VD, the British government was understandably anxious not to provoke a similar oppositional situation.

In particular, the Americans put increased pressure on the British government to tackle the problem of VD. The United States had taken a hard line against both VD and prostitution and was conducting a prolific propaganda campaign warning against the dangers of VD. It viewed with concern the perceived lack of action by the British government. The

British government was reluctant to introduce legislation that targeted women specifically, believing there would "be an outcry if a woman of good character was arrested."[13]

However, action needed to be taken, and in January 1943 the government introduced Defence Regulation 33B. The regulation made compulsory the examination and treatment of suspected carriers of VD who were named twice by a VD patient. It applied to both men and women, with the offense being refusal of treatment.[14] Although the language used in the regulation was gender neutral, in Northern Ireland as in the rest of Great Britain 33B impacted women more heavily than men.[15] The reports given by Charles Thomson, the medical superintendant of health (MSOH) for Belfast, illustrate how women were regarded as the principal source of infection and to blame for the spread of VD. In his report of June 1943, the only potential suspect in the spread of VD he referred to was a "female infector."[16] On the Belfast Public Health Department register of people named twice as contacts by those who had VD, all thirty-seven entries were women. Of those, nineteen included the woman's full name and address, and for the other eighteen the name and address were too vague to be of any use. Thomson believed that the lack of detail about the women on the register was owing in part to the fact that "male adventurers have already fortified themselves with more or less copious draughts of wine" and that when they began to display the symptoms of VD, the "gay Lothario[s] [were] unable to give a helpful statement as to who, how, when or where!"[17] As far as the MSOH was concerned, women were "infectors," "suspects," and a grave source of danger, whereas the men involved were merely "adventurers" and "gay lotharios."

As Davidson has contended, the "social epidemiology shaping the successive drafts of Regulation 33B remained clearly directed towards sexually active *females* and it was assumed that most informants would be servicemen who had dipped into this 'reservoir' of venereal infection."[18] The US Command in Northern Ireland similarly stated that although there were no red-light districts in Northern Ireland, and the level of prostitution was low, it "must be presumed that prostitutes of whatever degree are infected with one or more venereal diseases." The report went on to explain that "American personnel cohabiting with such persons do so in the full knowledge that those women, in all likelihood are infected." As the MSOH had also argued, the US Command blamed alcohol for male indiscretions: "[T]he influence of alcohol on the venereal rate is well known. Alcohol impairs a mans [sic] judgement to the extent that he will accept the services of the lowest woman of the area and completely disregard his personal safety."[19] The implication was that men's sexual activities were simply pleasure seeking, normal activities and acceptable aspects of natural male behavior, whereas sexually active women were predatory, dangerous, and a source of disease.

Under pressure from London, the Stormont government had from 1943 on increased publicity and propaganda about VD and its treatment. The Ministry of Home Affairs placed advertisements in newspapers between February and July 1943 detailing the opening times of VD clinics and giving the "ten plain facts about VD." In addition, the chief medical officer at the Ministry of Health approved the displaying of notices on hoardings or "suitable walls."[20] The issue of where it was acceptable to display VD posters and the problem of causing offense with VD propaganda and advertising had generated debate within the Public Health Committee of the Belfast Corporation through the 1930s.[21] In particular, the Public Health Committee was concerned about displaying notices in public toilets and the fact that the Ministry of Home Affairs prohibited the posting of such announcements.[22] It was not until 1942 that the corporation asked the ministry to amend the legislation and asked the MSOH for Belfast to prepare a draft notice for display.[23]

The advertisements in newspapers were deemed successful in generating interest and inquiries. A letter to the Ministry of Health in London from its Stormont counterpart reported that there had been a large number of inquires by both telephone and letter and that the VD clinic at the Royal Victoria Hospital in Belfast had seen an appreciable increase in the number of people coming for advice and treatment.[24] The number of new cases of VD and the total number of attendances for treatment of VD in Northern Ireland as a whole did increase during the war years; however, what is also interesting is the high level of those attending for treatment who did not have VD: on average, 55 percent of those attending for the whole of Northern Ireland during the war years 1939–45 and more than 60 percent for Belfast for the same period.[25] Although there are a number of arguable reasons why this proportion was so high, including the success of publicity about treatment centers, it is nonetheless evident that there must have been considerable ignorance about VD, how the diseases were spread, and what the symptoms were to cause so many people to believe wrongly that they were infected.

Charles Thomson, the MSOH for Belfast, recognized the need for greater publicity and in particular education about VD. He was a strong advocate of sex education for young people and believed that it was only by frank discussion and openness that VD rates would decline. Thomson countered the argument that increased education about VD would put "evil thoughts into the minds of the innocent" by suggesting that because adolescents were already discussing these issues, as far as he was concerned, it would be better to educate them properly. He argued against the suppression of facts and contended that a gust of fresh air was needed because "knowledge is power."[26] Thomson returned to the issue in his annual report the following year, 1944, and encouraged the Belfast Corporation to reaffiliate itself with the Health Education Central Council as a step on the way to reinvigorate the public-health propaganda campaign. Thomson reported how sex education be brought into schools by visiting experts had been discussed, but nothing more had been done about the issue.[27] He was a lone voice on this issue, and the idea of sex education in schools did not have popular support; it was not until 1987 that the aims and objectives of sex education were actually set out by the Department of Education in Northern Ireland.[28]

Moral issues were regarded largely as the churches' remit, and local and governmental authorities were unwilling to stray into areas that had the potential to cause controversy. In 1942, for example, following a discussion by the Belfast Corporation Committee of Public Health about VD propaganda, it was decided that one of the main strategies for publicity was for the MSOH to request that church leaders speak to their younger members about the issue.[29] As noted earlier, this idea did not sit well with the MSOH, Charles Thomson, who contended that although there had been "generations of eminent preachers and the example of countless saintly lives," VD still existed. He maintained that religion was important, but it was not enough, and that educating children and trusting them with knowledge about VD were of greater value.[30]

From the first attempts to establish VD treatment centers in 1917, the belief that Northern Ireland was largely free from VD had been expressed. Local councils were reluctant to implement legislation and set up treatment centers for something they believed was not a "common experience."[31] Mr. Murnaghan, a member of the Tyrone County Council, was an extremely vocal opponent of establishing treatment centers, and his solution for the "lepers" who had VD was for the government to purchase a plot of land somewhere in West Africa and deport them to be treated there.[32]

Into the Second World War, the belief that rates were low was still being expressed. With the planned extension of VD regulations to Northern Ireland in 1942, the Ministry of Home Affairs took the line that "while the trouble is not that serious in Northern Ireland, as we cannot prevent the English people making this regulation applicable here, there would be no point raising any difficulty about it."[33] There were still those who felt that although Northern Ireland was free from VD, it was vulnerable to the spread of infection from elsewhere. For example, in 1942 Mr. McGurk, member of Parliament for mid-Tyrone, asked Sir Dawson Bates, the minister for home affairs, whether "[i]n the view of the existence of VD in Great Britain he will take steps to ensure that every person coming into Northern Ireland from Great Britain will be subject to a medical examination at the port of embarkation?" The answer, unsurprisingly, was no.[34]

The arrival of large numbers of US troops in Northern Ireland from 1942 on gave a new dimension to VD prevention. As mentioned earlier, the US military was extremely active in its efforts to prevent the spread of VD, using a variety of methods of propaganda and providing its troops with prophylactics and access to early-treatment centers. However, these methods, in particular the issuing of prophylactics, met with opposition in Northern Ireland. The US authorities described the "prejudice amongst the civil population" in Northern Ireland that prevented the establishment of prophylactic stations at US bases there. The compromise was to use the name "Aid Station" and a green light rather than "Prophylactic Station." Before these stations were established, the US unit commanders in Northern Ireland were instructed to make available enough prophylactics to meet early demand. In addition, the headquarters of the US forces in Northern Ireland issued instructions that any man departing "upon such a mission" was to "carry in his pocket a piece of non-irritating toilet soap with which he will thoroughly wash his hands and all exposed parts immediately after sexual intercourse, whether or not he has used individual prophylaxis."[35]

British troops had established Early Treatment Stations prior to the US forces' arrival. They were located across Northern Ireland in military hospitals in Belfast and Londonderry and at Victoria Barracks in Belfast and St. Patrick's Barracks in Ballymena. However, the US military authorities were evidently not convinced about the effectiveness of the British Early Treatment Stations. They advocated that regardless of what other methods were employed, the American soldier should apply prophylaxis of the American type at the earliest opportunity. This treatment involved an injection of 2 percent protargol and thereafter an application of 10 percent calomel ointment.[36]

The Welfare Committee, which was responsible for the welfare of troops in Northern Ireland, was also concerned about VD rates. When considering what measures could be taken to improve the troops' health, the committee commented that "every endeavour is being made by the military authorities to reduce the incidence of VD and tighten up the conditions regarding medical treatment." However, they questioned whether more could be done by the civil authorities to "ensure that those who will be naughty will be clean?"[37]

Some US troops were nonetheless evidently making use of the readily available prophylactics. One contemporary observer recalled a report in an Armagh newspaper that described how troops were employed in the city with spiked sticks to pick up the litter of condoms. This litter was found to be particularly bad when the American troops were leaving the city.[38] Littering of condoms was a problem wherever troops were stationed, and as a Home Office circular issued on 17 July

1944 explained, "[C]ontraceptives are left in public places, private gardens, shop fronts, shelters etc., where they cannot but give offence to decent people."[39]

It is difficult to draw definite conclusions about the VD rate among troops in Northern Ireland during the Second World War. The Ministry of Home Affairs reported in 1943 that the number of soldiers who had contracted VD in Northern Ireland was "negligible" and that the area "is in a very satisfactory state so far as it [VD] is concerned."[40] However, a report from the British Troops in Northern Ireland in February 1942 indicated that the daily number of cases for VD in hospital was about one hundred for the army, navy, and air force. The weekly average of men hospitalized was recorded as between forty and fifty, of which two-thirds came from the army. These totals, the report claimed, were "somewhat higher than in the rest of the UK." It was suggested that this greater number was owing to men being far away from home and to the lack of entertainments and sports grounds.[41] The Reverend T. Gordon Ott, an Anglican chaplain attached to the Royal Canadian Navy in Londonderry, also commented on the relatively high rates of VD amongst navy troops. He noted in March 1945 that 20 percent of Royal Canadian Navy personnel in hospital were suffering from VD.[42] Although it is possible that the sailors may have contacted the disease elsewhere, as Keith Jeffery has suggested, "it seems likely that the majority of contacts were in Northern Ireland."[43] The US Command in Northern Ireland, however, suggested that for British troops in Northern Ireland the venereal rate was low, owing, it believed, to the "high moral standards of the inhabitants."[44] The rate for US army troops based in Northern Ireland was also supposedly low and compared favorably to other parts of the British Isles according to the US Medical Corps historian Colonel J. H. McNick.[45] These favorable comments about the rates of VD from the US military may have been influenced by the need to maintain friendly relations with Great Britain both during and after the war. There were relatively high civilian rates of VD in Northern Ireland during the Second World War, so it is probable that the troop rate was also high. The fact that there was a lack of publicity and public discussion about VD is likely to have contributed to the level of infection.

The most detailed figures available to determine the prevalence and incidence of VD in Northern Ireland are for those treated at the Royal Victoria and Mater Infirmo (Mater) hospitals in Belfast. These figures show that total attendances at both hospitals—that is, the number of cases under treatment for VD, which includes those who had previously attended the center, those who had stopped attending and had returned, and new cases—grew over the war years from 8,031 in 1939 to 12,080 in 1942 before a fall to 10,708 in 1944, then rose again in 1945 to 12,175 and continued to rise to 13,116 in 1946.[46] The number of new cases treated at both the Mater Hospital and the Royal Victoria follows a similar pattern, rising from 1,006 in 1939 to 1,150 in 1943, followed by a small fall in 1944 to 1,065, before rising to 1,209 in 1945 and 1,393 in 1946. There was also a general increase in those patients whom both hospitals treated and who gave their address as outside Belfast between 1939 and 1945. The most marked increase was among those who gave their address as "Port." This group rose in number from 48 in 1940 to 153 in 1942. During this period, the number of ships docked in Belfast increased rapidly, and the Belfast docks were vastly extended. From January 1942, there was a particular increase in the number of American ships docking in Northern Ireland, which may be linked to this increase in the number of those seeking treatment.[47]

It is clear that when compared with the situation in Scotland over a similar period, there was a marked lack of discussion and interest in VD in Northern Ireland. Davidson details the moves taken by the Department of Health for Scotland to revise VD provisions and to prepare for the challenges of war, whereas the only moves taken in Northern Ireland were those forced upon it by Westminster. Davidson also refers to the debates that took place among Scottish venereologists concerning legislation and treatment within the Scottish branch of the Medical Society for the Study of Venereal Diseases and the debates and opposition around Regulation 33B from women's organizations, the churches, and medical groups.[48] There was no equivalent medical society concerned with VD in Northern Ireland, and there is no evidence of debates among clinicians concerning VD. Furthermore, there was no public debate prompted by Regulation 33B. The reasons for this silence are unclear; it may have been a reflection of a more traditional conservative Northern Irish society, where issues of a sexual nature were not discussed, or the debate in Scotland may reflect the Scots' more interventionist approach and tradition of civic authoritarianism.[49] However, consideration must be taken of the economic situation in Northern Ireland. The Northern Ireland government was financially strapped, and the amount of money available for spending in areas such as health and social services remained virtually unchanged from 1922 to 1944.[50] This state of affairs resulted in these services' failure to develop at a rate similar to such services in the rest of the United Kingdom.[51] As Greta Jones has shown, tuberculosis services were similarly restricted in the interwar period in Northern Ireland owing to financial difficulties and local authorities' reluctance to increase their financial commitments.[52] It must be concluded that if TB treatment was restricted, the treatment of VD, which carried such moral stigma, would be farther down the priority list.

Notes

Select Bibliography

Index

Notes

Introduction

1. For the classic accounts of Irish medicine, see John F. Fleetwood, *The History of Medicine in Ireland* (Dublin: Skellig Press, 1983), and Ruth Barrington, *Health, Medicine, and Politics in Ireland, 1900–70* (Dublin: Institute of Public Administration, 1987); for a more social approach, see Tony Farmar, *Patients, Potions, and Physicians: A Social History of Medicine in Ireland 1654–2004* (Dublin: A. & A. Farmar, 2004).

2. Rosemary Cullen Owens's *A Social History of Women in Ireland 1870–1970* (Dublin: Gill & MacMillan, 2005) and Lindsey Earner-Byrne's *Mother and Child, Maternity in Dublin, 1922–71* (Manchester, UK: Manchester Univ. Press, 2007) give a gendered perspective on the trials facing women in twentieth-century Ireland. Margaret Preston's *Charitable Words: Women, Philanthropy, and the Language of Charity in Nineteenth-Century Dublin* (Westport, CT: Praeger, 2004) emphasizes the importance of women in philanthropy.

3. Greta Jones and Elizabeth Malcolm, eds., *Medicine, Disease, and the State in Ireland, 1650–1940* (Cork: Cork Univ. Press, 1999).

4. William Doolin, *Wayfarers in Medicine: Studies in the Progress and Triumph of Medicine* (London: Heinemann, 1947).

5. See also Greta Jones, *Captain of All These Men of Death: The History of Tuberculosis in Nineteenth and Twentieth Century Ireland* (Amsterdam: Rodolpi, 2001). The international perspective is best analyzed in Linda Bryder, *Below the Magic Mountain: A Social History of Tuberculosis in Twentieth Century Britain* (Oxford: Oxford Univ. Press 1988).

6. For an illuminating example of the difficulties facing Dublin in 1900 from a geographer's perspective, see Joseph Brady, "Dublin at the Turn of the Century," in *Dublin Through Space and Time*, edited by Joseph Brady and Anngret Simms, 221–81 (Dublin: Four Courts Press, 2001). The international perspective is provided in Marco Breschi and Lucia Pozzi, eds., *The Determinants of Infant and Child Mortality in Past European Populations* (Udine, Italy: Forum, 2004).

7. For more on this topic, see also Oonagh Walsh, "'Tales from the Big House': The Connaught District Lunatic Asylum in the Late Nineteenth-Century," *History Ireland* (Nov.–Dec. 2005): 21–25, and Oonagh Walsh, "A Lightness of Mind: Gender and Insanity in Nineteenth Century Ireland," in *Gender Perspectives in Nineteenth-Century Ireland,* edited by Margaret Kelleher and James H. Murphy, 159–67 (Dublin: Irish Academic Press, 1997).

8. For an outstanding introduction to this topic, see Mark Finnane, *Insanity and the Insane in Post-famine Ireland* (London: Croom Helm, 1981).

9. See also Peter McCandless, "'Curses of Civilization': Insanity and Drunkenness in Victorian Britain," *British Journal of Addiction* 79, no. 1 (Mar. 1984): 49–58.

10. For temperance in Ireland, see Elizabeth Malcolm, *Ireland Sober, Ireland Free* (Dublin: Gill & MacMillan, 1986).

11. For more on nurses and midwives in Ireland, see Margaret Ó hÓgartaigh, "Flower Power and 'Mental Grooviness': Nurses and Midwives in Ireland in the Early Twentieth Century," in *Women and Paid Work in Ireland, 1500–1930,* edited by Bernadette Whelan, 133–47 (Dublin: Four Courts Press, 2000); Margaret Ó hÓgartaigh, "Nurses and Teachers in the West of Ireland in the Late-Nineteenth and Early-Twentieth Centuries," in *Framing the West: Images of Rural Ireland, 1891–1920,* edited by Ciara Breathnach, 197–214 (Dublin: Irish Academic Press, 2007); Margaret Ó hÓgartaigh, "Irish Nurses in Post World War II England," in *Encyclopedia: Migration in Europe since the 17th Century,* edited by Klaus J. Blade, Pieter C. Emmer, Leo Lucassen, and Jochen Oltmer, 494–96 (Cambridge: Cambridge Univ. Press, 2011); Gerard M. Fealy, *A History of Apprenticeship Nurse Training in Ireland* (London: Routledge, 2006); Joseph Robbins, *Nursing and Midwifery in Ireland in the Twentieth Century* (Dublin: An Bord Altranais, 2000); and Pauline Scanlan, *The Irish Nurse: A Study of Nursing in Ireland, History and Education 1718–1981* (Drunshambo, Ireland: Drumlin, 1991).

12. For the varied roles of the Rotunda, the oldest lying-in hospital in Europe in the eighteenth century, see Gary Boyd, *Dublin 1745–1922: Hospitals, Spectacle, & Vice* (Dublin: Four Courts Press, 2006). The best introduction to the Rotunda can be found in Alan Browne, ed., *Masters, Midwives, and Ladies-in-Waiting: The Rotunda Hospital 1745–1995* (Dublin: A. & A. Farmar, 1995). For an international approach, see Hilary Marland and Anne Marie Rafferty, eds., *Midwives, Society, and Childbirth: Debates and Controversies in the Modern Period* (New York: Routledge, 1997).

13. See Ciara Breathnach, *A History of the Congested Districts Board of Ireland, 1891–1923: Poverty and Development in the West of Ireland* (Dublin: Four Courts Press, 2005).

14. See also Laurence M. Geary, *Medicine and Charity in Ireland, 1718–1851* (Dublin: Univ. College Dublin Press, 2004).

15. See also Mel Cousins, *The Birth of Social Welfare in Ireland 1922–52* (Dublin: Four Courts Press, 2003). For an excellent summary of nineteenth-century governmental

administration, see Virginia Crossman, *Local Government in Nineteenth-Century Ireland* (Belfast: Institute of Irish Studies, 1994).

16. See also Sandra McAvoy, "The Regulation of Sexuality in the Irish Free State 1929–35," in Jones and Malcolm, eds., *Medicine, Disease, and the State in Ireland,* 253–66.

17. Mark Finnane's work is most illuminating on this topic; see Mark Finnane, "The Carrigan Committee of 1930–1 and the 'Moral Condition of the Saorstát,'" *Irish Historical Studies* 33, no. 128 (Nov. 2001): 519–36. For the influence of the state, see Finola Kennedy, "The Suppression of the Carrigan Report," *Studies* 89, no. 356 (2000): 354–62, and Finola Kennedy, *Cottage to Crèche: Family Change in Ireland* (Dublin: Institute of Public Administration, 2001).

18. Greta Jones and Elizabeth Malcolm, "Introduction: An Anatomy of Irish Medical History," in Jones and Malcolm, eds., *Medicine, Disease, and the State in Ireland,* 9.

1. "I Was Right Glad to Be Rid of It": Dental Medical Practice in Eighteenth-Century Ireland

1. William Doolin, *Wayfarers in Medicine: Studies in the Progress and Triumph of Medicine* (London: Heinemann, 1947).

2. For a critical assessment of this interpretative model and for the impact of the new medical history, see Colin Jones, "Pulling Teeth in Eighteenth-Century Paris," *Past and Present* 166 (Feb. 2000): 120–22.

3. Roy Porter, "The People's Health in Georgian England," in *Popular Culture in England,* edited by Tim Harris (London: Macmillan 1995), 126. The different "types" Porter alludes to ranged across a spectrum that included the scientific or clinical, the quack or commercial, the magicoreligious, and the popular or folk. The existence of so many approaches meant not only that different forms of healing were appealed to, but also—because no one possessed the diagnostic insight to identify illness with precision, the therapies or medications to ensure recovery, or the infrastructure (human and material) to provide general care—that the individual or the family unit took primary responsibility for health provision. See James Kelly, "Domestic Medication and Medical Care in Late Early-Modern Ireland," in *Ireland and Medicine in the Seventeenth and Eighteenth Centuries,* edited by James Kelly and Fiona Clark, 109–36 (Burlington, VT: Ashgate, 2009). This home care was made possible during the eighteenth century by the proliferation of commercial nostrums: see James Kelly, "Health for Sale: Mountebanks, Doctors, Printers, and the Supply of Medication in Eighteenth-Century Ireland," *Proceedings of the Royal Irish Academy* 108C (2008): 75–113.

4. The text of the charter is to be found in the records of the Guild of Barbers, Surgeons, Apothecaries, and Perukemakers, MS 1447/1, Trinity College, Dublin (TCD),

and is reprinted in Charles A. Cameron, *History of the Royal College of Surgeons in Ireland* (Dublin: Fannin, 1886), 60–65.

5. Minutes of the Guild of Barbers, Surgeons, Apothecaries, and Perukemakers, 1706–57, MS 1447/8/1, and 1714–92, MS 1447/8/1, folios 1–4, TCD.

6. See Colin Jones, "French Dentists and English Teeth in the Long Eighteenth Century: A Tale of Two Cities and One Dentist," in *Medicine, Madness, and Social History,* edited by Roberta Bivins and John V. Pickstone (Basingstoke, UK: Palgrave Macmillan, 2007), 83–84.

7. A seven years' brief of the bills of mortality for the city and suburbs of Dublin, 1712–18, in Sir John Gilbert, ed., *Calendar of Ancient Records of Dublin,* 19 vols. (Dublin: Dublin Corporation, 1889–1944), 7:578. Doubts can reasonably be posed against these bills' accuracy. According to Archbishop William King, the person responsible for drawing up the bills in 1712 made up the figures (King to the clergy of Dublin, 20 Dec. 1712, King Papers, MS 750/4/1, 90, TCD). I thank Professor S. J. Connolly for this information.

8. *Dublin Gazette,* 6 Oct. 1733, 6 Apr. 1734, 5 Apr. 1735, 5 Apr. 1737, and 8 Apr. 1738.

9. Christine Hillam, "Introduction: Dental Practice in Europe at the End of the Eighteenth Century," in *Dental Practice in Europe at the End of the Eighteenth Century,* edited by Christine Hillam (Amsterdam: Rodolpi, 2003), 18–19, 25, 28; M. L. Legg, ed., *The Diary of Nicholas Peacock, 1740–51* (Dublin: Four Courts Press, 2005), 107.

10. Bishop Edward Synge to Alicia Synge, 31 May 1751, in M. L. Legg, ed., *The Synge Letters: Bishop Edward Synge to His Daughter Alicia, Roscommon to Dublin 1746–1752* (Dublin: Lilliput Press, 1996), 282.

11. Bishop Synge to Alicia Synge, 11 Oct. 1751, in Legg, *Synge Letters,* 384.

12. Liam Swords, *A Hidden Church: The Diocese of Achonry* (Dublin: Columba Press, 1997), 114; Bishop Synge to Alicia Synge, 16 Sept. 1752, in Legg, *Synge Letters,* 470.

13. Bishop Synge to Alicia Synge, 7 June 1750, in Legg, *Synge Letters,* 196.

14. Bishop Synge to Alicia Synge, [Sept. 1752], in Legg, *Synge Letters,* 466.

15. Bishop St. George to Bishop King, 18 Apr. 1701, King Papers, MS 1995–2008, folio 788, TCD; Synge to Alicia Synge, 31 May 1751, in Legg, *Synge Letters,* 467.

16. Legg, *Diary of Nicholas Peacock,* 175 and 205.

17. Bishop Synge to Alicia Synge, 29 Aug. 1752, in Legg, *Synge Letters,* 464.

18. Bishop William Nicolson to Edward Wake, 19 Jan. and 7 Feb. 1719, Wake Papers, MS 27, folios 205, 205–8, Gilbert Library, Dublin City Library.

19. Bishop Synge to Alicia Synge, 29 Aug. 1752, in Legg, *Synge Letters,* 464.

20. Basil Cozens-Hardy, ed., *The Diary of Silas Neville, 1767–88* (Oxford: Oxford Univ. Press, 1950), cited in Roy Porter and Dorothy Porter, *Patient's Progress: Doctors and Doctoring in Eighteenth-Century England* (Stanford, CA: Stanford Univ. Press,

1989), 104, and in Roy Porter, *Health for Sale: Quackery in England, 1660–1800* (Manchester, UK: Manchester Univ. Press, 1989), 54; Legg, *Diary of Nicholas Peacock*, 203, 205.

21. Porter and Porter, *Patient's Progress*, 51.

22. Legg, *Diary of Nicholas Peacock*, 27, 203.

23. French's story is told in Bishop Synge to Alicia Synge, 4 Oct. 1751, in Legg, *Synge Letters*, 380–81; Swords, *A Hidden Church*, 114.

24. John Beresford, ed., *The Diary of a Country Parson: The Reverend James Woodforde*, 4 vols. (Oxford: Oxford Univ. Press, 1926), 1:183, 2:212; Porter and Porter, *Patient's Progress*, 22; Legg, *Diary of Nicholas Peacock*, 175.

25. Elizabeth Fagan to Lord Fitzwilliam, 15 Nov. 1766, Pembroke Estate Papers, File 97/46/1/2/8/75, National Archives of Ireland, Dublin.

26. Bishop Synge to Alicia Synge, 29 Aug. 1752 and [Sept. 1752], in Legg, *Synge Letters*, 464, 469; Porter and Porter, *Patient's Progress*, 177.

27. The fees in England ranged from 2s.6d, which was the sum paid by Woodforde (Beresford, *Diary of a Country Parson*, 1:183, 2:212), to half a guinea "at least" for drawing a tooth (Porter and Porter, *Patient's Progress*, 68). A fee of half a guinea was deemed reasonable in Ireland (Bishop Synge to Alicia Synge, [Sept. 1752], in Legg, *Synge Letters*, 466).

28. Porter and Porter, *Patient's Progress*, 168–69; Bishop Synge to Alicia Synge, 11 Oct. 1751 and 29 Aug. 1752, in Legg, *Synge Letters*, 384, 464.

29. Kelly, "Health for Sale," 75; Porter and Porter, *Patient's Progress*, 7.

30. Kelly, "Health for Sale," 75.

31. Porter and Porter, *Patient's Progress*, 6–7; L. M. Cullen, *Anglo-Irish Trade, 1660–1800* (Manchester, UK: Manchester Univ. Press, 1968), 77, 101; Hillam, "Introduction," 16; Anne Hargreaves, "Dentistry in the British Isles," in Hillam, ed., *Dental Practice in Europe at the End of the Eighteenth Century*, 195; Jones, "Pulling Teeth in Eighteenth-Century Paris," 123. Per capita sugar consumption in Great Britain rose eightfold in the eighteenth century (Warren Harvey, "Some Dental and Social Conditions of 1696–1852 Connected with St Bride's Church, Fleet Street, London," *Medical History* 12 [1968], 70–71). Colin Jones also points out that the increased "demand for false teeth and artificial palates" ("Pulling Teeth in Eighteenth-Century Paris," 123) can be attributed to the impact of both venereal disease and its mercurial cures.

32. Hillam, "Introduction," 15, 25, 28; Hargreaves, "Dentistry in the British Isles," 187.

33. Minutes of the Guild of Barbers, Surgeons, Apothecaries, and Perukemakers, 1714–92, MS 1447/8/1, folios 1–5, TCD; Roy Porter, *Bodies Politic: Disease, Death, and Doctors in Britain, 1650–1900* (Ithaca, NY: Cornell Univ. Press, 2001), 196–97.

34. Minutes of the Guild of Barbers, Surgeons, Apothecaries, and Perukemakers, 1706–57, MS 1447/8/1, folios 4–5, 7, 12, 13, 36, 40, TCD.

35. Ibid., folio 44; *Reasons for Regulating the Practice of Surgery in the City of Dublin* [Dublin: n.p., 1703], 23.

36. *Reasons for Regulating the Practice of Surgery in the City of Dublin,* 15.

37. Bishop Synge to Alicia Synge, [Sept. 1752], in Legg, *Synge Letters,* 466–67.

38. See Andrew Sneddon, "Institutional Medicine and State Intervention in Eighteenth-Century Ireland," in *Ireland and Medicine in the Seventeenth and Eighteenth Centuries,* edited by James Kelly and Fiona Clark, 137–62 (Burlington, VT: Ashgate, 2009).

39. Hillam, "Introduction," 15, 27. The information on Fauchard in this and the following paragraphs is taken from B. W. Weinberger, "Early Dental Literature," *Bulletin of the Medical Library Association* 26 (1938): 222–47; Roger King, *The Making of the Dentiste, c. 1650–1760* (Aldershot, UK: Ashgate, 1998), 89–90, 97–146; Pierre Fauchard, *Le chirurgien dentiste ou triaté des dents,* 2 vols. (Paris: n.p., 1728); Jones, "Pulling Teeth in Eighteenth-Century Paris," 118–20; J. L. Angot, "Pierre Fauchard, 1677?–1761: Dental Expert and Master Surgeon of Saint-Come of Paris," *Clio-Med* (17 Mar. 1983): 207–21, accessed at http://www.ncbi.nlm.nih.gov/entrez/query/fcgi?c md=Retrieve&db+PubMed&list_uids+6; Claude Rousseau, "La prosthese au début du XVIIIeme siecle," accessed at http://bium.univ.paris5.fr/histmed/medica/odonto.htm.

40. Jones, "Pulling Teeth in Eighteenth-Century Paris," 120–35, esp. 134–35.

41. See James Kelly, *Sir Edward Newenham: Defender of the Protestant Constitution, 1734–1814* (Dublin: Four Courts Press, 2004), 25–26.

42. See, for example, Lancelot Coelson, *The Poor Mans Physician and Chyrurgion . . . with a Method of Drawing Teeth* (London: Printed by A. M. for Simon Miller at the Starre in St Pauls Church-yard, 1656).

43. Jones, "French Dentists and English Teeth," 81.

44. Significantly, the 1686 Dublin imprint was printed "for the author." Charles Allen, *The Operator for the Teeth, Shewing How to Preserve the Teeth and Gums from All the Accidents They are Subject To* (Dublin: For the Author, 1686).

45. Ibid.; *Reasons for Regulating the Practice of Surgery in the City of Dublin;* [Operator for the Teeth]: *Curious Observations in That Difficult Part of Chirurgy Relating to the Teeth, Shewing How to Preserve the Teeth and Gums from All Accidents They Are Subject to* (Dublin: n.p., 1687), 13, 25.

46. Hargreaves, "Dentistry in the British Isles," 182.

47. Robert Munter, *History of the Irish Newspaper, 1660–1760* (Cambridge: Cambridge Univ. Press, 1966), 56; *Flying Post* (Mar. 1708), 8, 29; *Dublin Gazette* (Oct. 1709), 4, 18.

48. *Dublin Weekly Journal,* 24 Jan. 1730; *Faulkner's Dublin Journal,* 17 July 1731; William Drennan to Martha McTier, 1789, in Jean Agnew, ed., *The Drennan–McTier Letters,* vol. 1 (Dublin: Women's History Project in association with the Irish Manuscripts Commission, 1998), 330.

49. *The Post Boy,* 9 May and 14 Nov. 1715.

50. *Flying Post,* 1 Apr. 1723; *Dublin Weekly Journal,* 26 Aug. 1727 and 23 Aug. 1729. It is noteworthy that Steel's dissatisfaction with silk thread was shared by Fauchard, who recommended gold wire or waxen thread.

51. *Faulkner's Dublin Journal,* 8 Apr. 1729; *Dublin Weekly Journal,* 23 Aug. 1729 and 22 Aug. 1730.

52. Ibid.; *Faulkner's Dublin Journal,* 4 Mar. and 8 Apr. 1729; Munter, *History of the Irish Newspaper,* 60.

53. Minutes of the Guild of Barbers, Surgeons, Apothecaries, and Perukemakers, 1706–57, MS 1447, folios 31, 33, 37, 38, 41, 52, 54, 56, TCD; H. F. Berry, "The Ancient Corporation of Barber-Surgeons, or Gild of St Mary Magdalene, Dublin," *Journal of the Royal Society of Antiquaries of Ireland* 33 (1903), 237; Kelly, "Health for Sale."

54. *Doctor Audouin's Last Legacies to the World* [Dublin: n.p., 1728]; James Kelly, *Gallows Speeches from Eighteenth-Century Ireland* (Dublin: Four Courts Press, 2001), 224–26.

55. *Dublin Intelligence,* 22 Sept. 1724; *Dickson's Dublin Postman,* 7 Dec. 1724; for Dickson's retailing endeavor, see Kelly, "Health for Sale."

56. *Dublin Intelligence,* 9 July 1726, 10 Sept. 1728, 16 Mar. 1731, and 4 June 1731; *Whitehall Gazette,* 3 Oct. and 8 Dec. 1726.

57. *Dublin Daily Advertizer,* 30 Nov. 1736; *Dublin Courant,* 26 Jan. 1748; *Esdall's Newsletter,* 23 Nov. 1749; *Pue's Occurrences,* 21 July 1753; Hargreaves, "Dentistry in the British Isles," 210.

58. Minutes of the Guild of Barbers, Surgeons, Apothecaries, and Perukemakers, 1706–57, MS 1447/8/1, folios 13, 14, 17, 31, 41, 43, 44, 52, 66, TCD; *Faulkner's Dublin Journal,* 25 July 1732.

59. Minutes of the Guild of Barbers, Surgeons, Apothecaries, and Perukemakers, 1706–57, MS 1447/8/1, folios 50, 52, 65, TCD; *Faulkner's Dublin Journal,* 4 Mar. 1729, 8 Apr. 1729, 24 Jan. 1730, 11 Sept. 1731, and 27 Jan. 1733; *Dublin Weekly Journal,* 7 Aug. 1731; *Dublin Evening Post,* 10 Dec. 1734; *Dublin Gazette,* 7 May 1737.

60. *Faulkner's Dublin Journal,* 11 Aug. 1730, 17 July 1731, 12 Feb. 1732, and 25 July 1732.

61. *Dublin Courant,* 14 Feb. 1747; *Dublin Weekly Journal,* 24 Jan. 1730; *Universal Advertiser,* 23 Sept. 1755.

62. Bishop Synge to Alicia Synge, 4 and 11 Oct. 1751, 16 Sept. 1752, in Legg, *Synge Letters,* 380–81, 384, 469, 470.

63. *Dublin Courant,* 14 Feb. 1747.

64. Bishop Synge to Alicia Synge, 4 Oct. 1751, in Legg, *Synge Letters,* 380.

65. Quoted in Vincenzo Guerini, *A History of Dentistry* (Philadelphia: Lea & Febiger, 1909), 266–67, cited in Legg, *Synge Letters,* 380.

66. Dr. Guiovani, *A Treatise on the Disorders of the Teeth and Gums, to Which Are Added Directions for Using the Liquid Paste* [Dublin: n.p., c. 1770].

67. Kelly, "Health for Sale"; Hillam, "Introduction," 24.

68. Kelly, "Health for Sale"; Hargreaves, "Dentistry in the British Isles," 188–90.

69. Weinberger, "Early Dental Literature," 223–24, 237–38; Jones, "French Dentists and English Teeth," 84–85.

70. *Universal Advertiser*, 22 Sept. 1753.

71. Friedrich Hoffmann, *A Treatise on the Teeth, Their Nature, Structure Formation, Beauty, Connection, and Use, in Which the Disorders Are Enumerated; and the Remedies Annexed*, 4th ed. (Dublin: n.p., 1760).

72. John Hunter, *The Natural History of the Human Teeth, Explaining Their Structure, Use, Formation, Growth, and Diseases* (London: J. Johnson, 1771); quote from Roy Porter, "The Eighteenth Century," in *Western Medical Tradition: 800 BC–AD 1800*, edited by L. I. Conrad, Michael Neve, Vivan Nutton, Roy Porter, and Andrew Were (Cambridge: Cambridge Univ. Press), 439; copies listed in *English Short Title Catalogue, 1473–1800*, 3rd ed. (London: Primary Source Microfilm, 2003).

73. Jones, "French Dentists and English Teeth," 83–84; Thomas Berdmore, *A Treatise on the Disorders and Deformities of the Teeth and Gums . . . the Whole Illustrated with Cases and Experiments, Intended for General Use* (Dublin: n.p., 1769).

74. Porter, *Health for Sale*, 147; Hillam, "Introduction," 16; Jones, "French Dentists and English Teeth," 86–87; *The Toilet Assistant: Or a Collection of the Most Simple and Approved Methods of Preparing Baths, Essences, Sweet Scented Waters, Pomatums, Powders, Perfumes, and Opiates for Preserving and Whitening the Teeth . . . in Letters to the Ladies* (Dublin: n.p., 1777).

75. *Freeman's Journal*, 5 May 1778.

76. *Freeman's Journal*, 7 Feb. 1771; *Hibernian Journal*, 28 Jan. 1778.

77. Porter, *Health for Sale*, 147; *Freeman's Journal*, 11 Nov. 1769, 26 May, 18 June, and 19 Dec. 1776; *Faulkner's Dublin Journal*, 11 Oct. 1777.

78. *Hibernian Journal*, 28 Jan. 1778 and 14 Jan., 6 Feb., and 6 Mar. 1782; Porter and Porter, *Patient's Progress*, 22–23.

79. Daniel Geale's account book, 1779–1803, MS 2286, folios 2, 16, National Library of Ireland, Dublin. Significantly, this amount was less than one-fifth the sum Geale paid a London practitioner in 1786 when he required dental care "while in England." I thank Dr. Lisa-Marie Griffith for this reference.

80. The first public record of the use of the term *dentist* dates from 1769, and it is the term employed to describe Edward Hudson, Jacob Hemet, H. Hart, and Mr. Davy in *Hibernian Journal*, 26 Jan. 1778 and 14 Jan. 1782; *Freeman's Journal*, 11 Nov. 1769, 25 May 1776, and 5 May 1778.

81. *Freeman's Journal*, 5 May 1778; *Hibernian Journal*, 14 Jan. 1782.

82. Kelly, "Health for Sale"; Hargreaves, "Dentistry in the British Isles," 212–13; *Freeman's Journal*, 22 Jan. 1771, 31 Mar. 1774, 23 May 1776, 1 Oct. 1782, 19 Dec.

1782, and 4 Dec. 1798; *Hibernian Journal,* 12 July 1780, 1 Sept. 1780, 18 May 1789, 1 Jan. 1790, 28 Feb. 1791, and 1 Aug. 1792.

83. Hargreaves, "Dentistry in the British Isles," 213; *Freeman's Journal,* 31 Mar. 1774, 19 Dec. 1782, and 4 Dec. 1798; *Hibernian Journal,* 17 Aug. 1789, 22 May 1790, and 2 Dec. 1794.

84. Bartholomew Ruspini, *A Treatise on Teeth, Wherein an Accurate Idea of Their Structure Is Given, and the Cause of Their Decay Pointed Out,* 1st ed. (London: n.p., 1768), 8th ed. (London: n.p., 1797); Hargreaves, "Dentistry in the British Isles," 186 and passim; *Hibernian Journal,* 8 May 1789, 17 Aug. 1789, and 4 Jan. and 1 Aug. 1792; *Cork Courier,* 18 Oct. 1794.

85. Porter, *Bodies Politic,* 198–99, plates 89–91; Hargreaves, "Dentistry in the British Isles," 198–200; Diana Donald, *The Age of Caricature: Satirical Prints in the Reign of George III* (London: Yale Univ. Press, 1996), 97–98.

86. *Hibernian Journal,* 25 Oct. 1790; *Cork Courier,* 29 Oct. 1794; *Dublin Evening Post,* 13 Oct. 1798.

87. *Freeman's Journal,* 22 Aug. and 5 Sept. 1793; *Hibernian Journal,* 23 Nov. 1792, 11 Mar. 1793, and 2 Dec. 1794; Hargreaves, "Dentistry in the British Isles," 257.

88. *Freeman's Journal,* 22 Aug. 1793.

89. *Dublin Morning Post,* 14 May 1785; *Hibernian Journal,* 25 Oct. 1790, 23 Nov. 1792, 11 Mar. 1793, 25 Jan. 1794, 5 May 1794, and 2 Dec. 1794; *Freeman's Journal,* 22 Aug. and 5 Sept. 1793, 27 Nov. 1794; Hargreaves, "Dentistry in the British Isles," 257.

90. *Clonmel Gazette,* 24 Mar. and 23 Oct. 1790; Hargreaves, "Dentistry in the British Isles," 176, 189, 190, 259–63.

91. Hargreaves, "Dentistry in the British Isles," 243 and 251; *Hibernian Journal,* 15 and 27 Jan. and 16 Apr. 1794; *Freeman's Journal,* 25 Feb. and 8 July 1794; *Cork Courier,* 8 and 29 Oct. and 1 Nov. 1794.

92. The quack element of dentistry can be identified in the advertisement of "Mr Braham, Dentist, 88 Dame Street," *Freeman's Journal,* 14 Feb. 1799.

93. Minutes of the Guild of Barbers, Surgeons, Apothecaries, and Perukemakers, 1714–92, MS 1447/8/2, folios 33, 34, 122, TCD; J. D. H. Widdess, *The Royal College of Surgeons in Ireland and Its Medical School, 1784–1984,* 3rd ed. (Dublin: Royal College of Surgeons, 1984), 4–10.

94. Widdess, *The Royal College of Surgeons,* 4–10.

95. Joan Lane, *A Social History of Medicine: Health, Healing, and Disease in England 1750–1950* (London: Routledge, 2001), 8; Porter and Porter, *Patient's Progress,* 23; Porter, *Health for Sale,* 61.

96. *Limerick Chronicle,* 18 Apr. 1829.

97. David McGowan, "A Story of Irish Extraction," *History of Dentistry Newsletter* 13 (Oct. 2003): 2–5, accessed at http://www.rcpsg.ac.uk/hdrg/2003Oct6.htm.

2. Women and Tuberculosis in Ireland

1. For the history of TB in the United States and Britain, see F. B. Smith, *The Retreat of Tuberculosis* (London: Croom Helm, 1988); Linda Bryder, *Below the Magic Mountain: A Social History of Tuberculosis in Twentieth Century Britain* (Oxford: Oxford Univ. Press, 1988); Michael Teller, *The Tuberculosis Movement: A Public Health Campaign in the Progressive Era* (New York: Greenwood Press, 1988); Georgina D. Feldberg, *Disease and Class: Tuberculosis and the Shaping of Modern North American Society* (New Brunswick, NJ: Rutgers Univ. Press, 1995); Barbara Bates, *Bargaining for Life: A Social History of Tuberculosis 1876 to 1938* (Philadelphia: Univ. of Pennsylvania Press, 1992).

2. An exception in Europe is Norway.

3. Greta Jones, *Captain of All These Men of Death: The History of Tuberculosis in Nineteenth and Twentieth Century Ireland* (Amsterdam: Rodolpi, 2001).

4. There are statistics for mortality in the early and mid–nineteenth century for Ireland, but, as in Britain, they are not always reliable. Collection of statistics of mortality improved significantly during the nineteenth century. Improvement in recordkeeping in Ireland was continuous, but an important landmark was the act setting up an Irish registrar general's office in 1863. Registration under this act was compulsory from 1864. An act in 1879, coming into force in 1880, improved registration procedures further.

5. Annual death rates from phthisis per 100,000 in England and Wales were, respectively, 270 per 100,000 living persons for men in 1851–60 and 290 for women. By 1871–80, the figures were 240 for men and 210 for women. In Ireland, the death rate for men in 1901–10 was 200 compared to 202 for women.

6. See Jones, *Captain of All These Men of Death,* 88 n. 26.

7. Donnell Deeny, *Tuberculosis in Ireland: A Thesis Presented for the Degree of Doctor of Medicine* (Belfast: Queen's Univ. of Belfast, 1945).

8. "Tuberculosis in Ireland," *National Tuberculosis Survey for the Medical Research Council of Ireland* (1954), table 2, p. 27.

9. Calculated for the years 1900, 1901, and 1902, the comparative death rate for men and women in Belfast was 293 men and 338 women per 100,000 living persons.

10. William Johnston, *The Modern Epidemic: A History of Tuberculosis in Japan* (Cambridge, MA: Harvard Univ. Press, 1995).

11. Joanna Bourke, *Husbandry to Housewifery: Women, Economic Change, and Housework in Ireland 1890–1914* (Oxford: Clarendon Press 1993).

12. C. D. Purdon, *Mortality of Flax Mill and Factory Workers and the Diseases They Labour Under,* pamphlet, Linenhall Library, Belfast, read to the annual meeting of the Association of Certifying Medical Officers of Great Britain and Ireland at Leeds, 1873.

13. *Report upon the Conditions of Work in Flax Mills and Linen Factories within the United Kingdom,* Parliamentary Papers (PP), 1893–94, vol. XVII, C. 7287.

14. *Report on Changes in the Employment of Women and Girls in Industrial Centres, Part 1: Flax and Jute Centres,* PP, 1898, vol. LXXXVIII, C. 8794.

15. *Report of the Belfast Health Commission to the Local Government Board* (Ireland), PP, 1908, vol. XXXI, Cd. 4128.

16. See Emily Boyle, "The Economic Development of the Irish Linen Industry 1825–1913," PhD diss., Queen's Univ. of Belfast, 1979.

17. Temperatures in the seventies and eighties Fahrenheit were common in the wet spinning sections and in the nineties in the dry spinning sections. Humidity in wet spinning led to condensation of water vapor, which wet clothes, as did splashes from the water that sprayed the machinery. Combined with the noise and labor, this moisture and heat led to the phenomenon known as "mill fever"—nausea and fainting—affecting new entrants to the mill.

18. An analysis of deaths from consumption in various occupations in Dublin appended to the 1871 census attributes 40 percent of deaths among dressmakers to phthisis—the largest mortality in any occupational category. (Male tailors are the next largest, with 35 percent of deaths from phthisis.) It was also recorded that 27 percent of female servants died from phthisis. However, from a modern statistical view, the samples in some cases are too small to make these figures entirely reliable. See Jones, *Captain of All These Men of Death,* 67 and 94.

19. Thomas Grimshaw (1839–1900), registrar general, established the connection with TB mortality and urbanization in 1885 in "Observations on the Relative Prevalence of Disease and the Relative Death Rates in Town and Country Districts in Ireland," *Transactions of the Academy of Medicine in Ireland* 111 (1885): 328–404, which he followed up with another study in 1887. Jones, *Captain of All These Men of Death,* 33–34.

20. Sheila Ryan Johansson, "Sex and Death in Victorian England: An Examination of Age and Sex Specific Death Rates, 1840–1910," in *Widening Sphere: The Changing Roles of Victorian Women,* edited by Martha Vicinus, 163–81 (Bloomington: Indiana Univ. Press, 1977).

21. Tuberculin tests indicate that up to 90 percent of the population in the early twentieth century had been exposed to the TB, though only a proportion went on to develop the disease fully. Among those who fell ill, some survived. Morbidity is the rate at which people fall ill, and mortality is the rate at which they die from that disease. The relationship between the two can shift over time. Morbidity might fall, for example, owing to the growth of natural resistance to a disease, even while mortality remains unaffected, or vice versa.

22. Richard Carmichael, *Essay on the Origin and Nature of Tuberculous and Cancerous Disease* (Dublin: Hodges and Smith, 1836), read to the Medical Section of the British Association for the Advancement of Science in 1836. Carmichael founded the

Dublin private medical school that goes by his name and was the first president of the Irish Medical Association.

23. Tables for mortality from phthisis in Dublin show a rate of 532 per 100,000 live persons for workhouse inmates compared with 102 and 170 for those designated as professional and middle class, respectively. Jones, *Captain of All These Men of Death,* appendix 4, p. 50.

24. Arthur Clarke, *Essays on the Exhibition of Iodine in Tubercular Consumption* (Dublin: A. Thom, 1836), v.

25. For a discussion of the cult of St. Therese in France, see David Barnes, *The Making of a Social Disease: Tuberculosis in Nineteenth Century France* (Berkeley: Univ. of California Press, 1995), 63–73.

26. Desmond Forristal, *Edel Quinn 1907–1944* (Dublin: Dominican Publications, 1994), 51.

27. See the extreme religiosity described by William J. Heaney in *Reminiscences of Our Lady of Lourdes Sanatorium in House of Courage* (Dublin: Clonmore and Reynolds, 1952).

28. Quoted in Jones, *Captain of All These Men of Death,* 165.

29. Van Morrison composed and sang "TB Sheets" around 1966 reputedly in memory of the death of a friend in Belfast.

30. Hospitals took the view that they could fill their wards up twice over with consumptives at the expense of patients with more treatable diseases. There were, however, hospitals specializing in chest diseases in the nineteenth century that accepted consumptives, such as Forster Green Hospital in Belfast. Some consumptives could also still be found in general wards. By the early twentieth century, the movement was under way to provide sanatorium and separate wards in hospitals and infirmaries for the tuberculosis patients, which led to the increasing segregation of the consumptive.

31. "Consumption of the Lung or Decline," in *Johnson and Oldham's Housekeeper's Almanac: A Manual of Domestic Medicine and the Treatment of Disease* (Dublin: n.p., July 1872), by Johnson and Oldham Druggist, 37 Grafton Street Dublin. The origin of their advice might well have been a number of medical texts, but in 1834 John T. Evans set out these basic principles in the article "Tuberculosis Treatment," *Dublin Journal of Medical Science* 2, no. 1 (1834): 3–19.

32. Patrick Logan, *Making the Cure: A Look at Irish Folk Medicine* (Dublin: Talbot Press, 1972). Logan mentions the drinking of a cup of linseed oil a day as a folk remedy against consumption.

33. Edward Barry, *Treatise on Consumption of the Lungs* (Dublin: Hodges and Smith, 1726); H. S. Purdon, "Cures for Consumption with Reference to Lady Wilde's 'Ancient Cure and Charms of Ireland,'" *Ulster Journal of Archaeology* 2, no. 10 (1904), 41. H. S. Purdon must be distinguished from his fellow medic C. D. Purdon, though they were probably from the same family.

34. H. S. Purdon also wrote *Notes on the Preservation of Health for Domestic Use* (Belfast: n.p., 1874), which listed the latest "scientific" cures for consumption and gave advice on the home nursing of the consumptive patient.

35. See Greta Jones, "Women and Eugenics in Britain: The Case of Mary Scharlieb, Elizabeth Sloan Chesser, and Stella Browne," *Annals of Science* 51 (1995): 481–502.

36. A reminiscence of medical work on TB in the 1940s refers to the cod liver oil regularly dispensed to TB sufferers by doctors who had long lost faith in it, but who regularly dispensed it anyway in the absence of anything else to offer patients. See Jones, *Captain of All These Men of Death*, 18.

37. David Rosner and Gerald Markowitz point out that the work environment received less attention from reformers than the domestic, though it played a major contribution to the spread of the disease. They attribute this neglect to politics. See David Rosner and Gerald Markowitz, *Deadly Dust: Silicosis and the Politics of Occupational Disease in the Twentieth Century* (Princeton, NJ: Princeton Univ. Press, 1991).

38. David Barnes regards the concentration on domestic hygiene as a way of avoiding more difficult and politically contentious issues of poverty, particularly in an era in France that saw a growing socialist and industrial threat. See Barnes, *The Making of a Social Disease*.

39. Most working-class homes did not have piped water until the twentieth century and only limited facilities for heating water or washing. Injunctions about nutritious and expensive patient diets and separate rooms for the sick similarly often did not take account of the realities of working-class income and accommodation. For domestic standards in Ireland, see Catriona Clear, *Women of the House: Women's Household Work in Ireland 1926–1961* (Dublin: Irish Academic Press, 2000).

40. Patricia Hollis, *Ladies Elect* (Oxford: Clarendon Press, 1987).

41. Dr. Alice Barry retired in 1946. For her career, see Margaret Ó hÓgartaigh, *Kathleen Lynn: Irishwoman, Patriot, Doctor* (Dublin: Irish Academic Press, 2006), chaps. 3 and 4.

42. For Dorothy Stopford-Price, see her book *An Account of 20 Years Fight Against TB,* (Oxford: Oxford Univ. Press, 1957), privately printed and held in the College of Surgeons Library, Dublin. For her career, see Margaret Ó hÓgartaigh, "Dorothy Stopford-Price and the Elimination of Childhood Tuberculosis," in *Ireland in the 1930s: New Perspectives,* edited by Joost Augusteijn, 67–82 (Dublin: Four Courts Press, 1999), and Margaret Ó hÓgartaigh, "Dorothy Stopford-Price (1890–1954)," in *Dictionary of Irish Biography,* edited by James McGuire and James Quinn, 299–300 (Cambridge: Cambridge Univ. Press, 2009).

43. Losing the main wage formed the basis of much of the radical campaign arising in the late 1930s and 1940s in the Irish Free State.

44. Sir Patrick Dun's Dispensary Casebook, in the library of the Royal College of Physicians of Ireland, cross-referenced with the 1901 census, National Archives of Ireland (NAI).

45. Textiles were considered to harbor TB germs so that laundries and even Ireland's linen exports were considered vulnerable to suspicions of spreading tuberculosis.

46. Economic activity of this kind was not always recorded in the census. Though a substantial number of women were recorded as engaged in the provision of food and lodging and commodities (in the Decennial Census of 1881, more than 18,000 women in Leinster and a similar number in Ulster were occupied in these two sectors), the number was small compared with that of women in domestic service (117,873 in Leinster and 111,731 in Ulster). However, it was probably an underestimate of this kind of economic activity, which tended to be intermittent and casual and therefore underreported.

47. Jacques Donzelot, *The Policing of Families* (New York: Pantheon, 1979),135.

48. See the discussion of Donzelot and women's preparedness to submit to medical authority in the case of the institutionalization of the mentally deficient in Greta Jones, *Social Hygiene in Twentieth Century Britain* (London: Croom Helm, 1986), 37–39.

49. For a discussion of these successes, see Jones, *Captain of All These Men of Death*, 231.

50. See Department of Local Government and Public Health, Questionnaire to TB Authorities and Medical Practitioners on the Adequacy of Treatment, 1941, File D102/15, NAI. It is probable that country areas in particular had low rates of registration. For Dublin, see letter from Charles Street Dispensary, File D34A/45, NAI.

51. There appears to be no significant difference between systems of compulsory and voluntary registration in the extent of "avoidance." Britain allowed for compulsory notification, and Linda Bryder records that in 1923 in Liverpool 22 percent of all deaths from TB were unregistered, and 47 percent of the registered were advanced cases. In Cumberland, a largely rural county of England, the rate of unregistered cases was 50 percent in 1935. See Bryder, *Below the Magic Mountain,* 210. Cultural and economic factors rather than compulsion appear to have played a large part in determining levels of registration.

52. Tuberculosis Authority of Northern Ireland (Belfast), Files TBA 1/1/3, TBA 1/1/4, TBA 6/3/3, Public Record Office of Northern Ireland (PRONI), Belfast.

53. "Statistical Analysis of Circumstances Relating to a Sample of 653 Tuberculous Patients Who Were Resident in the City of Dublin in 1944," table 15, p. 3, and "Statistical Analysis of Circumstances Relating to a Sample of 352 Residents of Dublin Who Died of TB" (1944), table 9, p. 2, both in Department of Local Government and Health, File D112/86, NAI.

54. Files of the Tuberculosis Authority of Northern Ireland, TBA 1/1/3, TBA 1/1/4, TBA 6/3/3, PRONI.

55. Family affection was mentioned by 14.5 percent of women and 6.5 percent of men. Economic hardship was mentioned by 16.6 and 16.5 percent, respectively.

Twenty-four percent of women as opposed to 28 percent of men gave dislike of the institution as the main reason for refusing treatment. Most of the remaining reasons given for refusal—not ill enough, wanted a particular sanatorium, would do better at home—are less than 5 percent of the total.

56. For example, the tone of the reports shows sympathy to women who cited the problems of family life as the reason for avoiding sanatorium care, but such reasons as a belief that one was not as ill as the doctor said or would get on better at home or a preference for alternative medicine were greeted with a great deal less sympathy. All government investigations of the reasons for refusing a sanatorium place must be treated with caution. Public-health officials were often exasperated with those they regarded as jeopardizing their own and others' health by refusal to enter a sanatorium, and this attitude may very well have led patients to cite what they felt were "acceptable" reasons.

57. See Heaney, *Reminiscences of Our Lady of Lourdes.*

58. See Susan Kelly, "Suffer the Little Children: Childhood Tuberculosis in the North of Ireland, c. 1865–1965," DPhil diss., Univ. of Ulster, 2008.

3. Infant and Child Mortality in Dublin a Century Ago

A previous version of this paper was published as "Infant and Child Mortality a Century Ago," in *The Determinants of Infant and Child Mortality in Past European Populations,* edited by Marco Breschi and Lucia Pozzi, 89–104 (Udine, Italy: Forum, 2004).

1. See Eilidh Garrett and Alice Reid, "Thinking of England and Taking Care: Family Building Strategies and Infant Mortality in England and Wales, 1891–1911," *International Journal of Population Geography* 1 (1995): 69–102; Frans van Poppel and Kees Mandemakers, "Differential Infant and Child Mortality in the Netherlands, 1812–1912: First Results of the Historical Sample of the Population of the Netherlands," in *Infant and Child Mortality in the Past,* edited by Alain Bideau, Bertrand Desjardins, and Hector Pérez Brignoli, 276–300 (Oxford: Oxford Univ. Press, 1997); George Alter, "Infant and Child Mortality in the US and Canada," in Bideau, Desjardins, and Pérez Brignoli, eds., *Infant and Child Mortality in the Past,* 91–108; Michael R. Haines, "Inequality and Childhood Mortality: A Comparison of England and Wales, 1911, and the United States, 1900," *Journal of Economic History* 45 (1985): 885–912; and S. H. Preston, Douglas Ewbank, and Mark Hereward, "Child Mortality Differences by Ethnicity and Race in the United States, 1900–1910," in *After Ellis Island: Newcomers and Natives in the 1910 Census,* edited by Susan Cotts Watkins, 35–82 (New York: Russell Sage Foundation, 1994).

2. The literature is voluminous. Modern assessments include Joseph P. O'Brien, *Dear Dirty Dublin: A City in Distress, 1899–1916* (Berkeley: Univ. of California Press, 1982); F. H. A. Aalen, "The Working-Class Housing Movement in Dublin, 1850–1920," in *The Genesis of Irish Planning 1880–1920,* edited by Michael J. Bannon, 131–88

(Dublin: Turoe Press, 1985); Mary E. Daly, "Social Structure of the Dublin Working Class, 1871–1911," *Irish Historical Studies* 22, no. 90 (1982): 121–33; Mary E. Daly, *The Deposed Capital: A Social and Economic History of Dublin, 1860–1914* (Cork: Cork Univ. Press, 1984); Mary E. Daly, "Working-Class Housing in Scottish and Irish Cities on the Eve of World War 1," in *Conflict, Identity, and Economic Development 1600–1939*, edited by S. J. Connolly, R. A. Houston, and R. J. Morris, 217–27 (Preston, UK: Carnegie Publishing, 1995); and Jacinta Prunty, *Dublin Slums, 1800–1925: A Study in Urban Geography* (Dublin: Irish Academic Press, 1998).

3. For example, see van Poppel and Mandemakers, "Differential Infant and Child Mortality in the Netherlands," 276–300; Werner Troesken, *Water, Race, and Disease* (Cambridge, MA: MIT Press, 2004).

4. Mary E. Daly, "Late Nineteenth and Early Twentieth-Century Dublin," in *The Town in Ireland: Historical Studies XIII*, edited by David Harkness and Mary O'Dowd (Belfast: Appletree Press, 1981), 237–38; *Report of the Royal Commissioners Appointed to Inquire into the Sewerage and Drainage of the City of Dublin* (1880), British Parliamentary Papers (BPP), vol. XVII, [2605], v; and Frederic W. Pim, "Preventable Diseases: Why Are They Not Prevented?" address delivered at the annual general meeting of the Dublin Sanitary Association, 30 Mar. 1892, 13.

5. In Dublin (as elsewhere), however, it was claimed that mains water may have exacerbated an already serious drainage and sewage problem for a time by prompting the spread of domestic flush toilets. Because many of the house drains were of poor quality, the rich may have been affected more than the poor to the extent that their houses ran an increased risk of infection, whereas the poor continued to rely on the ashpit and privy. See O'Brien, *Dear Dirty Dublin*, 19. Occasional high-profile fatalities from typhoid fever such as that of the Jesuit poet-professor Gerard Manley Hopkins at the age of forty-four in 1889 lent credence to the view that a proper sewerage system was a necessary complement to a clean water supply. See also Daly, "Late Nineteenth and Early Twentieth-Century Dublin," 238–41; Daly, *The Deposed Capital;* and Prunty, *Dublin Slums.*

6. O'Brien, *Dear Dirty Dublin.* 103. On Irish Americans, see Ewa Morawska, "Afterward: America's Immigrants in the 1910 Census Monograph: Where Can We Who Do It Differently Go from Here?" in Watkins, ed., *After Ellis Island,* 326–27.

7. See Derosas Renzo, "When Culture Matters: Differential Infant Mortality of Jews and Catholics in Nineteenth-Century Venice," *History of the Family: An International Quarterly* (forthcoming); Eilidh Garrett, Alice Reid, Kevin Schürer, and Simon Szreter, *Changing Family Size in England and Wales: Place, Class, and Demography, 1891–1911* (Cambridge: Cambridge Univ. Press, 2001), 153; L. Marks, *Model Mothers: Jewish Mothers and Maternity Provision in East London, 1870–1939* (Oxford: Oxford Univ. Press, 1994); U. O. Schmelz, *Infant and Early Childhood Mortality among the*

Jews of the Diaspora (Jerusalem: Institute of Contemporary Jewry, Hebrew Univ., 1971); and R. M. Woodbury, *Infant Mortality and Its Causes* (Baltimore: Williams & Wilkins, 1926).

8. Quoted in O'Brien, *Dear Dirty Dublin,* 102.

9. Cormac Ó Gráda, "Dublin Jewish Demography a Century Ago," *Economic and Social Review* 37, 2 (2006): 123–47; Cormac Ó Gráda, *Jewish Ireland in the Age of Joyce: A Socioeconomic History* (Princeton, NJ: Princeton Univ. Press, 2006), chap. 7.

10. Prunty, *Dublin Slums,* 343–46.

11. Elizabeth Bowen, *Seven Winters; Memories of a Dublin Childhood & Afterthoughts; Pieces on Writing* (New York: Knopf, 1962), 44.

12. Prunty, *Dublin Slums,* 154–57.

13. Including "civic" areas of the county (i.e., municipal boroughs, townships, and towns of two thousand people or more) changes the percentages to 40.6 percent in 1861, 33.8 percent in 1881, and 26.2 percent in 1911. In 1841, the percentage of families living in fourth-class accommodation was 46.9 percent. See *Census of Ireland, 1841* (Dublin: Her Majesty's Stationery Office, 1841), 21. Most fourth-class housing in urban Ireland consisted of one-room tenement apartments.

14. Daly, "Working-Class Housing in Scottish and Irish Cities," 218–20; O'Brien, *Dear Dirty Dublin,* chap. 3; F. H. A. Aalen, "Health and Housing in Dublin c. 1850–1921," in *Dublin, City and County: From Prehistory to Present,* edited by F. H. A. Aalen and Kevin Whelan (Dublin: Geography Publications, 1992), 296–97; and Prunty, *Dublin Slums.*

15. Daly, "Working-Class Housing in Scottish and Irish Cities," 226; and Prunty, *Dublin Slums,* 175.

16. Charles Cameron, Chief Medical Officer, City of Dublin, *Annual Report for the City of Dublin, 1913* (Dublin: Dublin Corporation, 1913), 127–28; Charles Cameron, Chief Medical Officer, City of Dublin, *Annual Report for the City of Dublin, 1914* (Dublin: Dublin Corporation, 1914), 82–83; Charles Cameron, Chief Medical Officer, City of Dublin, *Annual Report for the City of Dublin, 1906* (Dublin: Dublin Corporation, 1906); Aalen, "Health and Housing in Dublin c. 1850–1921," 293–94.

17. Fergus D'Arcy, "Wages of Labour in the Dublin Building Industry, 1667–1918," *Saothar: Journal of the Irish Labour History Society* 14 (1989): 17–34.

18. Fergus D'Arcy presents his annual general laborer series as a range. The "low" and "high" columns in the list given in this note are the five-year averages of the low and high ends of his range of wages (in pounds per annum); see D'Arcy, "Wages of Labour." The final column in the list is Bowley's index for the building industry in the United Kingdom, as reported in C. H. Feinstein, "New Estimates of Average Earnings in the United Kingdom, 1880–1913," *Economic History Review* 43, no. 4 (1990), 608–9.

Period	Low	High	United Kingdom
1880–84	28	30	87.0
1885–89	28	35	87.8
1890–94	29	38	82.3
1895–99	38	39	86.9
1900–1904	40	40	100.0
1905–1909	40	43	100.0
1910–14	41	46	101.1

Compare K. G. J. C. Knowles and D. J. Robertson, "Differences Between the Wages of Skilled and Unskilled Workers, 1880–1950," *Bulletin of the Oxford University Institute of Statistics* (Apr. 1951), appendix, table 1.

19. For example, see Liam Kennedy, "The Cost of Living in Ireland over Three Centuries c. 1660–1960," paper presented to the Historical National Accounts Group, Dublin, Jan. 2002.

20. Cameron, *Annual Report for the City of Dublin, 1913,* 127–28.

21. Thus excluding the presumably small number of burials in parish graveyards.

22. Daly, *The Deposed Capital,* 242.

23. Pim, "Preventable Diseases," 7.

24. Compare Aalen, "Health and Housing in Dublin c. 1850–1921," 85. The downward drift in Aalen's moving average is halted temporarily by a blip owing mainly to a measles epidemic in the late 1890s.

25. Using 2, 12, 29, 49, 69, and 85 years as age-group midpoints yields the following crude estimates of the expectation of life (in years):

Class	Mid-1880s	1900s	Increase
I	53.4	60.3	6.9
II	37.0	42.1	5.1
III	27.9	33.75	5.85
IV	31.8	32.25	0.45
Average	32.6	35.2	2.6

26. That mortality in the late 1890s was above trend does not alter this conclusion. See Robert I. Woods, *The Demography of Victorian England and Wales* (Cambridge: Cambridge Univ. Press, 2000).

27. Ibid., 279, citing Jacques Vallin, *La démographie* (Paris: La Découverte, 1991).

28. Woods, *The Demography of Victorian England and Wales,* 291, 295, 307; compare David Reher, "Back to the Basics: Mortality and Fertility Interactions during the Demographic Transition," *Continuity and Change* 14, no. 1 (1999): 9–31. The

impact of declining fertility on infant and child mortality in early-twentieth-century England is also stressed in Garrett et al., *Changing Family Size in England and Wales.*

29. Haines, "Inequality and Childhood Mortality," 888; P. A. Watterson, "Infant Mortality by Father's Occupation from the 1911 Census of England and Wales," *Demography* 25 (1988), 292; Samuel H. Preston and Michael Haines, *Fatal Years: Childhood Mortality in the United States in the Late Nineteenth Century* (Princeton, NJ: Princeton Univ. Press, 1991); and Garrett et al., *Changing Family Size in England and Wales.*

30. See John W. Budd and T. W. Guinnane, "Intentional Age-Misreporting, Age Heaping, and the 1908 Old Age Pensions Act in Ireland," *Population Studies* 45, no. 3 (1992): 497–518; and Cormac Ó Gráda, "The Greatest Blessing of All: The Old Age Pension in Ireland," *Past & Present* 175 (2002): 124–62.

31. Reher, "Back to the Basics," and Woods, *The Demography of Victorian England and Wales.*

32. For more on the township's origins, see Séamas Ó Maitiú, *Dublin's Suburban Towns* (Dublin: Four Courts Press, 2003).

33. For an evocative account of life in a working-class section of Pembroke a few decades after the period analyzed here, see Angeline Kearns Blain, *Stealing Sunlight: Growing Up in Irishtown* (Dublin: A. & A. Farmer, 2000).

34. More than 80 percent of the population of the island of Ireland was Catholic in 1911, and more than 90 percent of the area that would constitute the Irish Free State was Catholic in 1922. In the greater Dublin area that included the suburban townships of Pembroke, Rathmines, and Rathgar, the Catholic share was somewhat less (78.2 percent). Members of the Episcopalian Church of Ireland accounted for a further 16.7 percent of the population of this greater metropolitan area, Presbyterians 1.9 percent, Methodists 1.2 percent, and others (mainly other nonconformists) 2.1 percent.

35. However, this does not include instances whether either party changed religious affiliation beforehand to facilitate marriage.

36. There was either one male religious or one female religious per 180 inhabitants in Pembroke in 1911. Non-Catholics were proportionately better catered for in terms of male clergy, but there were ninety-three Catholic nuns.

37. See Timothy W. Guinnane, Carolyn Moehling, and Cormac Ó Gráda, *Fertility in South Dublin a Century Ago: A First Look,* Economic Growth Center Discussion Paper no. 838 (New Haven, CT: Economic Growth Center, Yale Univ., 2001).

38. Age exaggeration proved not to be a problem in Pembroke. Guinnane, Moehling, and Ó Gráda, "Fertility in South Dublin a Century Ago."

39. Preston and Haines, *Fatal Years;* Michael R. Haines and Samuel H. Preston, "The Use of the Census to Estimate Childhood Mortality: Comparisons from the 1900 and 1910 United States Census Public Use Samples," *Historical Methods* 30, no. 2 (Spring 1997): 77–97.

40. Garrett et al., *Changing Family Size in England and Wales.*

4. Cure or Custody: Therapeutic Philosophy
at the Connaught District Lunatic Asylum

1. In the sixty years between 1810 and 1870, twenty-two new district asylums had been built in Ireland; most were overcrowded within a few years of their opening.

2. In the mid–nineteenth century, W. A. F. Browne was breaking new ground at Montrose Asylum in Scotland. For example, he implemented one of the earliest systems of occupational therapy in Britain. See Andrew T. Scull, Charlotte MacKenzie, and Nicholas Hervey, *Masters of Bedlam: The Transformation of the Mad-Doctoring Trade* (Princeton, NJ: Princeton Univ. Press, 1996), 84–122; and Billy Gunn, "W. A. F. Browne and Scottish Psychiatry," PhD diss., Univ. of Aberdeen, 2008.

3. See Oonagh Walsh, "'Tales from the Big House': The Connaught District Lunatic Asylum in the Late Nineteenth-Century," *History Ireland* (Nov.–Dec. 2005): 21–25.

4. For a variety of discussions of the efficacy or otherwise of moral treatment, see Andrew Scull, *The Most Solitary of Afflictions: Madness and Society in Britain 1700–1900* (New Haven, CT: Yale Univ. Press, 1993); Edward Shorter, *A History of Psychiatry: From the Era of the Asylum to the Age of Prozac* (Toronto: Wiley, 1997); and Mark Michale and Roy Porter, eds., *Discovering the History of Psychiatry* (Oxford: Oxford Univ. Press, 1994).

5. *Bye-Rules and Regulations for the Government of the Connaught District Lunatic Asylum*, 1853, Connaught District Lunatic Asylum archives, Ballinasloe, County Galway. The Irish district asylums were nineteenth-century constructions and thus escaped the worst of the experimental "treatments" implemented in the eighteenth century in other countries. With the exception of William Saunders Halloran's adaptation of the "rotary machine" at Cork asylum, few Irish institutions utilized the often brutal mechanical devices intended to produce a cowed and passive patient body. See Oonagh Walsh, "Landscape and the Irish Asylum," in *Land and Landscape in Nineteenth-Century Ireland*, edited by Glenn Hooper and Úna Ní Bhroiméil, 157–61 (Dublin: Four Courts Press, 2008). For an international perspective on treatments, see Jan Goldstein, "Psychiatry," in *Companion Encyclopedia of the History of Medicine*, 237–34 (London: Routledge, 1993).

6. An entry from 7 February 1856 was typical:

> *Read* Matron's report stating that Ellen Pender night nurse had grossly neglected her duty on the 30th Jan. in leaving a servant who was in a most dangerous state without seeing her the whole night, and also refusing to attend the Infirmary where there were 13 patients very ill; when spoken to she was very impertinent. Also stating that Mary McDermott servant appointed deputy nurse last Board day was totally unfit for her situation.
>
> *Ordered* That Ellen Pender be reduced to Deputy Nurse, and Mary McDermott be dismissed.

From the minutes of the meeting of the Connaught District Lunatic Asylum Board of Governors, 7 Feb. 1856, asylum archives.

7. For a full discussion of the DLA's many implications, see Oonagh Walsh, "Lunatic and Criminal Alliances in Nineteenth-Century Ireland," in *Outside the Walls of the Asylum: The History of Care in the Community, 1750–2000*, edited by Peter Bartlett and David P. Wright, 132–52 (London: Athlone Press, 1999).

8. From Committal Warrant of a Dangerous Lunatic or a Dangerous Idiot, Act 18, 1852 (16 Vic., c.72).

9. J. Nugent's report, from the annual report of the Connaught District Lunatic Asylum for the year 1876, 11, asylum archives.

10. See, for example, Pamela Michael, *Care and Treatment of the Mentally Ill in North Wales, 1800–2000* (Cardiff: Univ. of Wales Press, 2003); Roy Porter and David Wright, eds., *The Confinement of the Insane: International Perspectives, 1800–1965* (Cambridge: Cambridge Univ. Press, 2003); and Akihito Suzuki, *Madness at Home: The Psychiatrist, the Patient, and the Family in England, 1820–1860* (Berkeley: Univ. of California Press, 2006).

11. The role of the asylum matron had been a contested one for many years in British and Irish institutions. Although the matrons were granted a great deal of authority over nursing staff and were part of the official "management team," their professional expertise, accumulated over several decades in post, was often resented by medical staff. See Elaine Showalter, *The Female Malady: Women, Madness, and English Culture, 1830–1980* (New York: Pantheon Books, 1985), 52–56.

12. Report of E. M. Courtenay, inspector of lunatics and commissioner of control, in *46th Report on the District, Criminal, and Private Lunatic Asylums in Ireland* (Dublin: n.p., 1897).

13. Hilary Marland, *Dangerous Motherhood: Insanity and Childbirth in Victorian Britain* (London: Palgrave, 2004), 148.

14. The effects of poverty and malnutrition as causative factors in the admission of women may also be seen in Wales. See Michael, *Care and Treatment,* chap. 7.

15. It is ironic that one of the best-known instances of such a "rest cure" was that applied to the writer Charlotte Perkins Gilman by her physician Dr. Weir Mitchell. The enforced inactivity and rich diet that drove Gilman's healthy narrator in *The Yellow Wallpaper* to insanity were the saving of debilitated and exhausted women elsewhere in the nineteenth century. See Charlotte Perkins Gilman, *The Yellow Wallpaper* (New York: Feminist Press, 1892).

16. 4029, Male Case Book 6, 85, Connaught District Lunatic Asylum archives.

17. See, for instance, *47th Report on the District, Criminal, and Private Lunatic Asylums in Ireland* (Dublin: n.p., 1898), 21.

18. Epilepsy is associated with certain types of mental illness but does not appear to be a predisposing factor.

19. 4067, Male Case Book 6, 169, Connaught District Lunatic Asylum archives.

20. 4076, Male Case Book 6, 197, ibid.

21. 4078, Male Case Book 6, 205, ibid.

22. *47th Report*, 9.

5. Gender and Criminal Lunacy in Nineteenth-Century Ireland

I am grateful for the financial support provided by the Wellcome Trust, London, and the expert advice from Dr. Art O'Connor at the Central Mental Hospital, Dundrum; Gregory O'Connor at the National Archives of Ireland; Dr. W. E. Vaughan at Trinity College, Dublin; and Dr. E. Margaret Crawford at Queen's University Belfast.

1. Joel P. Eigen, *Witnessing Insanity: Madness and Mad-Doctors in the English Court* (New Haven, CT: Yale Univ. Press, 1995); Ruth Harris, *Murders and Madness: Medicine, Law, and Society in the Fin de Siècle* (Oxford: Clarendon, 1989); Robert Menzies, "Contesting Criminal Lunacy: Narratives of Law and Madness in West Coast Canada 1874–1950," *History of Psychiatry* 12 (2001): 123–56; Roger Smith, *Trial by Medicine: Insanity and Responsibility in Victorian Trials* (Edinburgh: Edinburgh Univ. Press, 1981); Nigel Walker, *Crime and Insanity in England,* Vol. 2 (Edinburgh: Edinburgh Univ. Press, 1973).

2. For list of the statutes developed, see Pauline M. Prior, *Madness and Murder: Gender, Crime, and Mental Disorder in Nineteenth-Century Ireland* (Dublin: Irish Academic Press, 2008), 232.

3. *Report of the Select Committee on the Aged and Infirm Poor of Ireland, 1804,* HC 1803–1804 (109) iv.771; Arthur Williamson, "The Beginnings of State Care for the Mentally Ill in Ireland," *Economic and Social Review* 10, no. 1 (Jan. 1970): 281–90; T. P. C. Kirkpatrick, *History of the Care of the Insane in Ireland to the End of the Nineteenth Century* (Dublin: Dublin Univ. Press, 1931), 22.

4. Virginia Crossman, *Politics, Law, and Order in Nineteenth-Century Ireland* (Dublin: Gill and Macmillan, 1996), 194.

5. Williamson, "The Beginnings of State Care," 283.

6. *Report of the Select Committee on the Lunatic Poor in Ireland 1817*, HC 1817 (430) vii.1; Lunatic Asylums (Ireland) Act of 1817 (57 Geo. 3 c. 106); Lunacy (Ireland) Act of 1821 (1 & 2 Geo. 4 c. 33).

7. For a list of further legislation, see Williamson, "The Beginnings of State Care," 281 n. 3.

8. Mark Finnane, *Insanity and the Insane in Post-famine Ireland* (London: Croom Helm, 1981), table A, p. 227; Williamson, "The Beginnings of State Care," 288.

9. *Select Committee (HL) on the State of the Lunatic Poor in Ireland, Evidence,* xxv, HL 1843 (625) x.439.

10. For further discussion, see Ralph Partridge, *Broadmoor: A History of Criminal Lunacy and Its Problems* (London: Chatto and Windus, 1953); Walker, *Crime and Insanity in England*, 2:8.

11. *Annual Report on the District, Criminal and Private Lunatic Asylums in Ireland* (1893–94) (hereafter, *Asylums Report*, with date), HC 1893–94 (c.7125) xlvi.369, pp. 440–42. On women and crime statistics, see Kathleen Daly, *Gender, Crime, and Punishment* (New Haven, CT: Yale Univ. Press, 1994); Lorraine Gelsthorpe and Allison Morris, eds., *Feminist Perspectives in Criminology* (Milton Keynes, UK: Open Univ. Press, 1990); Frances Heidensohn, *Women and Crime*, 2nd ed. (Basingstoke, UK: Macmillan Press, 1996); Alido V. Merlo and Jocelyn M. Pollock, *Women, Law, and Social Control* (Boston: Allyn and Bacon, 1995); Sandra Walklate, *Gender and Crime: An Introduction* (London: Prentice Hall, 1995).

12. For further detail, see Prior, *Madness and Murder*, 35.

13. Finnane, *Insanity and the Insane*, 131–32.

14. *Census of Ireland, General Reports, 1841–1901* (Dublin: Her Majesty's Stationery Office, 1902). For discussion on the religious composition of the general population, see Roy F. Foster, *Modern Ireland 1600–1972* (London: Penguin, 1988), chap. 14.

15. Mary Daly, *Social and Economic History of Ireland since 1800* (Dublin: Educational Co., 1981); Joseph Lee, *The Modernization of Irish Society 1848–1918* (Dublin: Gill and Macmillan, 1973).

16. *Asylums Report* (1874), appendix F, table 7, p. 256, HC 1874 (c. 1004) xxvii.363.

17. Ibid., appendix F, table 10.

18. *Asylums Report* (1886), 571, HC 1886 (c. 4811) xxxiii.559.

19. Pat Gibbons, Niamh Mulryan, Angela McAleer, and Art O'Connor, "Criminal Responsibility and Mental Illness in Ireland 1850–1995: Fitness to Plead," *Irish Journal of Psychological Medicine* 16, no. 2 (1999), 52.

20. Pat Gibbons, Niamh Mulryan, and Art O'Connor, "Guilty but Insane: The Insanity Defence in Ireland 1850–1995," *British Journal of Psychiatry* 170 (1997), 447.

21. Pauline M. Prior, "Prisoner or Patient? The Official Debate on the Criminal Lunatic in Nineteenth-Century Ireland," *History of Psychiatry* 15 (2004): 177–92.

22. Eigen, *Witnessing Insanity;* Smith, *Trial by Medicine*.

23. S. W. North, "Insanity and Crime: Paper Read before the York Law Students' Society," *Journal of Mental Science* 32 (July 1886), 29. The *British Journal of Psychiatry* was originally founded in 1853 as the *Asylum Journal* and was known as the *Journal of Mental Science* from 1858 to 1963.

24. Ralph Partridge, *Broadmoor: A History of Criminal Lunacy and Its Problems* (London: Chatto and Windus, 1953), 1.

25. Criminal Lunatics Act of 1800 (39 & 40 Geo 3 c.94); Partridge, *Broadmoor*, 1.

26. For a full discussion of the case, see Richard Moran, *Knowing Right from Wrong: The Insanity Defense of Daniel McNaughtan* (New York: Free Press, 1981).

27. Quoted in ibid., 2.

28. Trial of Lunatics (Ireland) Act of 1883 (46 & 47 Vic., c.38), sec. 2.

29. Gibbons, Mulryan, and O'Connor, "Guilty but Insane," 468.

30. For further discussion of legal and medical involvement in court decisions, see Eigen, *Witnessing Insanity;* Harris, *Murders and Madness;* Smith, *Trial by Medicine;* Walker, *Crime and Insanity in England.*

31. Prior, *Madness and Murder,* table 2.3, p. 42 (for offenses), and appendix 1, p. 230 (for legal basis of admissions).

32. For further discussion on women who killed children, see ibid., chap. 5.

33. Merlo and Pollock, *Women, Law, and Social Control,* chap. 11.

34. Royal Irish Constabulary (RIC), *Return of Outrages 1838–1921,* Chief Secretary's Office (CSO), Irish Crime Records (ICR), Files CSO ICR1 and CSO ICR2, National Archives of Ireland (NAI), Dublin; police reports 1882–1921, Box 4, NAI; Carolyn A. Conley, *Melancholy Accidents: The Meaning of Violence in Post-famine Ireland* (Lanham, MD: Lexington Books, 1999).

35. Conley, *Melancholy Accidents;* Mark Finnane, "A Decline in Violence in Ireland? Crime, Policing, and Social Relations, 1860–1914," *Crime, History, and Societies* 1, no. 1 (1997): 51–70; Elizabeth Malcolm, *The Irish Policeman, 1822–1922: A Life* (Dublin: Four Courts Press, 2005); Ian O'Donnell, "Lethal Violence in Ireland, 1841–2003," *British Journal of Criminology* 45 (2005): 671–95; William Wilbanks, "Homicide in Ireland," *International Journal of Comparative and Applied Criminal Justice* 20, no. 1 (Spring 1996): 59–75.

36. For example, see Conley, *Melancholy Accidents,* table 4.1, p. 92.

37. RIC, *Return of Outrages 1838–1921,* Files CSO ICR1 and CSO ICR2, NAI; police reports 1882–1921, Box 4, NAI. For statistics on the same data, see Conley, *Melancholy Accidents,* 68.

38. *Asylums Report* (1854–55), 155, HC 1854–55 (1981) xvi.137.

39. See C. Lockhart Robertson, "A Case of Homicidal Mania, Without Disorder of the Intellect," *Journal of Mental Science* 9, no. 47 (Oct. 1863): 327–43.

40. Conley, *Melancholy Accidents,* table 4.1, p. 92.

41. *Asylums Report* (1864), 379, HC 1864 (3369) xxiii.317.

42. North, "Insanity and Crime," 166; Smith, *Trial by Medicine,* 10; David Yellowlees, "Case of Murder during Temporary Insanity Induced by Drinking or Epilepsy," *Journal of Mental Science* 29, no. 127 (Oct. 1883), 386.

43. Yellowlees, "Case of Murder," 386.

44. RIC, *Return of Outrages for 1868,* Homicides, 5, File CSO ICR1, NAI.

45. Ibid., Homicides, 8.

46. RIC, *Return of Outrages for 1892,* Homicides, 3, and *Return of Outrages for 1893,* 18, File CSO ICR2, NAI.

47. Conley, *Melancholy Accidents,* 69, 70.

48. *Cox's Criminal Law Cases, 1843–1900* (London: John Crockford, Law Times Offices, 1901); M. McDonnell Bodkin, *Famous Irish Trials* (Dublin: Blackhall, 1997).

49. North, "Insanity and Crime"; Yellowlees, "Case of Murder."

50. RIC, *Return of Outrages for 1883,* Homicides, 10, File CSO ICR2, NAI.

51. This case is fully discussed in Prior, *Murder and Madness,* chap. 4.

52. RIC, *Return of Outrages for 1870,* Homicides, 10, File CSO ICR1, NAI.

53. RIC, *Return of Outrages for 1887,* Homicides, 5, File CSO ICR2, NAI.

54. *Asylums Report* (1854–55), 17, HC 1854–55 (1981) xvi.137.

55. RIC, *Return of Outrages for 1838–1921,* Files CSO ICR1 and CSO ICR2, NAI; police reports 1882–1921, Box 4, NAI; *Death Book (Male) 1852–1932,* File GPB CN 5, NAI; This figure is not complete because details on crimes are available only from 1868, and the data do not include the Dublin area because the same level of detail was not available in the Dublin Metropolitan Police records.

56. Prior, *Madness and Murder,* chap. 4, tables 4.3 and 4.4.

57. RIC, *Return of Outrages for 1890,* Homicides, 5, File CSO ICR1; police reports 1882–1921, Box 4, NAI.

58. *Kilkenny Journal,* 16 July 1890, cited in Conley, *Melancholy Accidents,* 60.

59. RIC, *Return of Outrages for 1892,* Homicides, 8, NAI; police reports 1882–1921, Box 4, NAI.

60. RIC, *Return of Outrages for 1868,* Homicides, 8, File CSO ICR1; transfers from Dundrum to District Asylum 1891, Convict Record File (CRF), File Misc. 392/1891, NAI.

61. RIC, *Return of Outrages for 1892,* Homicides, 6; police reports 1882–1921, Box 4, NAI.

62. See Daly, *Gender, Crime, and Punishment;* Clarice Feinman, *Women in the Criminal Justice System* (Westport, CT: Praeger, 1994); Heidensohn, *Women and Crime;* Allison Morris, *Women, Crime, and Criminal Justice* (London: Blackwell, 1987); Carol Smart, *Women, Crime, and Criminology: A Feminist Critique* (London: Routledge and Kegan Paul, 1977); Walklate, *Gender and Crime.*

63. For discussion, see Merlo and Pollock, *Women, Law, and Social Control;* Elicka Peterson, "Murder as Self-Help: Woman and Intimate Partner Homicide," *Homicide Studies* 3, no. 1 (1999): 30–46.

64. Inez Bailey, "Women and Crime in Nineteenth-Century Ireland," MA thesis, National Univ. of Ireland, Maynooth, 1992; Sinead Jackson, "Gender, Crime, and Punishment in Late Nineteenth-Century Ireland," MA thesis, National Univ. of Ireland, Galway, 1999; Rena Lohan, "The Treatment of Women Sentenced to Transportation and Penal Servitude 1790–1898," MLitt thesis, Trinity College, Dublin, 1989.

65. Prior, *Madness and Murder,* tables 6.1, 6.2, 6.3, pp. 150–53.

66. Ibid.

67. For a full discussion of these family killings, see ibid., chap. 7.

68. For a full discussion of the Cleary case, see Angela Bourke, *The Burning of Bridget Cleary* (London: Pimlico Press, 1999).

69. CRF on Mary Rielly/Reilly, CRF 1891/R.7, NAI.

70. For further discussion on this case, see Pauline M. Prior, "Roasting a Man Alive: The Case of Mary Rielly, Criminal Lunatic," *Eire–Ireland* 41, nos. 1–2 (Spring–Summer 2006): 169–91.

71. Many court records (held as part of the public-record archive) were lost in a major fire at the Custom House, Dublin, in the 1920s.

72. Correspondence and appeals for the Stackpoole family, CSORP Series, File 2421/1853, NAI.

73. CRF on Margaret Sheil, CRF 1870/S.7, NAI.

74. For a full discussion of such cases, see Prior, *Madness and Murder,* chap. 4.

75. Feinman, *Women in the Criminal Justice System,* 4.

76. See Prior, *Madness and Murder,* chap. 8.

6. Between Habitual Drunkards and Alcoholics: Inebriate Women and Reformatories in Ireland, 1899–1919

1. Rules governing the operation of reformatories in Ireland under the act were approved by Parliament in May 1899: *Inebriates Act, 1898. General Regulations for the Management and Discipline of Certified Inebriate Reformatories in Ireland, 1–24,* HC 1899 (182) lxxix.565–89.

2. *Twenty-Third Report of the General Prisons Board, Ireland [GPBI], 1900–01* (Dublin: General Prisons Board, 1901), 16–17. For a discussion of the Ennis reformatory in the context of developments in the Irish prison system, see B. A. Smith, "Ireland's Ennis Inebriates Reformatory: A 19th-Century Example of Failed Institutional Reform," *Federal Probation* 53, no. 1 (Mar. 1989): 53–64.

3. *First Report of the Inspector for Ireland under the Inebriates Acts [IIIA], 1879 to 1900, for the Years 1903 and 1904,* 5, Cd. 2796, HC 1906 xvi.137.

4. *Third Report of the IIIA, for the Year 1906,* 5, Cd. 3835, HC 1908 xii.1153.

5. *Sixth Report of the IIIA, for the Year 1909,* 5, Cd. 5344, HC 1910 xxxvi.837. For a discussion of the inebriate reformatories that dismisses them as reflecting an "imperial" and "ascendancy" approach to Ireland, see George Bretherton, "Irish Inebriate Reformatories, 1899–1920: An Experiment in Coercion," *Contemporary Drug Problems* 13, no. 3 (Fall 1986): 473–507.

6. The inspector initially appointed was Sir George Plunkett O'Farrell, MD, who was succeeded in 1911 by a new lunacy inspector, Dr. Thomas I. Considine.

7. Elizabeth Malcolm, "Hospitals in Ireland," in *The Field Day Anthology of Irish Writing,* vols. 4–5: *Irish Women's Writing and Traditions,* edited by Angela Bourke, Mair'n N' Dhonneadha, Siobhan Kilfeather, Maria Luddy, Margaret MacCurtain,

Geraldine Meaney, Mary O'Dowd, and Clair Wills (Cork: Cork Univ. Press, 2002), 705; R. D. Cassell, *Medical Charities and Medical Politics: The Irish Dispensary System and the Poor Law, 1836–72* (Woodbridge, UK: Boydell Press, 1997), 109–29.

8. Elizabeth Malcolm, "'Ireland's Crowded Madhouses': The Institutional Confinement of the Insane in Nineteenth- and Twentieth-Century Ireland," in *The Confinement of the Insane: International Perspectives, 1800–1965,* edited by Roy Porter and David Wright (Cambridge: Cambridge Univ. Press, 2003), 318.

9. Helen Burke, *The People and the Poor Law in 19th-Century Ireland* (Littlehampton, UK: Women's Education Bureau, 1987), 163 and 243–56; John O'Connor, *The Workhouses of Ireland: The Fate of Ireland's Poor* (Dublin: Anvil Books, 1995), 177–78.

10. Patrick Carroll-Burke, *Colonial Discipline: The Making of the Irish Convict System* (Dublin: Four Courts Press, 2000), 104; *Twenty-Third Report of the GPBI, 1900–01,* 8–9.

11. Jane Barnes, *Irish Industrial Schools, 1868–1908: Origins and Development* (Dublin: Irish Academic Press, 1989), 48–49, 65.

12. Nial Osborough, *Borstal in Ireland: Custodial Provision for the Young Adult Offender, 1906–74* (Dublin: Institute of Public Administration, 1975), 7–12.

13. David Garland, *Punishment and Welfare: A History of Penal Strategies* (Aldershot, UK: Gower, 1985), 3–35, 217–18; Nobert Finzsch and Robert Jütte, eds., *Institutions of Confinement: Hospitals, Asylums, and Prisons in Western Europe and North America, 1500–1950* (Cambridge: Cambridge Univ. Press, 1996).

14. Samuel B. Woodward, *Essays on Asylums for Inebriates* (Worcester, Mass.: n.p., 1838).

15. Jim Baumohl, "Inebriate Institutions in North America, 1840–1920," in *Drink in Canada: Historical Essays,* edited by C. K. Warsh (Montreal: McGill-Queen's Univ. Press, 1993), 92–94. The inebriate institutions had even spread to Australia by 1872, when one opened in Melbourne, instigated by an Irish doctor, Charles McCarthy, and supported by an Irish politician, Charles Gavan Duffy. See *Notes of Evidence Taken by the Departmental Committee on the Treatment of Inebriates* (London: Eyre and Spottiswoode, 1893), 12–13.

16. R. M. McLeod, "The Edge of Hope: Social Policy and Chronic Alcoholism, 1870–1900," *Journal of the History of Medicine* 22 (1967): 218–26.

17. The select committee had two Irish members, both of whom were temperance advocates: Mitchell Henry, Home Rule member for County Galway, and Lord Claud Hamilton, Conservative member for County Tyrone. It heard evidence from one of the two Dublin coroners, William White, who linked excessive drinking to suicide, and from one of the two Irish lunacy inspectors, Dr. John Nugent, who linked it to insanity. *Report of the Select Committee on the Control and Management of Habitual Drunkards,* ii, 17–21, 57–62, HC 1872 (242) ix.418, 461–65, 501–6.

18. D. W. Gutzke, *Protecting the Pub: Brewers and Publicans Against Temperance* (Woodbridge, UK: Boydell and Brewer, 1989), 60–98.

19. Elizabeth Malcolm, *"Ireland Sober, Ireland Free": Drink and Temperance in Nineteenth-Century Ireland* (Dublin: Gill and Macmillan, 1986), 274–75.

20. McLeod, "The Edge of Hope," 231.

21. *Notes of Evidence*, 1–106.

22. For an important discussion of habitual criminals and habitual drunkards, see Martin J. Wiener, *Reconstructing the Criminal: Culture, Law, and Policy in England, 1830–1914* (Cambridge: Cambridge Univ. Press, 1990), 294–306.

23. "It is a truism that 'therapy' and 'discipline' are necessarily conflicting goals." Russell P. Dobash and Sue Gutteridge, *The Imprisonment of Women* (Oxford: Basil Blackwell, 1986), 130.

24. Office of the General Prisons Board, Dublin Castle, *Memorandum on the Inebriates Act, 1898* (Dublin: General Prisons Board, 1906), 10, my emphasis.

25. *Thirty-Third Report of the GPBI, 1910–11* (Dublin: General Prisons Board, 1911), 16–17 and 40–41.

26. Office of the General Prisons Board, *Memorandum on the Inebriates Act, 1898*, 12.

27. *Thirty-Third Report of the GPBI, 1910–11*, xv.

28. For the stages system of imprisonment, see Elizabeth Dooley, "Sir Walter Crofton and the Irish or Intermediate System of Prison Discipline," in *Criminal Justice History: Themes and Controversies from Pre-independence Ireland*, edited by Ian O'Donnell and Finbarr McAuley, 196–213 (Dublin: Four Courts Press, 2003).

29. Office of the General Prisons Board, *Memorandum on the Inebriates Act, 1898*, 11–15; *Twenty-Third Report of the GPBI, 1900–01*, 18.

30. Office of the General Prisons Board, *Memorandum on the Inebriates Act, 1898*, 16–17.

31. Geraldine Curtin, *The Women of Galway Jail: Female Criminality in Nineteenth-Century Ireland* (Galway: Arlen House, 2001), 71–84.

32. For interesting details of the refurbishment, see *Twenty-Third Report of the GPBI, 1900–01*, 92.

33. *Forty-Second Report of the GPBI, 1919–20* (Dublin: General Prisons Board, 1920), vi, 5.

34. G. B. Wilson, *Alcohol and the Nation* (London: Nicolson and Watson, 1940), 442.

35. In the Irish Free State, more women than men were committed to prison for drunkenness each year up until 1937. Thereafter, with a few exceptions, men outnumbered women. See Ian O'Donnell, Eoin O'Sullivan, and Deirdre Healy, eds., *Crime and Punishment in Ireland, 1922 to 2003: A Statistical Sourcebook* (Dublin: Institute of Public Administration, 2005), 82 and 198–209.

36. *Eleventh Report of the IIIA, Being for the Year 1914*, 4, 8, Cd. 7888, HC 1914–16 xxiv.58, 62.

37. *Fourteenth Report of the IIIA, Being for the Year 1917*, 3, Cd. 9114, HC 1918 x.669.

38. During the 1920s and 1930s, the Northern Ireland government was concerned about drunkenness, especially the numbers of women committed to Armagh jail for drink-related offenses, and considered establishing an inebriate reformatory. Ministry of Home Affairs, Inebriate Home and "Red Biddy" Committee, 1922–38, File HA/9/2/272, Public Record Office of Northern Ireland (PRONI), Belfast.

39. *Thirty-Third Report of the GPBI, 1910–11*, 40; *Thirty-Seventh Report of the GPBI, 1914–15* (Dublin: General Prisons Board, 1915), 37; *Fortieth Report of the GPBI, 1917–18* (Dublin: General Prisons Board, 1918), 20; *Forty-Second Report of the GPBI, 1919–20*, vi.

40. W. J. Forsythe, *Penal Discipline, Reformatory Projects, and the English Prison Commission, 1895–1939* (Exeter, UK: Univ. of Exeter Press, 1991), 78–80 and 238–39.

41. Certified inebriate reformatories, registers of admissions and discharges, St. Patrick's, Waterford, Aug. 1906 to Oct. 1913, and St. Brigid's, Wexford, Mar. 1910 to Oct. 1917, OLA 13/1, National Archives of Ireland (NAI); *Third Report of the IIIA, for the Year 1906*, 6/1154; *Eleventh Report of the IIIA, Being for the Year 1914*. The 1914 report appears to suggest that thirty-three councils were supporting inmates, but it seems that this number relates to councils that had agreed in principle to do so. The registers list only eighteen councils as actually subsidizing inmates.

42. Virginia Crossman, *Local Government in Nineteenth-Century Ireland* (Belfast: Institute of Irish Studies, Queen's Univ., 1994), 91–97; Bradley Kadel, "The Pub and the Irish Nation," *Social History of Alcohol and Drugs* 18 (2003), 71, 79–82.

43. Elizabeth Malcolm, *The Irish Policeman, 1822–1922: A Life* (Dublin: Four Courts Press, 2006), 127; Mark Finnane, "A Decline in Violence in Ireland? Crime, Policing, and Social Relations, 1860–1914," *Crime, History, and Societies* 1, no. 1 (1997), 57–58; Carolyn A. Conley, *Melancholy Accidents: The Meaning of Violence in Post-famine Ireland* (Lanham, MD: Lexington Books, 1999), 28–32.

44. *Notes of Evidence Taken by the Departmental Committee on the Treatment of Inebriates*, 78; *Report of the Departmental Committee Appointed to Inquire into the Operation of the Law Relating to Inebriates' Detention in Reformatories and Retreats*, 52, Cd. 4438, HC 1908 xii.918.

45. Malcolm, *"Ireland Sober, Ireland Free,"* 277–321.

46. *Fourth Report of the IIIA, for the Year 1907*, 6, Cd. 4371, HC 1908 xii.1186

47. *First Report of the IIIA, for the Years 1903 and 1904*, 5–7 and 137–39. Around two-thirds of the retreat's patients entered for only six months, which most experts at the time considered far too short a period to achieve any lasting good.

48. *Sixth Report of the IIIA, for the Year 1909*, 6/838.

49. Diarmaid Ferriter, *A Nation of Extremes: The Pioneers in Twentieth-Century Ireland* (Dublin: Irish Academic Press, 1999).

50. Malcolm, *"Ireland Sober, Ireland Free,"* 306–11.

51. O'Farrell complained in particular about the lack of grounds for essential outdoor work and recreation, but by the end of 1906, within nine months of opening, St. Patrick's was already operating with a deficit of more than £500, which a year later had risen to more than £950. *Third Report of the IIIA, for the year 1906,* 22/1170; *Fourth Report of the IIIA, for the Year 1907,* 12/1192.

52. For a handy summary of the various medical opinions, see Virginia Berridge, "The Society for the Study of Addiction, 1884–1988," *British Journal of Addiction,* special issue, 85, no. 8 (Aug. 1990): 999–1016.

53. *Report of the Departmental Committee,* 3/823.

54. Reed had published a book and convened a conference in 1906 on excessive drinking and shortcomings in the Irish liquor-licensing laws. See Andrew Reed, *The Temperance Problem and the Liquor Licensing Laws of Ireland* (Dublin: A. Thom, 1906).

55. Sir Andrew Reed, preface to H. N. Barnett, *Legal Responsibility of the Drunkard* (London: Baillière, Tindall and Cox, 1908), ix. For an influential address along similar lines to the British Medical Association's annual conference in Belfast in 1909, see T. N. Kelynack, "Recent Researches Regarding Alcohol and Alcoholism," *British Journal of Inebriety* 7, no. 2 (Oct. 1909): 107–13. For the linking of inebriety to insanity, see Peter McCandless, "'Curses of Civilization': Insanity and Drunkenness in Victorian Britain," *British Journal of Addiction* 79, no. 1 (Mar. 1984): 49–58.

56. Barnett, *Legal Responsibility of the Drunkard,* 14–15.

57. Wilson, *Alcohol and the Nation,* 442.

58. Lucia Zedner, *Women, Crime, and Custody in Victorian England* (Oxford: Clarendon Press, 1991), 222–31; Greta Jones, "Eugenics in Ireland: The Belfast Eugenics Society," *Irish Historical Studies* 28, no. 109 (May 1992): 81–95.

59. *Fourteenth Report of the IIIA, Being for the Year 1917,* 4–5/670–1. Some of Dr. Considine's tables differentiate by sex, but most unfortunately do not.

60. For an informative oral history of drinking among women and men in early-twentieth-century Dublin, see K. C. Kearns, *Dublin Pub Life and Lore: An Oral History* (Dublin: Gill and Macmillan, 1996).

61. *Twenty-Ninth Report of the GPBI, 1906–7* (Dublin: General Prisons Board, 1907), 135–39; Smith, "Ireland's Ennis Inebriates Reformatory," 62–63.

62. *Fourteenth Report of the IIIA, Being for the Year 1917,* 3/669.

63. *Thirteenth Report of the IIIA, Being for the Year 1916,* 6, Cd. 8602, HC 1917 xv.162; *Fourteenth Report of the IIIA, Being for the Year 1917,* 6/672.

64. Two state and inebriate reformatories for men and women that were attached to prisons operated in England up to the First World War, in addition to twelve certified reformatories. Of nearly 4,600 committals, 81 percent were female. Greg Hunt, James

Mellor, and John Turner, "Wretched, Hatless, and Miserably Clad: Women and the Inebriate Reformatories from 1900–13," *British Journal of Sociology* 40, no. 2 (June 1989), 245–46.

65. George Bretherton's 1986 article, which was republished in 2003, suffers from this problem as well as from unfamiliarity with the complexities of contemporary medical debates concerning chronic drunkenness. George Bretherton, "Irish Inebriate Reformatories, 1899–1920: A Small Experiment in Coercion," in O'Donnell and McAuley, eds., *Criminal Justice History*, 214–32.

66. For important initiatives in the treatment of alcoholism in Ireland and England during the 1940s, see Elizabeth Malcolm, *Swift's Hospital: A History of St. Patrick's Hospital, Dublin, 1746–1989* (Dublin: Gill and Macmillan, 1989), 277–78; B. Thom and Virginia Berridge, "'Special Units for Common Problems': The Birth of Alcohol Treatment Units in England," *Social History of Medicine* 8, no. 1 (Apr. 1995): 75–93.

7. Managing Midwifery in Dublin: Practice and Practitioners, 1700–1800

1. David Cressy, *Birth, Marriage, and Death: Ritual, Religion, and the Life-Cycle in Tudor and Stuart England* (Oxford: Oxford Univ. Press, 1997), 15–92; Patricia Crawford, "The Construction and Experience of Maternity in Seventeenth-Century England," in *Women as Mothers in Pre-industrial England,* edited by Valerie Fildes, 3–38 (London: Routledge 1990); Linda A. Pollock, "Embarking on a Rough Passage: The Experience of Pregnancy in Early Modern Society," in Fildes, ed., *Women as Mothers in Pre-industrial England,* 39–67; Adrian Wilson, "The Ceremony of Childbirth and Its Interpretation," in Fildes, ed., *Women as Mothers in Pre-industrial England,* 68–107; Adrian Wilson, "Participant or Patient? Seventeenth-Century Childbirth from the Mother's Point of View," in *Patients and Practitioners: Lay Perceptions of Medicine in Pre-industrial Society,* edited by Roy Porter, 129–44 (Cambridge: Cambridge Univ. Press, 1985); Clodagh Tait, "Safely Delivered: Childbirth, Wet-Nursing, Gossip-Feasts, and Churching in Ireland c. 1530–1690," *Irish Economic Social History* 30 (2003): 1–23.

2. A crotchet was a type of hook that was used to grasp the fetal skull in order to extract infants that had died in utero.

3. James Wolveridge, *Speculum Matrisis Hibernicum; or the Irish Midwives Handmaid* (London: E. Okes, 1670), 94; Percival Willughby, *Observations in Midwifery: As Also the Country Midwife's Opusculum or Vade Mecum,* edited by Henry Blenkinsop (Warwick, UK: n.p., 1863), reprint edited by John L. Thornton (Wakefield, UK: S. R. Publishers, 1972), 149–57; Maurice Lenihan, "The Fee-Book of a Physician of the Seventeenth Century," *Journal of the Royal Society of Antiquaries of Ireland* 9 (1867), 22, 27, 165, 150, 242.

4. Jean Donninson, *Midwives and Medical Men: A History of Inter-professional Rivalries and Women's Rights* (London: Heinemann Educational, 1977), 42–61; Adrian

Wilson, *The Making of Man-Midwifery: Childbirth in England 1660–1770* (London: Univ. College of London Press, 1995), 53–59.

5. Donnison, *Midwives and Medical Men,* 3.

6. Alan G. R. Smith, *Science and Society in the Sixteenth and Seventeenth Centuries* (London: Thames and Hudson, 1972), 134–49.

7. Laurence Brockliss, "Science, Universities, and Other Public Spaces," in *Eighteenth Century Science,* vol. 4 of *The Cambridge History of Science,* edited by Roy Porter, 44–86 (Cambridge: Cambridge Univ. Press, 2003).

8. Willughby, *Observations in Midwifery,* introduction and vii; Donninson, *Midwives and Medical Men,* 21–41.

9. Donninson, *Midwives and Medical Men,* 42–62.

10. J. H. Aveling, *The Chamberlens and the Midwifery Forceps* (London: J. & A. Churchill, 1882), 215–26; Walter Radcliffe, *The Secret Instrument: The Birth of the Midwifery Forceps* (London: Heinemann Medical Books, 1947), 17–18.

11. François Mauriceau, *The Diseases of Women with Child and in Child-Bed,* translated by Hugh Chamberlen (London: John Darby, 1672), 208.

12. It is not clear when this marriage took place. I am grateful to Robert Mills, archivist at the College of Physicians, Dublin, for access to the file "Family of Walker and their connection with Dr Peter Chamberlen" in the Kirkpatrick Collection in this archive.

13. *Dublin Weekly Journal,* 11 Mar. 1731.

14. H. Drinkwater, "The Modern Descendants of Dr. Peter Chamberlen," *Liverpool Medico-Chirurgical Journal* 36 (1916): 98–105; R. W. Innes Smith, *English-Speaking Students of Medicine at the Univ. of Leyden* (London: Oliver and Boyd, 1932), 140; and Laetitia Pilkington, *Memoirs of Laetitia Pilkington, 1712–1750* (London: R. Griffiths, 1748), 30.

15. Charles A. Cameron, *History of the Royal College of Surgeons in Ireland* (Dublin: Fannin, 1886), 69–103, 111–15.

16. *Dublin Journal* (July 1762): 24–27.

17. W. J. Reader, *Professional Men: The Rise of the Professional Classes in Nineteenth-Century England* (London: Weidenfeld & Nicolson, 1966), 33–34.

18. Hilary Marland, ed., *The Art of Midwifery: Early Modern Midwives in Europe* (London: Routledge, 1993); Doreen Evenden, *The Midwives of Seventeenth-Century London* (Cambridge: Cambridge Univ. Press, 2000).

19. Justine Siegmund, *The Court Midwife,* translated by Lynne Tatlock (Chicago: Univ. of Chicago Press, 2005); Hilary Marland, trans., *"Mother and Child Were Saved": The Memoirs (1693–1740) of the Friesen Midwife Catherina Schrader* (Amsterdam: Rodolpi, 1987); Duncan Stewart, "The Caesarean Operation Done with Success by a Midwife," *Medical Essays and Observations* 5, no. 38 (1747): 360–62.

20. Thomas R. Forbes, *The Midwife and the Witch* (New Haven, CT: Yale Univ. Press, 1966), 131. The first municipal ordinances are believed to be those in the Hebammenordnung of Regensburg, Germany, dating from 1452. For regulation, see David Harley, "Provincial Midwives in England: Lancashire and Cheshire, 1660–1760," in Marland, ed., *The Art of Midwifery,* 31, 34.

21. P. F. Moran, *History of the Catholic Archbishops of Dublin, since the Reformation* (Dublin: J. Duffy, 1864), 444; Daniel McCarthy, ed., *Collections on Irish Church History from the Manuscripts of the Late Very Reverend Laurence Renehan,* vol. 1 (Dublin: C. M. Warren, 1861), 429–30; *Articles Given in Charge to Be Inquired upon and Presented Too, by the Churchwardens, Side-men, Quest-men, and Inquisitors in Every Parish within the Province of Armagh, in the Course of the Metropoliticall Visitation of the Same, in This Present Yeare Begun, by the Most Reverend Father in God, Christopher, by the Mercy of God, Lord Archbishop of Ardmagh, Primate and Metropolitane of All Ireland* (Dublin: n.p., 1623), one page only, item 19; *Articles to Be Inquired of by the Church-Wardens and Questmen of Every Parish in the Next Visitation, to Be Made by the Right Reverend Father in God John, (Leslie) Bishop of Clogher* (Dublin: n.p., 1667), 3–10; the charge given by Narcissus Marsh, lord archbishop of Dublin, to his clergy at his primary visitation, 27 June 1694, Cathedral Church of St. Patrick's, Dublin, 26; William Keatinge Clay, ed., *Liturgical Services: Liturgies and Occasional Forms of Prayer Set Forth in the Reign of Queen Elizabeth* (Cambridge: Cambridge Univ. Press, 1847), 206–9; *The Book of Common Prayer and Administration of the Sacraments and Other Rites and Ceremonies of the Church of England* (London: n.p., 1641), section on public and private baptism; Francis Proctor, *A History of the Book of Common Prayer,* 17th ed. (London: n.p., 1871), 388.

22. The Catholic Church did not license midwives. Regulation took the form of decrees and instructions to parish priests to oversee the implementation of these decrees (see note 21). The Church of Ireland granted licenses to both midwives and physicians following the swearing of an oath. Richard Caulfield, *Annals of St. Fin Barre's Cathedral, Cork* (Cork: Purcell & Co., 1871), 46–47; Richard Caulfield, "Midwives," *Notes and Queries,* 2nd series, 2 (Jan. 1861): 59; Richard Garnet, *The Book of Oaths and Severall Forms Thereof Both Ancient and Modern* (London: For W. Lee, M. Walbancke, D. Pakeman, and G. Bedle, 1649), 284–90.

23. National Men's meeting at Dublin, 1671–88, File 1/2YM1, 47 (Epistle 12/9/1677), Swanbrook House, Dublin.

24. Evenden, *The Midwives of Seventeenth-Century London,* 174–75.

25. Thomas Forbes, "The Regulation of English Midwives in the 18th and 19th centuries," *Medical History* 15 (1971): 352–62. See also John R. Guy, "The Episcopal Licensing of Physicians, Surgeons, and Midwives," *Bulletin of the History of Medicine*

56, no. 4 (1982): 528–54; Ian Mortimer, "Diocesan Licensing and Medical Practitioners in South-West England 1660–1780," *Medical History* 48 (2004): 49–68.

26. N. B. White, "A Lycence and Oath of a Midwife, Granted to a Midwife, Mrs. Elliot, by the Bishop of Ossary, in 1740," *Journal of the Kilkenny and South East of Ireland Archaeological Society* 5 (1864–66), 412–13.

27. Dr. McKenna's Visitation Notes, c. 1785, Diocese of Cloyne, File U.181, no. 25, Cork Archives Institute.

28. *Statuta dioecesana per Provincium Dubliniensem, observanda et a Daniel Murray [Archbishhop of Dublin]*, 1831, 86, collection not cataloged, Dublin Diocesan Archives.

29. *Journal of the Royal College of Physicians of Ireland* 1 (1971), 73, Royal College of Physicians of Ireland (RCPI), Dublin.

30. Copy of the Charter of the Kings and Queens College of Physicians of Ireland (1692), 44, RCPI.

31. *Register of Licentiates in Midwifery of King and Queen's College of Physicians of Ireland,* RCPI.

32. Ibid.

33. *Declaration on Admission as Licentiate in Midwifery,* single certificate, not cataloged, RCPI.

34. T. C. P. Kirkpatrick, *History of the Medical Teaching in Trinity College* (Dublin: Hanna and Neale, 1912), 117; J. D. H. Widdess, *History of the Royal College of Physicians of Ireland* (Edinburgh: E. & S. Livingstone, 1963), 66; *Journal of the Royal College of Physicians* 2 (1972), 146.

35. Roy Porter, "A Touch of Danger: The Man-Midwife as Sexual Predator," in *Sexual Underworlds of the Enlightenment,* edited by G. S. Rousseau and Roy Porter, 206–24 (Manchester, UK: Manchester Univ. Press, 1987).

36. Phillip Thicknesse, *Man-Midwifery Analysed* (London: n.p., 1765), 5–10; Francis Foster, *Thoughts on the Times, but Chiefly on the Profligacy of Our Women, and Its Causes* (London: C. Parker & J. Bew, 1779), 78–92: John Blunt, *Man-Midwifery Dissected* (London: S. W. Fores, 1793), 66–93.

37. Fielding Ould, *A Treatise of Midwifery in Three Parts* (Dublin: Oli Nelson, 1742), 34.

38. William Wilde, "Illustrious Physicians and Surgeons in Ireland, no. II, Bartholomew Mosse, M.D.," *Dublin Quarterly Journal of Medical Science* 15, no. 2 (1846), 567.

39. Quoted in ibid. No attempt was made to record the life and work of Bartholomew Mosse after his death. Dr. Fleetwood Churchill presented a paper marking Mosse's achievements at a meeting of the Obstetrical Society in 1842. The details in that paper were taken from a manuscript by Benjamin Higgins, who was the first secretary of the Lying-in Hospital's board of governors and registrar from 1760.

40. Women were recommended by the Protestant ministers or churchwardens from 1745. The arrangement was formalized when the hospital relocated to Great Britain Street, when women attended the hospital on Mondays, Wednesdays, and Fridays to have their letters of recommendation signed by the master. Minutes of the proceedings of the Board of Governors of the Lying-in Hospital of Dublin, 3 Feb. 1758, Dublin 22, Box 23, National Archives of Ireland (NAI), Dublin. Catholic women started to be recommended shortly afterward.

41. Registry of patients admitted to the Lying-in Hospital in George's Lane, from its opening 15 March 1745 until November 1756, Dublin 22, Box 23, NAI.

42. For a discussion on maternal mortality in the early modern period, see Roger Schofield, "Did the Mothers Really Die? Three Centuries of Maternal Mortality," in *The World We Have Gained: Histories of Population and Social Structure,* edited by Lloyd Bonfield, Richard Smith, and Keith Wrightson (Oxford: Oxford Univ. Press, 1986), 259–60.

43. Quoted in Wilde, "Illustrious Physicians," 578.

44. Minutes of the proceedings of the Board of Governors of the Lying-in Hospital of Dublin, Dec. 1756–Feb. 1798, Dublin 22, Box 23, vol. 1, p. 2, NAI.

45. On the history of the Rotunda Hospital, see T. P. C. Kirkpatrick, *The Book of the Rotunda Hospital* (London: Adlard & Bartholomew Press, 1913); O'Donel T. D. Browne, *The Rotunda Hospital, 1745–1947* (Edinburgh: E & S. Livingstone, 1947); Ian Campbell Ross, ed., *Public Virtue, Public Love: The Early Years of the Dublin Lying-in Hospital* (Dublin: O'Brien Press, 1986); and Alan Brown, ed., *Masters, Midwives, and Ladies-in-Waiting: The Rotunda Hospital 1745–1995* (Dublin: A. & A. Farmar, 1995).

46. Ould, *A Treatise of Midwifery,* 4.

47. Ibid., 71.

48. Ibid., 79.

49. Thomas Southwell, "Remarks on Some of the Errors Both in Anatomy and Practice Contained in the Late Treatise of Midwifery, Published by Fielding Ould, Man-Midwife," 1742, *Haliday Pamphlets* 165/6, 9–14, 19–22, Royal Irish Academy (RIA), Dublin.

50. Widdess, *History,* 66.

51. E. Ashworth Underwood, *Boerhaave's Men at Leyden and After* (Edinburgh: Edinburgh Univ. Press, 1977), 122–23. In the space of ten years (1741–51), Smellie taught more than nine hundred male pupils. See William Smellie, *A Treatise on the Theory and Practice of Midwifery,* 3 vols. (Edinburgh: n.p., 1784), 1:i and viii.

52. Aquilla Smith, "Illustrious Physicians and Surgeons in Ireland No. III, David McBride M.D.," *Dublin Quarterly Journal of Medical Science* (Feb. 1847): 281–90.

53. David McBride, *Miscellanea Medica* (1749–60), Dublin 22, Bundle 13, not paginated, NAI.

54. Ibid., cases 132 and 141.

55. Ibid., case 147. Placenta praevia was first noted as "unavoidable haemorrhage" in 1775; eclampsia was recognized in 1813; see Irvine Loudon, *Death in Childbirth: An International Study of Maternal Care and Maternal Mortality 1800–1950* (Oxford: Oxford Univ. Press, 1992), 100 and 87, respectively.

56. McBride, *Miscellanea Medica,* cases 36, 74, 77.

57. Smith, "Illustrious Physicians," 287.

58. Jo Murphy-Lawless, "Images of 'Poor' Women in the Writings of Irish Men Midwives," in *Women in Early Modern Ireland,* edited by Margaret MacCurtain and Mary O' Dowd, 291–303 (Edinburgh: Edinburgh Univ. Press, 1991).

59. Adrian Wilson, "The Politics of Medical Improvement in Early Hanoverian London," in *The Medical Enlightenment of the Eighteenth Century,* edited by Andrew Cunningham and Roger French, 13–15 (Cambridge: Cambridge Univ. Press, 1990); Roy Porter, "The Gift Relation: Philanthropy and Provincial Hospitals in Eighteenth-Century England," in *The Hospital in History,* edited by Lindsay Granshaw and Roy Porter, 149–78 (London: Routledge, 1989); Lindsay Granshaw, "The Rise of the Modern Hospital in Britain," in *Medicine in Society,* edited by Andrew Wear, 197–218 (Cambridge: Cambridge Univ. Press, 1992); Margaret Connor Versluysen, "Midwives, Medical Men, and 'Poor Women Labouring of Child': Lying-in Hospitals in Eighteenth-Century London," in *Women, Health, and Reproduction,* edited by Helen Roberts, 18–49 (London: Routledge & Kegan Paul, 1981); Margaret Pelling, "Medical Practice in Early Modern England: Trade or Profession?" in *The Professions in Early Modern England,* edited by Wilfred Prest, 90–128 (London: Croom Helm, 1987).

60. Joseph Clarke, "An Account of a Disease Which, Until Lately, Proved Fatal to a Great Number of Infants in the Lying-in Hospital, with Observations on Its Causes and Prevention," *Transactions of the Royal Irish Academy* 3 (1789): 89–109; Joseph Clarke, "Remarks on the Causes and Cure of Some Diseases of Infancy," *Transactions of the Royal Irish Academy* 6 (1789): 3–14; Joseph Clarke, "On Bilious Colic and Convulsions in Early Infancy," *Transactions of the Royal Irish Academy* 11 (1797): 121–30.

61. William Dease, *Observations in Midwifery, Particularly on the Different Methods of Assisting Women in Tedious and Difficult Labours* (Dublin: J. Williams, L. White, W. Wilson, P. Byrne, and J. Cash, 1783); Joseph Clarke, "Observations on Puerperal Fever; More Especially As It Has of Late Occurred in the Lying-in Hospital of Dublin," in *Medical and Philosophical Commentaries,* edited by Andrew Duncan, 299–324 (Philadelphia: T. Dobson, 1783–95).

62. *Freeman's Journal,* 29 Dec. 1769–1 Jan. 1779; William Collum, *Reasons Against Lectures in the Lying-in Hospital* (1770), Haliday Pamphlets no. 354, RIA; Frederick Jebb, *A View of the Schemes at Present under Consideration of the Governors of the Lying-in Hospital* (1771), Haliday Pamphlets no. 354, RIA.

63. Smellie, *A Treatise on the Theory and Practice of Midwifery,* 1:430–34.

64. G. L'E. Turner, "Eighteenth-Century Scientific Instruments and Their Makers," in Porter, ed., *Eighteenth Century Science*, 521–25.

65. *Dublin Journal*, 13–17 July 1762.

66. Wilson, *Making of Man-Midwifery*, chap. 14; Audrey Eccles, *Obstetrics and Gynaecology in Tudor and Stewart England* (London: Croom Helm, 1982), 119–24; Hilary Marland and Anne Marie Rafferty, eds., *Midwives, Society, and Childbirth: Debates and Controversies in the Modern Period* (London: Routledge, 1997), 1–14.

8. Lady Dudley's District Nursing Scheme and the Congested Districts Board, 1903–1923

1. In this essay, "West of Ireland" describes the congested areas/districts of Donegal, Roscommon, Leitrim, Sligo, Mayo, Galway, Kerry, and West Cork.

2. There is one notable exception: Bridget N. Hedderman, *Glimpses of My Life in Aran: Some Experiences of a District Nurse in These Remote Islands, off the West Coast of Ireland*, Part 1 (Bristol, UK: Wright, 1917). Part 2 was never published; this account was intended to give an insight into the daily grind of public-health nursing, but it is unfortunately bereft of personal details and dates.

3. For an example of such photographs, see Margaret Ó hÓgartaigh, "Nurses and Teachers in the West of Ireland in the Late-Nineteenth and Early-Twentieth Centuries," in *Framing the West: Images of Rural Ireland, 1891–1920*, edited by Ciara Breathnach, 197–214 (Dublin: Irish Academic Press, 2007)4. For perceptive discussions of the professionalization of nursing and the role of philanthropy, see Siobhan Nelson, *Say Little, Do Much: Nursing, Nuns, and Hospitals in the Nineteenth Century* (Philadelphia: Univ. of Pennsylvania Press, 2003); Margaret H. Preston, *Charitable Words: Women, Philanthropy, and the Language of Charity in Nineteenth-Century Dublin* (Westport, CT: Praeger, 2004); and Gerard M. Fealy, *A History of Apprenticeship Nurse Training in Ireland* (London: Routledge, 2006).

5. R. B. McDowell, *The Irish Administration, 1801–1914* (London: Routledge, 1964), 60.

6. Ibid., 53; *Nursing Record*, 6 Feb. 1890, 72. District nursing is the practice of administering to patients in their homes and has its origins in Liverpool.

7. The *Irish Homestead* was founded by Sir Horace Plunkett in 1895 and continued as a weekly journal until 1925. It was a mouthpiece for the Irish Agricultural Organisation Society, founded in 1894. The Dudley committee took over the running of the Foxford center in 1907.

8. Lady Dudley's Scheme for the Establishment of District Nurses in the Poorest Parts of Ireland, *First Annual Report* (Dublin: n.p., 1904), 6–7, National Library of Ireland (NLI), Dublin. For the Dudley nurses' impact on the local community, see

Ó hÓgartaigh, "Nurses and Teachers in the West of Ireland." For the Dudley Estate Archives, see the Dudley Archives & Local History Service, Coseley, West Midlands, United Kingdom.

9. For development of system up to 1851, see Laurence M. Geary, *Medicine and Charity in Ireland, 1718–1851* (Dublin: Univ. College Dublin Press, 2004).

10. John F. Fleetwood, *The History of Medicine in Ireland* (Dublin: Skellig Press, 1983), 168.

11. Letter to the editor, *Irish Times,* 31 Dec. 1903.

12. Ruth Barrington, *Health, Medicine, and Politics in Ireland, 1900–70* (Dublin: Institute of Public Administration, 1987), 10–11.

13. Lady Dudley's Scheme, *First Annual Report* (Dublin: n.p., 1904), 12. The annual reports of the Dudley scheme are held at the National Library of Ireland, Dublin.

14. Commission of Inquiry on Better Care, Relief, and Treatment of Poor Who Are Lunatic, Idiotic or Imbecile in Mind (1878–79), midwifery evidence of Mr. Horsley, sixty-one, and the evidence of Captain George O'Callaghan, Tulla, County Clare, Parliamentary Papers (PP), C. 2239, 157.

15. *Report as to the Practice of Medicine and Surgery by Unqualified Persons in the United Kingdom* (London: Medical Council, Unqualified Practitioners, 1910), PP, Cd. 5422, vol. XLIII, 5, 22. Roy Porter's analysis of quacks in the England has yet to be rivaled by a study of the Irish context; see Roy Porter, "The Language of Quackery in England, 1660–1800," in *The Social History of Language,* edited by P. Burke and R. Porter, 73–104 (Cambridge: Cambridge Univ. Press, 1987).

16. Porter, "The Language of Quackery," 74.

17. Fleetwood, *The History of Medicine in Ireland,* 163.

18. Barrington, *Health, Medicine, and Politics in Ireland,* 7–8. Barrington also argues that the further duty of medical officer of health created a conflict for doctors, and "the arrangement did little to improve environmental conditions for public health since the obligations of the MOH often conflicted with the interests of private practice."

19. Hedderman, *Glimpses of My Life in Aran,* 83.

20. Micks later became CDB secretary.

21. William L. Micks, *Balfour Papers,* Add., 49817, folios 124–25, British Library, London.

22. Hedderman, *Glimpses of my Life in Aran,* 9.

23. Lady Dudley's Scheme, *First Annual Report,* 15.

24. *British Journal of Nursing* (16 Sept. 1905): 233.

25. The 1851 figures are derived from a paper delivered by Laurence M. Geary at an Economic and Social Research Council–funded workshop on welfare regimes in Ireland 1850–1921, 20 Feb. 2008, Oxford Brookes, UK.

26. For information on superannuation of those describing themselves as "midwives" in workhouse hospitals, see *Thirtieth Annual Report of the Local Government*

Board for Ireland, for the Year Ending 31st March 1902 (1903), PP, Cd. 1606. The extent to which such nurses could be categorized as midwives is questionable.

27. *British Journal of Nursing* (16 Sept. 1905): 233.

28. For a thorough analysis of Anglican social conscience, see Oonagh Walsh, *Anglican Women in Dublin: Philanthropy, Politics, and Education in the Early Twentieth Century* (Dublin: Univ. College Dublin Press, 2005).

29. Joseph Robbins, *Nursing and Midwifery in Ireland in the Twentieth Century* (Dublin: An Bord Altranais, 2000), 12; Robert Dingwall, Anne Marie Rafferty, and Charles Webster, *An Introduction to the Social History of Nursing* (London: Routledge, 1988), 181.

30. See Pauline Scanlan, *The Irish Nurse: A Study of Nursing in Ireland, History and Education 1718–1981* (Drunshambo, Ireland: Drumlin, 1991), 79. St. Patrick's became affiliated with the Irish branch of the QVJIN in 1890. Lady Dudley's Scheme, *First Annual Report*, 3.

31. Arthur J. Balfour established the CDB to deal with regionally specific rural poverty along the western seaboard. For further analysis of the CDB's work, see Ciara Breathnach, *A History of the Congested Districts Board of Ireland, 1891–1923: Poverty and Development in the West of Ireland* (Dublin: Four Courts Press, 2005), and William L. Micks, *An Account of the Constitution, Administration, and Dissolution of the Congested Districts Board of Ireland, 1891–1923* (Dublin: Eason & Son, 1925).

32. Quoted in *British Journal of Nursing* (18 Aug. 1906), 126.

33. For further information on the Parish Committee Scheme, see Breathnach, *A History of the Congested Districts Board of Ireland*, 131–36.

34. CDB, *Sixth Annual Report* (Dublin: CDB, 1897), 27. The CDB's annual reports were returned to Parliament and are available as British PP until 1922, and thereafter two annual reports were returned to Saorstát Éireann.

35. I am grateful to Ivor Hamrock, local history librarian, Mayo County Library, for information on the Achill Disaster Fund. The fund was collected to alleviate suffering following an accident in June 1894 when thirty-two young seasonal migrants drowned; the hooker they were traveling in capsized on its way to Westport. CDB, *Seventh Annual Report* (Dublin: CDB, 1898), 37; CDB, *Eighth Annual Report* (Dublin: CDB, 1899), 30; CDB, *Ninth Annual Report* (Dublin: CDB, 1900), 44.

36. Lady Dudley's Scheme, *First Annual Report*, 3. This amount covered "rents and taxes, salary, uniform allowance, board wages and an allowance for the keep of a servant, and fire and lighting."

37. Ibid.

38. CDB, *Fourteenth Annual Report* (Dublin: CDB, 1905), 41.

39. Lady Dudley's Scheme, *Second Annual Report* (Dublin: n.p., 1905), 8.

40. CDB, *Fifteenth Annual Report* (Dublin: CDB, 1906), 33. In 1901, the board gave its coffee stall at Roundstone to the Galway Temperance Association.

41. Lady Dudley's scheme, *Second Annual Report,* 13.

42. *British Journal of Nursing* (15 July 1905): 53. Lady Dudley's Scheme, *Fourth Annual Report* (Dublin: n.p., 1907), 19. Descriptions such as the following routinely appeared in the annual reports: "There is at present a district on the coast of Co Galway, near the region of Costello Bay, which is known to the Committee as being in urgent need of the services of a nurse. It is one of the poorest and most thickly populated of the Congested Districts. It is many miles from the nearest dispensary relief. The poor people of this locality send constant appeals for help in sickness to the nurse established in the neighbouring district on the coast, but the distances are too great, and the work in her own neighbourhood too constant for it to be possible for her to respond to these calls."

43. Lady Dudley's Scheme, *Fourth Annual Report,* 11–12.

44. Lady Dudley's Scheme, *Eighteenth Annual Report* (Dublin: n.p., 1921), 10.

45. Lady Dudley's Scheme, *Fourth Annual Report,* 12.

46. CDB, *Twenty-Third Annual Report* (Dublin: CDB, 1915), 21.

47. CDB, *Sixteenth Annual Report* (Dublin: CDB, 1907), 34.

48. CDB, *Twentieth Annual Report* (Dublin: CDB, 1912), 31.

49. Lord Dudley became governor-general in Australia, and while there Lady Dudley initiated a district nursing scheme in the outback. See Trudy Yuginovich, "A Potted History of 19th-Century Remote-Area Nursing in Australia and, in Particular, Queensland," *Australian Journal of Rural Health* 8 (2000): 63–67.

50. Lady Dudley's Scheme, *Seventh Annual Report* (Dublin: n.p., 1910), 7.

51. CDB, *Twentieth Annual Report,* 31.

52. Comment included in Lady Dudley's Scheme, *Eighth Annual Report* (Dublin: n.p., 1910), 12.

53. Comment included in Lady Dudley's Scheme, *First Annual Report,* 8.

54. Comment included in Lady Dudley's Scheme, *First Annual Report,* 3–10. Excerpt of an account written by Thomas Lawler, parish priest of Kilorglin.

55. Comment included in Lady Dudley's Scheme, *Ninth Annual Report* (Dublin: n.p., 1911), 16.

56. Reports to the Local Government Board in Ireland respecting outbreak of fever in Swinford Union, County Mayo (1880), 277-I, vol. LXII, 271, 275, 1–12, National Archives of Ireland, Dublin.

57. Commission of Inquiry on Better Care, Relief, and Treatment of Poor Who Are Lunatic, Idiotic, or Imbecile in Mind, 1878–79, PP, C. 2239, 114.

58. Hedderman, *Glimpses of My Life in Aran,* 80.

59. Ibid.

60. Late-nineteenth-century newspaper adverts highlight a vast array of patent medicines making spurious curative claims.

61. Letter dated 29 Feb. 1903, in Lady Dudley's Scheme, *First Annual Report,* 14.

62. Lady Dudley's Scheme, *Tenth Annual Report* (Dublin: n.p., 1913), 15.

63. Comment included in ibid., 15.

64. Account included in Lady Dudley's Scheme, *Eighth Annual Report,* 13.

65. Quoted in E. Morrison, "A District Nurse among the Poor," *New Ireland Review* (Mar. 1909): 24–31. For further cases of unqualified nurses working in Union hospitals, see *Report from Commissioners, Inspectors, and Poor Law Reform Commissioners,* 1906, PP, Cd. 3204, vol. LII. See also Scanlan, *The Irish Nurse,* 67–68, where Scanlan cites cases of pauper inmates working as nursing assistants in workhouse hospitals.

66. Maria Luddy, *Women and Philanthropy in Nineteenth-Century Ireland* (Cambridge: Cambridge Univ. Press, 1995), 49–50.

67. Lady Dudley's Scheme, *Fourth Annual Report,* 13.

68. Quoted in *British Journal of Nursing* (17 Nov. 1906), 398.

69. *Royal Commission on the Poor Laws and Relief of Distress: Report on Ireland,* 1909, PP, Cd. 4630, vol. XXXVIII.

70. Lady Dudley's Scheme, *Eighth Annual Report,* 4.

71. Hedderman, *Glimpses of My Life in Aran,* preface.

72. Lady Dudley's Scheme, *Third Annual Report,* 10.

73. Lady Dudley's Scheme, *Fourth Annual Report,* 9.

74. Lady Dudley's Scheme, *Eighth Annual Report,* 6.

75. Lady Dudley's Scheme, *Ninth Annual Report,* 10. For further information on how the National Insurance Act applied to Ireland, see W. Dudley Edwards, "The National Insurance Act, 1911 (Part I): As Applying to Ireland," *Journal of the Statistical and Social Inquiry Society of Ireland* 12, no. 92 (1911–12): 569–82.

76. Lady Dudley's Scheme, *Twelfth Annual Report* (Dublin: n.p., 1915), 8–9.

77. Lady Dudley's Scheme, *Thirteenth Annual Report* (Dublin: n.p., 1916), 1.

78. Letter in File 614L3, Ireland Catalogue (IR), National Library of Ireland (NLI); Lady Dudley's Scheme, *Fourth Annual Report,* 12.

79. Robbins, *Nursing and Midwifery in Ireland in the Twentieth Century,* 11.

80. Lady Dudley's Scheme, *Eleventh Annual Report* (Dublin: n.p., 1914), 10.

81. Lady Dudley's Scheme, *Twenty-Sixth Annual Report* (Dublin: n.p., 1928), 6.

82. Barrington, *Health, Medicine, and Politics in Ireland,* 12.

83. CDB, Minutes of Proceedings, 29 May 1923. These houses were sold during the 1980s under the auspices of the Charitable Bequests of Ireland.

84. Dáil Éireann, debates, Dec. 1922, vols. II–XIII, 2–13; June 1974 letter from Brendan Corish, then *tánaiste* (deputy prime minister) and minister for health, IR 614L3, NLI. "I have noted, with regret that your Committee has found it necessary to terminate the activities of the lady Dudley's Nursing Scheme. As Minister for Health I would like to express my thanks to the committee for the invaluable work that has been performed by the Lady Dudley nurses in the home nursing field since the foundation of the scheme. I am pleased to know that the nurses employed by your committee have

now been transferred to services of the health boards and I am glad that my department has been able to help in the matter."

85. Saorstát Éireann, *Report of the Commission on the Relief of the Sick and Destitute Poor Including the Insane Poor* (Dublin: n.p., 1927), File R27, IR 66, NLI.

9. "The Wages of Sin Is Death": Lock Hospitals, Venereal Disease, and Gender in Prefamine Ireland

A version of this paper was presented at the annual conference of the Economic and Social History Society of Ireland, Queen's Univ., Belfast, 17 Nov. 2006. I am grateful to those who attended for their helpful comments. Since the completed paper was submitted to the editors of the current volume, Maria Luddy's important study *Prostitution and Irish Society, 1800–1940* (Cambridge: Cambridge Univ. Press, 2007), has been published, and her work deals comprehensively with many of the issues raised in my paper.

1. T. P. C. Kirkpatrick, "Syphilis and the State," *Dublin Journal of Medical Science* 145 (1918): 339–57. See also David Fleming, "Public Attitudes to Prostitution in Eighteenth-Century Ireland," *Irish Economic and Social History* 32 (2005): 1–18.

2. Carmel Quinlan, *Genteel Revolutionaries: Anna and Thomas Haslam and the Irish Women's Movement* (Cork: Cork Univ. Press, 2002), 75–76.

3. In relation to Ireland, see in particular ibid., 75–107; Elizabeth Malcolm, "'Troops of Largely Diseased Women': VD, the Contagious Diseases Acts, and Moral Policing in Late Nineteenth-Century Ireland," *Irish Economic and Social History* 26 (1999): 1–14; Maria Luddy, "Prostitution and Rescue Work in Nineteenth-Century Ireland," in *Women Surviving: Studies of Irish Women's History in the 19th and 20th Centuries,* edited by Maria Luddy and Cliona Murphy, 51–84 (Dublin: Poolbeg Press, 1990); Maria Luddy, "Women and the Contagious Diseases Acts 1864–1886," *History Ireland* (Spring 1993): 32–34; Maria Luddy, "'Abandoned Women and Bad Characters': Prostitution in Nineteenth-Century Ireland," *Women's History Review* 6 (1997): 485–503.

4. *The Census of Ireland for the Year 1851,* Part III: *Report on the Status of Disease,* British Parliamentary Papers (BPP) [1765] 1854, vol. LVIII, 1, 92.

5. *A Report upon Certain Charitable Establishments in the City of Dublin* (Dublin: n.p., 1809), appendix 6. The etymon of the word *lock,* when referring to venereal disease, is uncertain. It may have originated with a hospital for venereal disease in Southwark, originally a lazar house for the care of lepers, probably as specially isolated. According to Gary A. Boyd, "[T]he generic term 'lock' hospital derived from the French *locques,* the bandages applied to lepers' sores." Gary A. Boyd, *Dublin 1745–1922: Hospitals, Spectacle, & Vice* (Dublin: Four Courts Press, 2006), 149.

6. *Lancet,* 4 Mar. 1826, reprinted in Erinensis, *The Sketches of Erinensis: Selections of Irish Medical Satire, 1824–1836,* edited by Martin Fallon (London: Skilton & Shaw, 1979), 110–11.

7. John F. Devane, *A History of St John's Hospital, Limerick* (N.p.: n.p., 1970), 6.

8. William J. Geary, "Report of St John's Fever and Lock Hospitals, Limerick," *Dublin Journal of Medical Science* 11 (1837), 384.

9. *Report from the Select Committee on the Irish Miscellaneous Estimates*, BPP 1829 (342), vol. IV, 127, 179–81.

10. *A Report upon Certain Charitable Establishments in the City of Dublin*, 3.

11. *Report from the Select Committee on the Irish Miscellaneous Estimates*, 176–79.

12. These concerns did not dissipate over time. A century after Crampton and Renny's investigation, a prominent Dublin venereologist commented that the chief difficulty in any venereal disease clinic was to get patients to complete their treatment. T. P. C. Kirkpatrick, "The Work of a Venereal Disease Treatment Centre," *Irish Journal of Medical Science*, 5th series, no. 15 (June 1923), 153–54.

13. *A Report upon Certain Charitable Establishments in the City of Dublin*, 3 and appendixes 23 and 26.

14. *Lancet*, 4 Mar. 1826, reprinted in Erinensis, *The Sketches of Erinensis*, 110–12. This same commentator suggested that the soldiers "function was to restrict movement between the male and female wards, to keep Venus and Cupid at arms length" (ibid.).

15. *A Report upon Certain Charitable Establishments in the City of Dublin*, appendixes 6–10; General Lock Hospital Board Book 1792, 22 Oct. 1792; Minute Book 1820–1826, 20 May 1820; Governors' Minute Book 1826–1838, 9 July 1831, all in Westmoreland Lock Hospital (WLH) Papers, Royal College of Physicians of Ireland (RCPI), Dublin.

16. *A Report upon Certain Charitable Establishments in the City of Dublin*, 4.

17. Ibid., 7

18. *Report from the Select Committee on the Irish Miscellaneous Estimates*, 172. The governors of the hospital were aware of the problem. On 23 March 1819, some months prior to Crampton and Renny's investigation, the governors noted in the minutes that unrestricted access had given rise to "much inconvenience and confusion" in the institution and ordered that in future visitors would not be admitted without written permission from one of the medical staff or by the special permission of the steward. Ibid., 179.

19. Quotes from Renny and Crampton's report in these paragraphs come from ibid., 172–74.

20. *Report from the Select Committee on Dublin Hospitals; Together with the Proceedings of the Committee, Minutes of Evidence, Appendix and index*, BPP 1854 (338), vol. XII, iv.

21. Ibid., 4–5.

22. T. P. C. Kirkpatrick, *The History of Doctor Steevens' Hospital, Dublin, 1720–1920* (Dublin: Univ. College Dublin Press, 1924), 186–92.

23. *Copy of a Letter from the Under Secretary to the Lord Lieutenant of Ireland to the Commissioners Appointed to Report on Certain Charitable Institutions in Dublin,* BPP 1842 (337), vol. XXXVIII, 7, 90.

24. Minute Book 1820–1826, May 20, 1820, WLH Papers, RCPI.

25. Governors' memorial to the lord lieutenant, 3 Feb. 1838, in *Copy of a Letter from the Under Secretary to the Lord Lieutenant of Ireland,* 54. It appears that the governors overestimated their success in weaning nurses from their partiality to alcohol. Luddy, "Prostitution and Rescue Work in Nineteenth-Century Ireland," 107.

26. *Lancet,* 4 Mar. 1826, reprinted in Erinensis, *The Sketches of Erinensis,* 110–112.

27. *Charitable Institutions, Dublin; Reports of Commissioners Appointed by the Lord Lieutenant to Inquire into Certain Charitable Institutions in the City of Dublin, viz. 1. Lying-in Hospital, 2. Doctor Steevens' Hospital, 3. Fever Hospital, Cork Street, 4. Incurables, 5. Westmoreland Lock Hospital, 6. House of Industry,* BPP 1830 (7), vol. XXVI, 1, 65–74.

28. Ibid., "Supplemental Observations of the Governors of the Westmoreland Lock Hospital," appendix 6, 93–94.

29. *A Report upon Certain Charitable Establishments in the City of Dublin,* 10–11. See also Joseph Archer, *Statistical Survey of the County of Dublin, with Observations on the Means of Improvement* (Dublin: Graisberry & Campbell, 1801), 125. The 1851 census records seventeen penitentiaries or reformatories, accommodating 450 individuals on the night of 30 March 1851. *The Census of Ireland for the Year 1851,* Part III: *Report on the Status of Disease* (Dublin: Her Majesty's Stationery Office, 1852), 108. For these institutions, see in particular Maria Luddy, *Women and Philanthropy in Nineteenth-Century Ireland* (Cambridge: Cambridge Univ. Press 1995), 109–48; Luddy, "Prostitution and Rescue Work in Nineteenth-Century Ireland"; Jacinta Prunty, *Dublin Slums, 1800–1925: A Study in Urban Geography* (Dublin: Four Courts Press, 1998), 267–70.

30. *A Selection of Hymns, Used in the Chapel of the Lock Penitentiary, Dorset Street* (Dublin: n.p., 1799), 14, hymn 14.

31. *Charitable Institutions, Dublin,* 67.

32. *Copy of a Letter from the Under Secretary to the Lord Lieutenant of Ireland,* 40.

33. Ibid.

34. *Report from the Select Committee on Dublin Hospitals,* 9.

35. *Report from the Select Committee on the Irish Miscellaneous Estimates,* 13.

36. Ibid., 12.

37. *Report from the Select Committee on Dublin Hospitals,* iv, 10–11, 19.

38. *Copy of a Letter from the Under Secretary to the Lord Lieutenant of Ireland,* 53–56.

39. *Report from the Select Committee on Dublin Hospitals,* iv. See also Sir James Pitcairn, Inspector-General of Hospitals, "On the State of Health of the Army Serving in This Country," 10 May 1852, WLH Papers, RCPI; "Copies of Communications Between the Treasury and the Irish Government on the Subject of the Grants to Westmoreland Lock Hospital," in *City of Dublin, During the Years 1852 and 1853,* BPP 1852–53 (421), vol. XCIV, 3–4.

40. *Report of the Commissioners Appointed to Inquire into the Hospitals of Dublin, with Appendices,* BPP 1856 [2063], vol. XIX, 115, 10.

41. Ibid., 6 and 9.

42. See, for instance, *Thirty-First Annual Report of the Board of Superintendence of Dublin Hospitals, with Appendices* (Dublin: n.p., 1889), 5; *Fifty-First Annual Report of the Board of Superintendence of Dublin Hospitals, with Appendices* (Dublin: n.p., 1909), 6.

43. Quoted in Devane, *A History of St John's Hospital,* 13.

10. "Sickness," Gender, and National Health Insurance in Ireland, 1920s to 1940s

1. See Ruth Barrington, *Health, Medicine, and Politics in Ireland, 1900–1970* (Dublin: Institute of Public Administration, 1987), for the reasons behind this. On the development of the national health insurance system in this period, see Mel Cousins, *The Birth of Social Welfare in Ireland 1922–52* (Dublin: Four Courts Press, 2003).

2. The rates are those applicable from 1920. The maximum rate of sickness benefit was payable only where two years contributions had been paid. Where at least twenty-six weeks contributions had been paid, a reduced benefit of nine shillings per week for men and seven shillings and sixpence for women was payable.

3. See Arthur S. Comyns Carr, William H. Stuart Garnett, and James H. Taylor, *National Insurance* (London: MacMillan, 1912). On the adoption of the legislation, see Bentley B. Gilbert, *The Evolution of National Insurance in Great Britain: The Origins of the Welfare State* (London: Joseph, 1966).

4. A lump-sum maternity benefit was payable to insured women and in respect of wives of insured men.

5. Given the very different manner in which the figures were compiled, it would be unwise to compare the administrative data on numbers insured under the national health insurance scheme with census data in other than very general terms.

6. See Cousins, *The Birth of Social Welfare in Ireland,* 43–44.

7. Ibid., 47.

8. On the financial structures of national health insurance in the United Kingdom, see Noel Whiteside, "Private Agencies for Public Purposes," *Journal of Social Policy* 12, no. 2 (1983): 165–94; Noel Whiteside, "Regulating Markets: The Real Costs of

Poly-centric Administration under the National Health Insurance Scheme (1912–46)," *Public Administration* 75 (1997): 467–85; and Noel Whiteside, "Private Provision and Public Welfare: Health Insurance Between the Wars," in *Before Beveridge: Welfare before the Welfare State,* edited by David Gladstone, 26–42 (London: Institute of Economic Affairs, 1999).

9. Similar concerns emerged in the United Kingdom. See Bentley B. Gilbert, *British Social Policy 1914–1939* (Ithaca, NY: Cornell Univ. Press, 1970), 286–300; and Whiteside, "Private Agencies for Public Purposes," 175–79. For a detailed discussion, see Noel Whiteside, "Counting the Cost: Sickness and Disability Amongst Working People in an Age of Industrial Recession, 1919–39," *Economic History Review* (1987): 228–46, in particular 232–37.

10. Women's National Health Association, *Sláinte: The Journal of the Women's National Health Association of Ireland* (1936): 29 (henceforth WNHA, *Sláinte*). The WNHA published *Sláinte,* meaning "Health" in Irish, published annually from 1911 to 1961. The WNHA was a volunteer organization established by Lady Aberdeen in 1907 in order to reduce the incidence of TB in Ireland.

11. There was a significant discontinuity in membership between 1927 and 1928, when total membership, having risen consistently since 1923, fell by some 100,000 in one year. This decline appears to relate to the noncontinuance of the National Health Insurance (Prolongation of Insurance) Act of 1921 beyond 1927. It was estimated that this would affect some 90,000 members, although the government argued that many members did "not exist," having died or emigrated or otherwise passed out of insurance. See Dáil Éireann, debates, Nov. 1927, vol. XXI, col. 909–918, 4; Seanad Éireann, debates, Nov. 1927, vol. X, col. 11–18, 16. Perhaps surprisingly this discontinuity appears to have made little difference in the gender breakdown of those insured.

12. This fall in the claim level occurred, in particular, after 1933, and it is unclear whether it was related to improved administration by the unified society, improved economic conditions for insured workers, or a combination of both (or indeed other) factors.

13. Ruairi Ó Brolcháin, "Examination of the Sickness Experience for the Year 1935 of Persons Insured under the National Health Insurance Acts," *Journal of the Statistical and Social Inquiry Society of Ireland* 16 (1938–40): 53–72.

14. Ó Brolcháin, "Examination of the Sickness Experience," 54.

15. Ó Brolcháin also reports that the incidence of sickness and disablement varied significantly by county and by occupation. Unfortunately, however, he reports the data only for men. Ibid.

16. *Report on the Investigation of the Sickness Claims Experience of the Unified Society,* 1935–37, File IA91/53 (Department of Social Welfare file), National Archives of Ireland (NAI). The report was not published but was laid before the Oireachtas.

17. Set out in the National Health Insurance (Valuation) Regulations, 1936.

18. See Gilbert, *British Social Policy*, 297–99.

19. *Report on the Investigation of the Sickness Claims Experience of the Unified Society* (1935–37), File IA91/53, NAI.

20. *Actuarial Report on the Financial Position of the National Health Insurance System*, File S.12457, NAI.

21. Ibid.

22. Seán MacEntee to Secretary of the Department of Local Government and Public Health, 13 Jan. 1942, File IA91/53, NAI. On MacEntee, see Tom Feeney, *Seán MacEntee: A Political Life* (Dublin: Irish Academic Press, 2008).

23. P. J. Keady to Seán MacEntee, 29 Jan. 1942,, File IA91/53, NAI.

24. See Cousins, *The Birth of Social Welfare in Ireland*, 99–103.

25. Hence the frequent use of height data as a proxy for health status.

26. Married women insured under the national health insurance acts make up a very small proportion of the total population of married women in Ireland.

27. Cumann an Arachais Náisiúnta ár Shláinte (National Health Insurance Society), *Secretary's Report Year 1944* (Dublin: Department of Social and Family Affairs, 1944), introduction. The Department of Social and Family Affairs was renamed the Department of Social Protection in 2010. The NHIS suggests that the preponderance of claims by women for dental and optical benefits "may be due, to some extent, to the adaptability of these benefits to adornment."

28. Tony Fahey, "Why Did Women Have Higher Mortality Rates Than Men in Early Twentieth Century Rural Ireland?" paper presented at the meeting of the Economic and Social Research Institute, Dublin, 9 Nov. 2000, 4–5.

29. Ibid., 10. Fahey notes that 299 women's deaths (or only 1.4 percent of total women's deaths) were recorded in 1926 as having occurred in childbirth. Maternal mortality *was* higher for women in childbearing years (9.9 percent of total deaths), but this number can be compared to, for example, 12 percent in the same age group in the Netherlands in 1931.

30. Ibid., 21.

31. Roy C. Geary, "The Mortality from Tuberculosis in Saorstat Éireann: A Statistical Study," *Journal of the Statistical and Social Inquiry Society of Ireland* 14 (1929–30), 67. Fahey points out that these data possibly overstated the mortality advantages of domestic servants, but he concludes that it is likely that death rates among domestic servants were genuinely low; Fahey, "Why Did Women Have Higher Mortality Rates."

32. Separate data on the claims experience of domestic servants are not recorded, but given that domestic servants make up more than 50 percent of the single women group, their experience is unlikely to differ significantly from the group as a whole. The claims experience for domestic female servants is significantly worse than for single women in the United Kingdom. Although this comparison does not take account of issues such as differences in the occupational composition of this group, it is still

interesting given that the mortality data would suggest that domestic servants should have been among the healthiest groups—that is, a different UK composition should favor rather than disadvantage the comparison with Ireland.

33. James C. Riley, *Sick, Not Dead: The Health of British Workingmen during the Mortality Decline* (Baltimore: Johns Hopkins Univ. Press, 1997).

34. John E. Murray, "Social Insurance Claims as Morbidity Estimates: Sickness or Absence?" *Social History of Medicine* 16, no. 2 (2003), 237.

35. Quoted in WNHA, *Sláinte* (1935), 81.

36. See a broadly similar comment on the level of sickness claims among British women in Whiteside, "Counting the Cost," 238–9.

37. See Cousins, *The Birth of Social Welfare in Ireland*, 64. Single women could qualify if they had dependants or had been insured for at least one year in the four years prior to the claim.

38. Wage rate quoted in Cormac Ó Gráda, *Ireland: A New Economic History* (Oxford: Oxford Univ. Press, 1994), 436.

39. In contrast, Bentley Gilbert argues that the British-approved societies, concerned about their financial viability, played a significant role in the passage of the UK legislation that saw a cut in married women's benefits in 1932. Gilbert, *British Social Policy,* 297–99.

40. It is interesting to note that the annual reports of the NHIS secretary to its Committee of Management indicate that the NHIS's statistical department carried out a wide range of statistical studies. These studies unfortunately do not appear to be extant, and I have been unable to establish the fate of the NHIS files.

41. On the White Paper, see generally Cousins, *The Birth of Social Welfare in Ireland,* and Sophia Carey, *Social Security in Ireland 1939–1952* (Dublin: Irish Academic Press, 2007).

42. Department of Social Welfare, *Social Security,* 21. Note that divorce was not legal in Ireland until 1995.

43. See James Deeny's study of disability claims in the 1960s: *The Irish Worker: A Demographic Study of the Labour Force in Ireland* (Dublin: Institute of Public Administration, 1971), 57–75.

44. See *Comptroller and Auditor General Report 1990* (Dublin: Her Majesty's Stationery Office, 1999), 133–50; Department of Social Welfare, *The Incidence of Women on Long Term Disability Benefit* (Dublin: Her Majesty's Stationery Office, 1994), a report to the Public Accounts Committee; Richard O'Leary, "Female Workers on Long-Term Sickness Benefit in the Republic of Ireland," *Social Policy and Administration* 32, no. 3 (1998): 245–62.

45. O'Leary, "Female Workers on Long-Term Sickness Benefit," 258.

46. Noel Whiteside, "Unemployment and Health: An Historical Perspective," *Journal of Social Policy* 17, no. 2 (1988), 29.

11. "A Perpetual Nightmare": Women, Fertility Control,
the Irish State, and the 1935 Ban on Contraceptives

1. Minutes of Geoghegan Committee meeting, 31 May 1933, File D/JUS H247/41D,
National Archives of Ireland (NAI), Dublin.

2. On contemporary methods, see Hera Cook, *The Long Sexual Revolution:
English Women and Contraception 1800–1975* (Oxford: Oxford Univ. Press, 2004),
122–42; and on the survival of traditional methods in Britain, see Kate Fisher, *Birth
Control, Sex, and Marriage in Britain 1918–1960* (Oxford: Oxford Univ. Press, 2006).

3. Office of Revenue Commissioners, handwritten memorandum, 3 Sept. 1934,
signed "Tim Cleary," File D/JUS H247/41E, NAI. The word transcribed as "sprang" is
difficult to decipher.

4. Submission from the Secretary to the Department of Posts and Telegraphs, 10
May 1926, File D/JUS 7/2/17, NAI. Prosecutions information in legal advice to the
Geoghegan Committee, File D/JUS H 247/41D, NAI.

5. "Correspondence," *British Medical Journal* (30 July 1921), 169.

6. Gibbon FitzGibbon, "Birth Control," *British Medical Journal* 2, no. 3165 (27
Aug. 1921), 338.

7. Issues arise regarding the reliability of Irish demographic statistics and the methods of analysis applied to them, but several scholars have produced valuable microstud-
ies. See Cormac Ó Gráda and Niall Duffy, "The Fertility Transition in Ireland and
Scotland c. 1880–1930," in *Conflict, Identity, and Economic Development: Ireland
and Scotland, 1600–1939*, edited by S. J. Connolly, R. A. Houston, and R. J. Morris,
89–102 (Preston, UK: Carnegie Publishing, 1995). They examined 1911 census returns
for Clare, Tyrone, and the Dublin suburb Rathgar, using Clare as the "model population," and suggested that more than "one fifth of rural Irishwomen who married in
their twenties were controllers [controlled the family finances]" (101). For an urban
microstudy, see Timothy W. Guinnane, Carolyn Moehling, and Cormac Ó Gráda, *Fertility in South Dublin a Century Ago: A First Look*, Discussion Paper no. 838 (New
Haven, CT: Economic Growth Centre, Yale Univ., Nov. 2001), a study of 1911 census
results for the Pembroke District of Dublin. It implies that a range of factors, including
social class, religion, place of birth, and even street of residence, may have influenced
decisions on limiting fertility.

8. On effectiveness of various birth-control methods, see Cook, *The Long Sexual Revolution*, 139–42, and Carmel Quinlan, *Genteel Revolutionaries: Anna and
Thomas Haslam and the Irish Women's Movement* (Cork: Cork Univ. Press, 2002),
25–52. Thomas Haslam's writings on birth control are an excellent source on nineteenth-century knowledge.

9. Return headed "Prosecutions under Obscene Publications Act 1857," with 17
May 1926 confidential note from Gárda Commissioner's Office, File D/JUS 7/2/11, NAI.

10. FitzGibbon, "Birth Control," 338.

11. Ibid., 338.

12. Dáil Éireann (House) debate, 1 Aug. 1934, vol. LIII, col. 2017–2020. Marie Stopes listed "good domestic makeshift" barrier methods, including sponges or powder puffs soaked in oils, butter, or Vaseline and vinegar or lemon juice as useful douches; Marie Stopes, *Birth Control To-Day: A Practical Handbook for Those who Want to Be Their Own Masters in This Vital Matter* (London: J. Bale, 1934), 53–71.

13. Corby retired in 1925.

14. Henry Corby, "Birth Control and Economy," *The Practitioner* (July 1923), 62–73.

15. Vincent McNabb, "The Ethics and Psychology of Neo-Malthusian Birth-Control," *Catholic Medical Guardian* 2, no. 5 (Jan. 1924), 12–16, originally a paper delivered in Dublin in 1923 and reprinted in *The Problem of Undesirable Printed Matter: Suggested Remedies. Evidence of the Catholic Truth Society of Ireland Presented to the Departmental Committee of Enquiry, 1926* (Dublin: n.p., 1926), 8–14, copy in File D/JUS 7/1/2, NAI.

16. Memorandum and 6 June 1930 letter signed J. P. Walsh, Secretary, Department of Foreign Affairs, File D/T S3250A, NAI. Two Evil Literature Committee members were Protestants—Professor W. E. Thrift, TD, of Trinity College, Dublin, and Reverend T. Sinclair Stevenson, a Church of Ireland clergyman. Three were Catholic—Robert Donovan, professor of English literature at University College, Dublin; Reverend James Dempsey, parish priest of Clontarf, Dublin; and Thomas J. O'Connell, TD, of the Irish National Teachers' Organisation.

17. *A Practical Treatise on Birth Control by an Eminent London Physician* (London: S. Seymour, n.d.), 11, File D/JUS 7/2/9, NAI; S. Seymour was a manufacturing chemist.

18. *Report of the Committee on Evil Literature* (Dublin: n.p., 1926), 13–15, 19, 15.

19. Seanad Éireann (Senate) debates, 11 Apr. 1929, vol. XII, col. 55–71.

20. For example, see the materials in File D/JUS H315/7, NAI.

21. *Encyclical Letter from the Bishops with Resolutions and Reports* (London: n.p., 1930), 91, 85–87.

22. Canon James Blennerhassett Leslie MA, "The Lambeth Conference Report: An Appreciation," *Church of Ireland Gazette* (19 Sept. 1930), 517.

23. Pius XI, "On Christian Marriage," *Casti Connubii* (1933), 28.

24. *Irish Times*, 16 Feb. 1931.

25. "'Molula,' a Call for Catholic Action: The Medical School of Trinity College," *Catholic Bulletin* 21, no. 2 (Feb. 1931): 139–43. Dermot Keogh suggests that the author was Catholic Action activist Father Edward Cahill. See Dermot Keogh, *The Vatican, the Bishops, and Irish Politics 1919–1939* (Cambridge: Cambridge Univ. Press, 1986), 64.

26. *Irish Chemist and Druggist* (Aug. 1931), 228, and *Chemist and Druggist* (25 July 1931), 91.

27. Memorandum marked "Returned by Professor O'Sullivan 24/3/31," File D/T S2547B, NAI.

28. W. T. Cosgrave to Joseph MacRory, 28 Mar. 1931, File D/T S2547B, NAI.

29. Tony Farmar, *Holles Street 1894–1994: The National Maternity Hospital—a Centenary History* (Dublin: A. & A. Farmar, 1994), 86–87, 100.

30. The impact of sectarian medical ethics on employment prospects in Britain had been a concern since 1928: see Dáil debates, 8 June 1928, col. 350, and letters to the editor, *Irish Independent,* 20 Dec. 1930, signed Thomas Hennessy (former secretary of the Irish section of the British Medical Association and Cumann na nGaedheal back-bencher) and James J. Gorham, MD.

31. Bethel Solomons, "The Prevention of Maternal Morbidity and Mortality," *Irish Journal of Medical Science* 6 (1933), , 174, 175.

32. Bethel Solomons, "The Dangerous Multipara," *Lancet* (7 July 1934): 8–11.

33. Carrigan Committee members were William Carrigan, KC; Reverend John Hannon, a Jesuit and Church of Ireland dean of Christ Church Cathedral, Dublin; Very Reverend H. B. Kennedy; surgeon Francis Morrin; Dublin Union poor-law commissioner Mrs. Jane Power; and matron of the Coombe maternity hospital Miss V. O'Carroll.

34. *Carrigan Report* (1931), 36–37, File D/T S5998, NAI.

35. Ibid., 37, 41, and minutes of Geoghegan Committee meeting, 31 May 1933, File D/JUS H247/41D, NAI.

36. Members of the Geoghegan Committee were James Geoghegan, Minister for Justice; Attorney General Conor Maguire; William Davin (Labour); Desmond Fitzgerald (Cumann na nGaedheal); James Fitzgerald-Kenney (Cumann na nGaedheal); T. D. James Dillon (independent); and Dublin University doctor of divinity and professor of philosophy William Edward Thrift. The committee survived the fall of the Cumann na nGaedheal government and Fianna Fáil's election victories in 1932.

37. Department of Justice Memorandum to Executive Council, 9 Nov. 1933, File D/JUS 8/20, NAI.

38. "Heads for the Bill," 1931, File D/JUS H 247/41D, NAI.

39. Department of Justice Memorandum to Executive Council, 9 Nov. 1933.

40. This position was equivalent to Ireland's modern-day office of *tánaiste* (deputy prime minister). O'Kelly quoted in Keogh, *The Vatican, the Bishops, and Irish Politics,* 203.

41. Quoted in ibid.

42. Cabinet Minutes, Cab. 7/95, 8 Dec. 1933, item 1, File D/T S6489, NAI.

43. In Committee secretary J. E. Duff to James Geoghegan, 14 Feb. 1934, File D/JUS 8/20, NAI.

44. Minutes of Geoghegan Committee meeting, 19 June 1934, File D/JUS 8/20, NAI.

45. Dáil debate, 1 Aug. 1934, vol. LIII, col. 2017–20.

46. Senate debate, 9 Feb. 1935, vol. XIX, col. 1249–53.

47. *Chemist and Druggist* (21 Mar. 1936), 337.

48. June 1936 case listed in documents relating to Charles Brocklebank in June 1944, Court of Criminal Appeal no. 83 of 1944 and no. 18 of 1945, NAI.

49. Michael Solomons, *Pro Life? The Irish Question* (Dublin: Lilliput Press, 1992), 6. See also Greta Jones, "Marie Stopes in Ireland: The Mother's Clinic in Belfast, 1936–1947," *Social History of Medicine* 5, no. 2 (1992): 255–77.

50. Caitriona Clear, *Women of the House: Women's Household Work in Ireland 1926–1961* (Dublin: Irish Academic Press, 2000), 122.

51. See Lindsey Earner-Byrne, *Mother and Child: Maternity and Child Welfare in Dublin, 1922–60* (Manchester, UK: Manchester Univ. Press, 2007), 222–23.

12. "A Probable Source of Infection": The Limitations of Venereal Disease Policy, 1943–1951

1. Fanning minute, 4 July 1951, File DH B135/26, National Archives of Ireland (NAI), Dublin.

2. Dr. Steevens' Hospital served schemes in Dublin city borough and counties Kildare and Wicklow, and Sir Patrick Dun's Hospital served Dublin county. Monaghan was served in principle by a dispensary in Clones, a small town in County Monaghan. *Report of the Interdepartmental Committee of Inquiry Regarding Venereal Disease* (Dublin: n.p., 1926), 6, File DT S4183, NAI. Ruth Barrington notes that the local authorities along the east coast were most active owing to the extent of local recruitment into the British army. Ruth Barrington, *Health, Medicine, and Politics in Ireland, 1900–1970* (Dublin: Institute of Public Administration, 1987), 81.

3. Department of the Taoiseach, File DF S72/11/26, NAI.

4. *Report of the Interdepartmental Committee of Inquiry Regarding Venereal Disease*, 23–24. See also Susannah Riordan, "Venereal Disease in the Irish Free State: The Politics of Public Health," *Irish Historical Studies* 35, no. 139 (May 2007): 345–64. The army's disinfection policy remained in force during the emergency. Tom Garvin's suggestion that condoms were issued in the army during the 1920s and that the practice was discontinued under Fianna Fáil stems from a confusion between the prohibition on prophylactics under the Criminal Law Amendment Act of 1935 and the army's policy of chemical prophylaxis. Tom Garvin, *Preventing the Future: Why Was Ireland so Poor for so Long?* (Dublin: Gill and MacMillan, 2004), 71. Senator Oliver St. John Gogarty raised the argument that the 1935 prohibition would lead to increased rates of venereal infection, but the Department of Local Government and Public Health later denied this suggestion, pointing to the decrease in cases between 1935 and 1939. Seanad Éireann (Senate) debate, 6 Feb. 1935, Parliamentary Papers (PP), vol. XIX, 1253–54; Deeny memorandum, 11 Oct. 1947, File DH B135/10, NAI.

5. *Report of the Interdepartmental Committee of Inquiry Regarding Venereal Disease*, 8–12.

6. "Memorandum on the Report of the Interdepartmental Committee on Venereal Disease," File DT S4183, NAI.

7. Riordan, "Venereal Disease in the Irish Free State." For an alternative interpretation, see Philip Howell, "Venereal Disease and the Politics of Prostitution in the Irish Free State," *Irish Historical Studies* 33, no. 131 (May 2003): 320–41.

8. O'Sullivan memorandum, 15 June 1951, File DH B136/26, NAI.

9. Seamus Ó Siothcháin to James McElligott, 5 Jan. 1948, File DF S72/11/26, NAI.

10. John Whyte, *Church and State in Modern Ireland 1923–70* (Dublin: Gill & MacMillan, 1971), 129.

11. McDonnell memorandum, 13 July 1934, File DH B135/13, NAI.

12. Department of Local Government and Public Health, *Reports* (Dublin: Department of Local Government and Public Health, 1930–45).

13. Unsigned letter on behalf of James Hurson, 2 May 1932, File DH B135/11, vol. I, NAI.

14. Notably in Cork and Westmeath; see *Irish Times*, 4 July 1944, and *Westmeath Independent*, 9 Sept. 1944.

15. "General Report on the Army for the Year Apr. 1, 1942 to Mar. 31, 1943," 42, Military Archives, Cathal Brugha Barracks, Dublin; *Medical Report: V.D.*, 7 June 1944, File DH B135/11, vol. I, NAI. Lice and flea infestations were also a problem in the confined and makeshift accommodation provided at the turf camps. See James Deeny, *To Cure and to Care: Memoirs of a Chief Medical Officer* (Dublin: Glendale Press, 1989), 65. For the turf scheme, see Mary E. Daly, *The Buffer State: The Historical Roots of the Department of the Environment* (Dublin: Institute of Public Administration, 1997), 263–70.

16. Anonymous letter, File DH B135/11, vol. I, NAI. The description of the creamery worker's symptoms suggests he was suffering from scabies.

17. James Hughes, Dáil Éireann (House) debate, 20 June 1944, PP, vol. XCIV, 1568; Liam O Buachalla, Seanad Éireann debate, 5 July 1944, PP, vol. XXVIII, 1588. It was argued in the Department of Local Government and Public Health that the proposal "would require such a thorough medical examination that it would be impossible to have it carried out without a general outcry." Sterling Berry memorandum, 1 Aug. 1944, File DT B135/11, vol. I, NAI.

18. Unattributed and untitled article, *Journal of the Medical Association of Éire* 10, no. 57 (Mar. 1942), 32.

19. J. C. Cherry, "The Control of Venereal Disease in Ireland," *Irish Journal of Medical Science* 6, no. 210 (June 1943), 170.

20. This public discussion included broadcasts on BBC radio and advertisements in the (generally uncooperative) press. Richard Davenport-Hines, *Sex, Death, and*

Punishment: Attitudes to Sex and Sexuality in Britain since the Renaissance (London: Collins, 1990), 266–67.

21. McQuaid donated £3,000 to this project. He later brought pressure to bear on other Dublin voluntary hospitals to admit venereal disease patients. See John Cooney, *John Charles McQuaid: Ruler of Catholic Ireland* (Syracuse, NY: Syracuse Univ. Press, 1999), 154, and Garvin, *Preventing the Future*, 71.

22. *Irish Times*, 26 May 1944.

23. Untitled article, *Journal of the Medical Association of Éire* 14, no. 84 (June 1944): 68–69. The article's author was anonymous, and although the journal's editorial also addressed venereal disease, it disavowed responsibility for the original author's views.

24. Dáil Éireann debate, 20 June 1944, PP, vol. XCIV, 824; *Irish Times*, 22 June 1944.

25. This initiative was prompted by correspondence from the Church of Ireland Temperance Society. John Jones to James Hurson, 12 Apr. 1944; McWeeney and Sterling Berry minutes, [Apr. 1943], File DH B135/11, vol. I, NAI.

26. James Hurson to Louis Fitzgerald, 26 Nov. 1945, File DH B135/2, NAI.

27. Garvin memorandum, 24 July 1944, and Fanning memorandum, 31 July 1944, File DH B135/2, NAI.

28. "Notes of Conference Held in Department on Sept. 15, 1944," File DH B135/12, NAI; Deeny minute, 2 Nov. 1944, File DH B135/2, NAI. Deeny took up his position on 1 Oct. 1944. Deeny, *To Cure and to Care*, 65. Deeny's appointment followed shortly upon the announcement made by the US minister to Ireland David Gray that some sodium penicillin would soon be made available to the Medical Research Council. The penicillin would thence be made available to the teaching hospitals in Dublin, Cork, and Galway. Unattributed and untitled article, *Journal of the Medical Association of Éire* 15, no. 87 (Sept. 1944), 25.

29. Lysaght memorandum, [May 1944], File DT B135/2, NAI.

30. "Draft Scheme for the Control and Treatment of Venereal Disease," [May 1945], File DH B135/2, NAI. This scheme was agreed between Deeny, Fanning, and the principal officers of the department's Public Health and Public Assistance sections, M. A. Lang and John Garvin.

31. Davenport-Hines, *Sex, Death, and Punishment*, 268; Roger Davidson, *Dangerous Liaisons: A Social History of Venereal Disease in Twentieth-Century Scotland* (Amsterdam: Rodolpi, 2000), 211–14.

32. "Draft Scheme for the Control and Treatment of Venereal Disease." The scheme was later expanded to include payments for practitioners who conducted or arranged follow-up cerebrospinal fluid tests in cases of syphilis. Martin Collins to James McElligott, 16 Sept. 1946, File DH B135/2, NAI.

33. Lang minute, 14 Aug. 1945, File DH B135/2, NAI.

34. D. J. Maher to M. A. Kiely, 28 Sept. 1945 and 7 Dec. 1945, File DF S72/11/45, NAI.

35. M. A. Kiely to Louis Fitzgerald, 8 Dec. 1945, DF S72/11/45, NAI.

36. Fitzgerald memorandum, 9 Jan. 1946, File DF S72/11/45, NAI.

37. James Hurson to Louis Fitzgerald, 26 Nov. 1945, File DH B135/2, NAI.

38. In his report of a conversation with C. F. Dowling of the Department of Local Government and Public Health, D. J. Maher of the Department of Finance noted that, "as to the problem of educating the public, I understand from Mr Dowling that the Church authorities were recently approached and that they voiced strong opposition to the launching of a widespread publicity campaign such as is conducted in other countries." D. J. Maher to M. A. Kiely, 7 Dec. 1945, File DF S72/11/45, NAI. According to Fitzgerald, "Dr. Deeny admitted that the failure to get authority for a publicity campaign wd. fundamentally weaken all their efforts but said that clerical objections had carried the day in his dept." Fitzgerald memorandum, 9 Jan. 1946, File DF S72/11/45, NAI.

39. Sandra McAvoy's suggestion that publicity was prohibited under the Censorship of Publications Act of 1929 is mistaken because the powers of public bodies to advertise venereal disease schemes were expressly excluded from that act. See Sandra L. McAvoy, "The Regulation of Sexuality in the Irish Free State 1929–35," in *Medicine, Disease, and the State in Ireland 1650–1940*, edited by Greta Jones and Elizabeth Malcolm (Cork: Cork Univ. Press, 1999), 264. See also Dáil Éireann debate, 18 Oct. 1928, PP, vol. XXVI, 608–9, and 24 Oct. 1928, 833.

40. Ryan was appointed the first minister of a separate Department of Health in January 1947.

41. Venereal diseases and tuberculosis became classified as "infectious diseases" for the first time under the 1948 regulations, although Ward and Ryan had earlier specified the intention of doing so.

42. Section 38 (1), No. 28/1947. See also section 29 (1), public-health bill, 1945, File DT S13444B, NAI. Section 38 was not dropped as Greta Jones suggests. Greta Jones, *Captain of All These Men of Death: The History of Tuberculosis in Nineteenth and Twentieth Century Ireland* (Amsterdam: Rodolpi, 2001), 105. For the controversy, see Barrington, *Health, Medicine, and Politics in Ireland*, 168–75, and Eamonn McKee, "Church–State Relations and the Development of Irish Health Policy: The Mother-and-Child Scheme, 1944–53," *Irish Historical Studies* 25, no. 98 (Nov. 1986): 167–69.

43. Dáil Éireann debate, 23 May 1928, PP, vol. XXIII, 1857.

44. Dáil Éireann debate, 11 Apr. 1929, PP, vol. XXIX, 199. See also the debate of 30 Apr. 1931, PP, vol. XXXVIII, 586.

45. Dáil Éireann debates, Mar. 28, 1946, PP, vol. C, 760; and 3 Apr. 1946, PP, vol. C, 1154.

46. Ward provided the Dáil with a list of the diseases to which he intended to apply the bill's various provisions. Dáil Éireann debate, 28 Mar. 1946, PP, vol. C, 714–19.

47. Dáil Éireann debate, 1 May 1947, PP, vol. CV, 1958.

48. Dáil Éireann debate, 12 June 1947, PP, vol. CVI, 1687.

49. "Statement of the Irish Hierarchy on the Health Act, 1947," 7 Oct. 1947, File DT S13444 I, NAI. See Whyte, *Church and State in Modern Ireland*, 140–55, and Barrington, *Health, Medicine, and Politics in Ireland*, 181–93.

50. John A. Horgan to Archbishop John Charles McQuaid, 6 Oct. 1952, and McQuaid note, Department of Health File, Dublin Diocesan Archives.

51. "Discussion Between the Táiniste, the Minister for Health, and the Archbishop of Dublin, the Archbishop of Cashel, the Bishop of Ferns, the Bishop of Galway, and the Bishop of Cork on Dec. 10, 1952," File DT S13444 I, NAI; "Report of Meeting on 6 Oct. 1952" and "Report of Meeting on Dec. 10, 1952," Department of Health File, Dublin Diocesan Archives.

52. Barrington, *Health, Medicine, and Politics in Ireland*, 169–70.

53. Dáil Éireann debate, 4 Apr. 1946, PP, vol. C, 1255.

54. Dr. Martin Brennan, Dáil Éireann debate, 13 Dec. 1945, xcviii, 1907. The Medical Association of Éire also approved of the infectious disease proposals. Barrington, *Health, Medicine, and Politics in Ireland*, 170.

55. Dáil Éireann debate, 12 June 1947, PP, vol. CVI, 1676–77. The provision specifically permitting the taking of blood samples was later removed by ministerial amendment. Dáil Éireann debate, 27 June 1947, PP, vol. CVII, 491–93.

56. In March 1946, following Christian Scientist representations to President Éamon De Valera, Ward agreed to omit sections of the bill that might be interpreted as permitting the medical or surgical treatment of patients without their consent and to include a section explicitly prohibiting such an interpretation. His willingness to do so suggests that compulsory treatment had never been a priority. Seamus Ó Suilleabhain to Maurice Moynihan, 5 Mar. 1946, File DT S13444 C, NAI.

57. Department of Local Government and Public Health, *Report 1940–41* (Dublin: Department of Local Government and Public Health, 1941), 34–35.

58. Ibid.

59. Kenny report, 21 Apr. 1943, File DH B135/26, NAI.

60. Lysaght memorandum, 3 Jan. 1944, and Daly memorandum, 10 Jan. 1944, File DH B135/26, NAI. The location of the complainant was not specified.

61. James Hurson to garda commissioner, 30 July 1943, File DH B135/26, NAI.

62. Lysaght memorandum, 3 Jan. 1944, and Daly memorandum, 10 Jan. 1944.

63. Edward Drum to James Hurson, 14 Oct. 1946, File DH B135/26, NAI.

64. Deeny memorandum, 24 Oct. 1946, File DH B135/26, NAI.

65. Garvin memorandum, 25 Oct. 1946, File DH B135/26, NAI.

66. McDonagh report, 7 Nov. 1946, File DH B135/26, NAI.

67. Department of Health, *Outline of Proposals for the Improvement of the Health Services* (Dublin: Department of Health, 1947), 16, 27–29.

68. Dáil Éireann debate, 6 July 1948, PP, vol. CXI, 2265.

69. P. Raymond Oliver, "The Problem of Defaulters in the Treatment of Syphilis," *Journal of the Medical Association of Éire* 24, 139 (May 1949): 72–73.

70. *Irish Times*, 21–25 July 1949.

71. Dáil Éireann debate, 1 July 1949, PP, vol. CXVI, 1811.

72. Kingston report, 16 May 1949; Moore minute, 17 May 1949; and Fanning minute, 29 Aug. 1949; all in File DH B135/26, NAI.

73. MacArdle minute, 24 May 1949, File DH B135/26, NAI.

74. Hensey minute, 24 May 1949, File DH B135/26, NAI.

75. Legal Section memorandum, 11 Nov. 1949, DH B135/26, NAI.

76. O'Sullivan minute, 1 Feb. 1950, File DH B135/26, NAI.

77. Fanning minute, 4 July 1951, DH B135/26, NAI. It is noteworthy that Browne tried to divest himself of this function under the 1950 health bill, but that the provision was not incorporated into the Health Act of 1953. "Explanatory Memorandum," 10 Oct. 1949, File DT S13444 G, NAI; "Proposed Legislation on the Health Services," 15 Oct. 1952, File DT S13444 H, NAI.

78. Fanning minute, 4 July 1951.

79. *Irish Times*, 10 Apr. 1950.

80. Kiely minute, 28 May 1951, File DF S72/11/45, NAI.

81. O'Sullivan memorandum, 15 June 1951.

82. McKeever memorandum, 23 Aug. 1952, File DH B135/26, NAI.

83. Kirby minute, 27 Sept. 1952, File DH B135/26, NAI.

84. O'Sullivan memorandum, 15 June 1951. Deeny's scheme had included the routine Wassermann testing of expectant women in the Dublin voluntary hospitals without their knowledge. The scheme was not put into operation. "Notes on Chargeability of Cost of Obtaining Samples from Certain Classes of Persons with a View to Testing for Venereal Disease," 16 June 1945, File DH B135/2, NAI. Wassermann test results may have been less reliable in Ireland than elsewhere. In 1945 or 1946, Deeny sent identical blood samples to be tested at the three laboratories employed for this purpose and discovered a 20 percent plus or minus difference in the results. His subsequent confrontation with the laboratories was unproductive. Deeny, *To Cure and to Care*, 99–101.

85. O'Sullivan memorandum, 15 June 1951.

13. Prophylactics and Prejudice: Venereal Diseases in Northern Ireland during the Second World War

1. For example, Elizabeth Malcolm, "'Troops of Largely Diseased Women': VD, the Contagious Diseases Acts, and Moral Policing in Late Nineteenth Century Ireland," *Irish Economic and Social History* 26 (1999): 1–14; Philip Howell, "Venereal Disease and the Politics of Prostitution in the Irish Free State," *Irish Historical Studies* 33, no.

131 (2003): 320–41; Sandra L. McAvoy, "The Regulation of Sexuality in the Irish Free State, 1929–35," in *Medicine, Disease, and the State in Ireland, 1650–1940,* edited by Greta Jones and Elizabeth Malcolm, 253–266 (Cork: Cork Univ. Press, 1999).

2. For the discussion of VD at the governmental level, see Peter Baldwin, *Contagion and the State in Europe, 1930–1930* (Cambridge: Cambridge Univ. Press, 1999). Recent examples of regional studies include Roger Davidson, *Dangerous Liaisons: A Social History of Venereal Disease in Twentieth-Century Scotland* (Amsterdam: Rodolpi, 2000); Anna Lundberg, "Passing the 'Black Judgement': Swedish Social Policy on Venereal Disease in the Early Twentieth Century," in *Sex, Sin, and Suffering: Venereal Disease and European Society since 1870,* edited by Roger Davidson and Lesley A. Hall, 29–43 (London: Routledge, 2001).

3. Ida Blom, "Sexuality and Public Policy: Prevention of VD in Scandinavia c. 1900–1950," paper presented at the Fourth Conference of the International Federation for Research in Women's History, Queens Univ., Belfast, Aug. 2003.

4. Roger Davidson, "'Great Scourge': Approaches to the History of Venereal Diseases in Modern European Society," unpublished paper, Feb. 2003. My thanks to the author for providing me with a copy of this paper.

5. See, for example, Jonathan Bardon, *A History of Ulster* (Belfast: Blackstaff Press, 1992), 515; Patrick Buckland, *The Factory of Grievances: Devolved Government in Northern Ireland, 1921–39* (Dublin: Gill and MacMillan, 1979), 37–38.

6. Mary Harris, *The Catholic Church and the Foundation of the Northern Irish State* (Cork: Cork Univ. Press, 1993), 175.

7. For more on the establishment of treatment centers in Northern Ireland, see Leanne McCormick, *Regulating Sexuality: Women in Twentieth Century Northern Ireland* (Manchester, UK: Manchester Univ. Press, 2009), chap. 4.

8. The names "Londonderry" and "Derry" refer to the same place; the choice of name is dictated by contemporary source usage.

9. Minutes of County of Londonderry VD Committee meetings, 1942–46, Local Authority Records, County Londonderry Borough Council, File LA/5/9AK/2, Public Record Office of Northern Ireland (PRONI), Belfast.

10. For more on the issues surrounding VD treatment in the Irish Free State, see Maria Luddy, *Prostitution and Irish Society, 1800–1940* (Cambridge: Cambridge Univ. Press, 2007), 184–209.

11. See, for example, Lucy Bland, "'Cleansing the Portals of Life': The Venereal Disease Campaign in the Early Twentieth Century," in *Crises in the British State, 1880–1930,* edited by Mary Langan and Bill Schwarz, 192–208 (London: Hutchinson, 1985); Suzanne Buckley, "The Failure to Resolve the Problem of Venereal Disease among the Troops in Britain during WW1," in *War and Society: A Yearbook of Military History,* vol. 2, edited by Brian Bond and Ian Roy, 65–85 (London: Croom Helm, 1977); Lesley Hall, "'War Always Brings It On': War, STD, the Military, and the Civilian Population

in Britain, 1850–1950," in *Medicine and Modern Warfare*, edited by Roger Cooter, Mark Harrison, and Steve Sturdy, 205–23 (Amsterdam: Rodolpi, 1999).

12. For more on the CDAs' impact, see Judith Walkowitz, *Prostitution and Victorian Society: Women, Class, and the State* (Cambridge: Cambridge Univ. Press, 1982).

13. Minutes of Home Office meeting, 29 Oct. 1942, Foreign Office Records, Foreign Office Political Department General Correspondence, United States File No. 33, United States Forces in the United Kingdom, File FO/371/34124, National Archives Kew (NA).

14. David Reynolds, *Rich Relations: The American Occupation of Britain, 1942–45* (London: Harper Collins, 1996), 205, includes citation to Defence Regulation 33B.

15. For more on the impact of 33B in Great Britain, see Leslie Hall, "Venereal Diseases and Society in Britain from the Contagious Diseases Acts to the National Health Service," in Davidson and Hall, eds., *Sex, Sin, and Suffering*, 120–37.

16. Medical Superintendant of Health (MSOH), Belfast, *Annual Report of Health* (1943), Local Authority Records, Belfast Corporation, File LA7/9DA/28, pp. 2–5, PRONI.

17. Ibid.

18. Roger Davidson, "'Fighting the "Deadly Scourge': The Impact of World War II on Civilian Health Policy in Scotland," *Scottish Historical Review* 75 (1999), 78.19. General Orders of the Headquarters of the United States Army, Northern Ireland Forces, 2 Feb. 1945, Cabinet Records, Civil Defence, File CAB/9CD/225/6, No. 31, PRONI.

20. Minutes of Public Health Committee meeting, Belfast Corporation, 20 Apr. 1943, Local Authority Records, Belfast Corporation, File LA7/9AA/20, PRONI.

21. Minutes of Public Health Committee meeting, Belfast Corporation, 1934–39, Local Authority Records, Belfast Corporation, File LA7/9AA/18–19, PRONI. Similar debates concerning placing posters in toilets also took place in Glasgow in the same period. See Davidson, *Dangerous Liaisons*, 138.

22. Minutes of Public Health Committee meeting, Belfast Corporation, 9 Jan. 1934, Local Authority Records, Belfast Corporation, File LA/7/9AA/18, PRONI.

23. Minutes of Public Health Committee meetings, Belfast Corporation, 21 Apr. 1942 and 30 June 1942, Local Authority Records, Belfast Corporation, File LA/7/9AA/20, PRONI.

24. Ministry of Health, Stormont, to Ministry of Health, Whitehall, 16 Mar. 1943, Ministry of Health and Local Government, VD Publicity and Propaganda, File HLG/1/2/2, PRONI.

25. MSOH, Belfast, *Annual Report of Health* (1939–45), Local Authority Records, Belfast Corporation, File LA7/9DA/28, PRONI.

26. MSOH, Belfast, *Annual Report of Health* (1943), 2–5.

27. MSOH, Belfast, *Annual Report of Health* (1944), Local Authority Records, Belfast Corporation, File LA7/9DA/28, pp. 2–5, PRONI.

28. Department of Education, Northern Ireland (1987), Circular no. 45. For more on the issue of sex education in contemporary Northern Ireland, see Audrey Simpson, "A Sociological Analysis of the Theory and Practice of Sex Education in Post-primary Schools in Northern Ireland," PhD diss., Univ. of Ulster, 2001.

29. Minutes of Public Health Committee meeting, Belfast Corporation, 8 Sept. 1942, Local Authority Records, Belfast Corporation, File LA/7/9AA/20, PRONI.

30. MSOH, Belfast, *Annual Report of Health* (1943), 2–5.

31. "Tyrone County Council Meeting," *Derry Journal*, 14 Feb. 1919.

32. Quoted in ibid.

33. Ministry of Home Affairs, Stormont, to Robert Gransden, Cabinet Secretariat, Stormont, 16 Apr. 1942, Cabinet Records, correspondence concerning the frequency, provision for, and treatment of venereal disease, 1922–42, File CAB/9B/23/1, PRONI.

34. Mr. McGurk and Sir Dawson Bates, House of Commons debates, 21 Apr. 1942, Northern Ireland Parliament.

35. General Orders of the Headquarters of the United States Army, Northern Ireland Forces, 2 Feb. 1945, Cabinet Records, Civil Defence, File CAB/9CD/225/6, No. 31, PRONI.

36. Ibid.

37. Special Committee Meeting of Welfare Committee 1942, Cabinet Records, Civil Defence, Entry of America into the War, File CAB/9CD/225/19, PRONI.

38. Derrick Gibson-Harries, *Life-line to Freedom: Ulster in the Second World War* (Lurgan, Northern Ireland: Ulster Society, 1990), 61.

39. Home Office Circular no. 202, 17 July 1944, Cabinet Records, Civil Defence, Entry of America into the War, Relationships Between the Civil Population and Members of the Armed Forces, File CAB/9CD/225/18, PRONI.

40. Ministry of Home Affairs, Stormont, to Robert Gransden, Cabinet Secretariat, Stormont, 16 Apr. 1942.

41. Appendix, 7 Feb. 1942, Cabinet Records, notes compiled from the war diary of various branches of the British Troops in Northern Ireland, War Diary "A," July 1941–May 1942, File CAB/3A/49, PRONI.

42. Cited in Keith Jeffery, "Canadian Sailors in Londonderry: A Study in Civil–Military Relations, 1942–45," unpublished paper, n.d., 42. My thanks to the author for giving me access to this paper.

43. Ibid., 43.

44. General Orders of the Headquarters of the United States Army, Northern Ireland Forces, 2 Feb. 1945, Cabinet Records, Civil Defence, File CAB/9CD/225/6, No. 31, PRONI.

45. Cited in A. S. McNulty, *The Colonies, the Medical Services of the Ministry of Pensions, Public Health in Scotland, Public Health in Northern Ireland,* vol. 2 of *His-*

tory of the Second World War: United Kingdom Medical Series: The Civilian Health and Medical Services (London: Her Majesty's Stationery Office, 1955), 399.

46. MSOH, Belfast, *Annual Report of Health* (1939–45).

47. Brian Barton, *Northern Ireland in the Second World War* (Belfast: Ulster Historical Foundation, 1995), 98–99

48. Davidson, "Fighting the "Deadly Scourge," 74, 75.

49. Ibid., 96.

50. Mary E. Daly, *A Social and Economic History of Ireland since 1800* (Dublin: Educational Co., 1981), 206.

51. Arthur Green, *Devolution and Public Finance: Stormont 1921–1972* (Glasgow: Centre for the Study of Public Policy, Univ. of Strathclyde, 1979), 7.

52. Greta Jones, *Captain of All These Men of Death: The History of Tuberculosis in Nineteenth and Twentieth Century Ireland* (Amsterdam: Rodolpi, 2001), 132.

.

Select Bibliography

Barnes, David. *The Making of a Social Disease: Tuberculosis in Nineteenth Century France*. Berkeley: Univ. of California Press, 1995.

Barrington, Ruth. *Health, Medicine, and Politics in Ireland, 1900–70*. Dublin: Institute of Public Administration, 1987.

Boyd, Gary. *Dublin 1745–1922: Hospitals, Spectacle, & Vice*. Dublin: Four Courts Press, 2006.

Boyle, Emily. "The Economic Development of the Irish Linen Industry 1825–1913." PhD diss., Queen's Univ. of Belfast, 1979.

Brady, Joseph. "Dublin at the Turn of the Century." In *Dublin Through Space and Time*, edited by Joseph Brady and Anngret Simms, 221–81. Dublin: Four Courts Press, 2001.

Breathnach, Ciara, ed. *Framing the West: Images of Rural Ireland 1891–1920*. Dublin: Irish Academic Press, 2007.

———. *A History of the Congested Districts Board of Ireland, 1891–1923: Poverty and Development in the West of Ireland*. Dublin: Four Courts Press, 2005.

Breschi, Marco, and Lucia Pozzi, ed. *The Determinants of Infant and Child Mortality in Past European Populations*. Udine: Forum Press, 2004.

Browne, Alan, ed. *Masters, Midwives, and Ladies-in-Waiting: The Rotunda Hospital 1745–1995*. Dublin: A. & A. Farmar, 1995.

Bryder, Linda. *Below the Magic Mountain: A Social History of Tuberculosis in Twentieth Century Britain*. Oxford: Oxford Univ. Press, 1988.

Burke, Helen. *The People and the Poor Law in 19th-Century Ireland*. Littlehampton, UK: Women's Education Bureau, 1987.

Cameron, Charles A. *History of the Royal College of Surgeons*. Dublin: Fannin, 1910.

———. *History of the Royal College of Surgeons in Ireland*. Dublin: Fannin, 1886.

Campbell Ross, Ian, ed. *Public Virtue, Public Love: The Early Years of the Dublin Lying-in Hospital*. Dublin: O'Brien Press, 1986.

Clear, Caitriona. *Women of the House: Women's Household Work in Ireland 1926–1961*. Dublin: Irish Academic Press, 2000.

Coakley, Davis. *Irish Masters of Medicine*. Dublin: Town House, 1992.

Cooney, John. *John Charles McQuaid: Ruler of Catholic Ireland*. Syracuse, NY: Syracuse Univ. Press, 1999.

Cousins, Mel. *The Birth of Social Welfare in Ireland 1922–52*. Dublin: Four Courts Press, 2003.

Crossman, Virginia. *Local Government in Nineteenth-Century Ireland*. Belfast: Institute of Irish Studies, Queen's Univ.1994.

Cullen Owens, Rosemary. *A Social History of Women in Ireland 1870–1970*. Dublin: Gill & Macmillan, 2005.

Davidson, Roger. *Dangerous Liaisons: A Social History of Venereal Disease in Twentieth-Century Scotland*. Amsterdam: Rodolpi, 2000.

Deeny, James. *To Cure and to Care: Memoirs of a Chief Medical Officer*. Dublin: Glendale Press, 1989.

Dempsey, Mary. "The Birth of a Mission." *History Ireland* 14, no. 4 (July–Aug. 2006): 25–29.

Earner-Byrne, Lindsey. *Mother and Child: Maternity and Child Welfare in Dublin, 1922–60*. Manchester, UK: Manchester Univ. Press, 2007.

Eccles, Audrey. *Obstetrics and Gynaecology in Tudor and Stewart England*. London: Croom Helm, 1982.

Farmar, Tony. *Holles Street 1894–1994: The National Maternity Hospital—a Centenary History*. Dublin: A. & A. Farmar, 1994.

———. *Patients, Potions, and Physicians: A Social History of Medicine in Ireland 1654–2004*. Dublin: A. & A. Farmar, 2004.

Fealy, Gerard. *A History of Apprenticeship Nurse Training in Ireland*. London: Routledge, 2006.

Feldberg, Georgina. *Disease and Class: Tuberculosis and the Shaping of Modern North American Society*. New Brunswick, NJ: Rutgers Univ. Press, 1995.

Finnane, Mark. "The Carrigan Committee of 1930–1 and the 'Moral Condition of the Saorstát.'" *Irish Historical Studies* 33, no. 128 (Nov. 2001): 519–36.

———. *Insanity and the Insane in Post-famine Ireland*. London: Croom Helm, 1981.

Finney, Patrick, and Patrick O Brien. *Moral Problems in Hospital Practice*. St Louis: B. Herder, 1922.

Fitzpatrick, David. *The Two Irelands, 1912–1939*. Oxford: Oxford Univ. Press, 1998.

Fleetwood, John F. *The History of Medicine in Ireland*. Dublin: Skellig Press, 1983.

Fleming, David. "Public Attitudes to Prostitution in Eighteenth-Century Ireland." *Irish Economic and Social History* 32 (2005): 1–18.

Fuller, Louise. *Irish Catholicism Since 1950: The Undoing of a Culture*. Dublin: Gill & Macmillan, 2002.

Geary, Laurence M. *Medicine and Charity in Ireland, 1718–1851*. Dublin: Univ. College Dublin Press, 2004.

Hayes, Bernadette, and Pauline M. Prior. *Gender and Health Care in the UK: Exploring the Stereotypes*. London: Palgrave, 2003.

Horgan-Ryan, Siobhan. "The Development of Nursing in Ireland, 1898–1920." PhD diss., Univ. College Cork, 2004.

Howell, Philip. "Venereal Disease and the Politics of Prostitution in the Irish Free State." *Irish Historical Studies* 33, no. 131 (May 2003): 320–41.

Hug, Chrystel. *The Politics of Sexual Morality In Ireland*. New York: St. Martin's Press, 1999.

Johnston, William. *The Modern Epidemic: A History of Tuberculosis in Japan*. Cambridge, MA: Harvard Univ. Press, 1995.

Jones, Greta. *Captain of All These Men of Death: The History of Tuberculosis in Nineteenth and Twentieth Century Ireland*. Amsterdam: Rodolpi, 2001.

———. "Eugenics in Ireland: The Belfast Eugenics Society." *Irish Historical Studies* 28, no. 109 (May 1992): 81–95.

———. "Marie Stopes in Ireland: The Mother's Clinic Belfast, 1936–1947." *Social History of Medicine* 5, no. 2 (1992): 255–77.

———. *Social Hygiene in Twentieth Century Britain*. London: Croom Helm, 1986.

Kelly, James. "The Emergence of Scientific and Institutional Medical Practice in Ireland, 1650–1800." In *Medicine, Disease, and the State in Ireland, 1650–1800*, edited by Greta Jones and Elizabeth Malcolm, 21–39. Cork: Cork Univ. Press, 1999.

———. *Gallows Speeches from Eighteenth-Century Ireland*. Dublin: Four Courts Press, 2001.

Kelly, Mary. "From Workhouse to Hospital: The Role of the Irish Workhouse in Medical Relief to 1921." MA thesis, Univ. College Galway, 1972.

Kenneally, James. *The History of American Catholic Women*. New York: Crossroad, 1990.

Kennedy, Finola. *Cottage to Crèche: Family Change in Ireland*. Dublin: Institute of Public Administration, 2001.

———. "The Suppression of the Carrigan Report." *Studies* 89, no. 356 (2000): 354–62.

Keogh, Dermot. *The Vatican, the Bishops, and Irish Politics 1919–1939*. Cambridge: Cambridge Univ. Press, 1986.

King, Roger. *The Making of the Dentiste, c. 1650–1760*. Aldershot, UK: Ashgate, 1998.

Kirkpatrick, T. P. C. *The History of Doctor Steevens' Hospital, Dublin, 1720–1920*. Dublin: Univ. College Dublin Press, 1924.

Legg, M. L., ed. *The Diary of Nicholas Peacock, 1740–51*. Dublin: Four Courts Press, 2005.

———, ed. *The Synge Letters: Bishop Edward Synge to His Daughter Alicia, Roscommon to Dublin 1746–1752*. Dublin: Lilliput Press, 1996.

Loudon, Irvine. *Death in Childbirth: An International Study of Maternal Care and Maternal Mortality 1800–1950*. Oxford: Oxford Univ. Press, 1992.

Luddy, Maria. "'Abandoned Women and Bad Characters': Prostitution in Nineteenth-Century Ireland." *Women's History Review* 6 (1997): 485–503.

———. *Women and Philanthropy in Nineteenth-Century Ireland*. Cambridge: Cambridge Univ. Press, 1995.

Magill, Isabel. "A Social History of T.B. in Belfast." DPhil diss., Univ. of Ulster, 1995.

Marland, Hilary, ed. *The Art of Midwifery in Europe: Early Modern Midwives in Europe*. London: Routledge, 1993.

———, trans. *"Mother and Child Were Saved": The Memoirs (1693–1740) of the Friesen Midwife Catherina Schrader*. Amsterdam: Rodolpi, 1987.

Marland, Hilary, and Anne Marie Rafferty, ed. *Midwives, Society, and Childbirth: Debates and Controversies in the Modern Period*. New York: Routledge, 1997.

McAvoy, Sandra. "Before Cadden: Abortion in Mid-Twentieth-Century Ireland." In *The Lost Decade: Ireland in the 1950s*, edited by Dermot Keogh, Finbarr O'Shea, and Carmel Quinlan, 147–63. Cork: Cork Univ. Press, 2004.

————. "The Regulation of Sexuality in the Irish Free State 1929–35." In *Medicine, Disease, and the State in Ireland 1650–1940*, edited by Greta Jones and Elizabeth Malcolm, 253–66. Cork: Cork Univ. Press, 1999.

McCandless, Peter. "'Curses of Civilization': Insanity and Drunkenness in Victorian Britain." *British Journal of Addiction* 79, no. 1 (Mar. 1984): 49–58.

McGowan, David. "A Story of Irish Extraction." *History of Dentistry Newsletter* 13 (Oct. 2003): 2–5. Available at http://www.rcpsg.ac.uk/hdrg/2003 Oct6.htm.

McKee, Eamonn. "Church–State Relations and the Development of Irish Health Policy: The Mother-and-Child Scheme, 1944–53." *Irish Historical Studies* 25, no. 98 (Nov. 1986): 167–69.

Murray, James. *Galway: A Medico-social History*. Galway: Kenny's, 1996.

Murray, John E. "Social Insurance Claims as Morbidity Estimates: Sickness or Absence?" *Social History of Medicine* 16, no. 2 (2003): 225–45.

Ó Gráda, Cormac. "The Greatest Blessing of All: The Old Age Pension in Ireland." *Past & Present* 175 (2002): 124–62.

————. *Ireland: A New Economic History 1780–1939*. Oxford: Oxford Univ. Press, 1995.

————. "New Evidence on the Fertility Transition in Ireland 1880–1911." *Demography* 28, no. 4 (1991): 535–48.

Ó Gráda, Cormac, and Niall Duffy. "Fertility Control in Marriage in Ireland a Century Ago." *Journal of Population Economics* 8 (1995): 423–31.

Ó hÓgartaigh, Margaret. "Dorothy Stopford-Price and the Elimination of Childhood Tuberculosis." In *Ireland in the 1930s: New Perspectives*, edited by Joost Augusteijn, 67–82. Dublin: Four Courts Press, 1999.

————. "Flower Power and 'Mental Grooviness': Nurses and Midwives in Ireland in the Early Twentieth Century." In *Women and Paid Work in Ireland, 1500–1930*, edited by Bernadette Whelan, 133–47. Dublin: Four Courts Press, 2000.

————. *Kathleen Lynn: Irishwoman, Patriot, Doctor*. Dublin: Irish Academic Press, 2006.

————. "Nurses and Teachers in the West of Ireland in the Late-Nineteenth and Early-Twentieth Centuries." In *Framing the West: Images of Rural Ireland, 1891–1920*, edited by Ciara Breathnach, 197–214. Dublin: Irish Academic Press, 2007.

Osborough, Nial. *Borstal in Ireland: Custodial Provision for the Young Adult Offender, 1906–74*. Dublin: Institute for Public Administration, 1975.

Pollock, Linda. "Embarking on a Rough Passage: The Experience of Pregnancy in Early Modern Society." In *Women as Mothers in Pre-industrial England: Essays in Memory of Dorothy McLaren*, edited by Valerie Fildes, 39–67. London: Routledge, 1990.

Porter, Roy. *Bodies Politic: Disease, Death, and Doctors in Britain, 1650–1900*. Ithaca, NY: Cornell Univ. Press, 2001.

———. *Health for Sale: Quackery in England, 1660–1800*. Manchester, UK: Manchester Univ. Press, 1989.

———. *Quacks: Fakes and Charlatans in English Medicine*. Gloucestershire, UK: Tempus, 2000.

Preston, Margaret. *Charitable Words: Women, Philanthropy, and the Language of Charity in Nineteenth-Century Dublin*. Westport, CT: Praeger, 2004.

Preston, Samuel H., and Michael Haines. *Fatal Years: Childhood Mortality in the United States in the Late Nineteenth Century*. Princeton, NJ: Princeton Univ. Press, 1991.

Prior, Pauline M. *Madness and Murder: Gender, Crime, and Mental Disorder in Nineteenth-Century Ireland*. Dublin: Irish Academic Press, 2008.

Proctor, Francis. *A History of the Book of Common Prayer*. 17th ed. London: n.p., 1871.

Prunty, Jacinta. *Dublin Slums, 1800–1925: A Study in Urban Geography*. Dublin: Irish Academic Press, 1998.

Reynolds, Joseph. *Grangegorman: Psychiatric Care in Dublin since 1815*. Dublin: Institute of Public Administration, 1992.

Riordan, Susannah. "Venereal Disease in the Irish Free State: The Politics of Public Health." *Irish Historical Studies* 35, no. 139 (May 2007): 345–64.

Robbins, Joseph. *Nursing and Midwifery in Ireland in the Twentieth Century*. Dublin: An Bord Altranais, 2000.

Scanlan, Pauline. *The Irish Nurse: A Study of Nursing in Ireland, History and Education 1718–1981*. Drunshambo, Ireland: Drumlin, 1991.

Smith, F. B. *The Retreat of Tuberculosis*. London: Croom Helm, 1988.

Stopford-Price, Dorothy. *An Account of 20 Years Fight Against TB*. Oxford: Oxford Univ. Press, 1957.

Walsh, Oonagh. "A Lightness of Mind: Gender and Insanity in Nineteenth Century Ireland." In *Gender Perspectives in Nineteenth-Century Ireland*, edited by Margaret Kelleher and James H. Murphy, 159–67. Dublin: Irish Academic Press, 1997.

———. "Lunatic and Criminal Alliances in Nineteenth-Century Ireland." In *Outside the Walls of the Asylum: The History of Care in the Community 1750–2000,* edited by Peter Bartlett and David P. Wright, 132–52. London: Athlone Press, 1999.

———. "'Tales from the Big House': The Connaught District Lunatic Asylum in the Late Nineteenth-Century." *History Ireland* (Nov.–Dec. 2005): 21–25.

Whyte, J. H. *Church and State in Modern Ireland 1923–1970.* Dublin: Gill & Macmillan, 1971.

Wilson, Adrian. *The Making of Man-Midwifery: Childbirth in England 1669–1770.* Cambridge, MA: Harvard Univ. Press, 1995.

———. "Participant or Patient? Seventeenth Century Childbirth from the Mother's Point of View." In *Patients and Practitioners: Lay Perceptions of Medicine in Pre-industrial Society,* edited by Roy Porter, 129–44. Cambridge: Cambridge Univ. Press, 1985.

Index

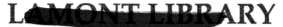

LAMONT LIBRARY

HARVARD COLLEGE, CAMBRIDGE, MA 02138

(617) 495-2452